Health Education

Health Education

Creating Strategies for School and Community Health

SECOND EDITION

Glen G. Gilbert
East Carolina University

Robin G. Sawyer
University of Maryland, College Park

JONES AND BARTLETT PUBLISHERS

Sudbury, Massachusetts

BOSTON   LONDON   SINGAPORE

World Headquarters

Jones and Bartlett Publishers
40 Tall Pine Drive
Sudbury, MA 01776
978-443-5000
info@jbpub.com
www.jbpub.com

Jones and Bartlett Publishers
Canada
6339 Ormindale Way
Mississauga, Ontario
CANADA L5V 1J2

Jones and Bartlett Publishers
International
Barb House, Barb Mews
London W6 7PA
UK

Production Credits
Sponsoring Editor: Suzanne Jeans
Associate Editor: Amy Austin
Senior Production Editor: Lianne Ames
Manufacturing Buyer: Therese Bräuer
Design: Clarinda Company
Editoral Production Service: Clarinda Company
Typesetting: Clarinda Company
Cover Design: Anne Spencer
Printing and Binding: Malloy Lithographing
Cover Printing: Malloy Lithographing

ISBN-13: 978-0-7637-1334-8
ISBN-10: 0-7637-1334-1

Library of Congress Cataloging-in-Publication Data
Gilbert, Glen G. (Glen Gordon), 1946-
  Health education : creating strategies for school and community
health / Glen G. Gilbert, Robin G. Sawyer.—2nd ed.
    p. cm.
  Includes bibliographical references and index.
  ISBN 0–7637–1334–1
    1. Health Education—United States. I. Sawyer, Robin G. II. Title.
RA440.5 .G48 2000
6139.0719073—dc21   00–024685

We dedicate this book to
Evelyn, Rosemarie, Jessica, Jennifer, and Jeffrey Gilbert
and
Anne Anderson-Sawyer, Katherine, Emily, Meg
and Gillian Sawyer

Contents

Chapter 3	**SELECTING AN INTERVENTION/METHOD**	**45**

Chapter 4	**PRESENTATION AND UNIT PLAN DEVELOPMENT**	**80**

Chapter 5	**METHODS OF INSTRUCTION/INTERVENTION**	**104**

Chapter 6   PERSONAL COMPUTERS AND THE INTERNET   175

Foreword

Surviving to a second edition is a lot like getting academic tenure. Like tenure, a second edition acknowledges a successful beginning. It recognizes recognition. It gives some license to push the envelope beyond the now conventional boundaries (regarding strategy and methods selection in health education) staked out by the first edition. With this right to push the boundaries comes the competition, emulation, and—alas—critiques that groundbreaking books stimulate. But the good news is that others have intensified their research on the development and tailoring of methods in health education; a book on intervention mapping has emerged; and the field is paying more critical attention to the gap between planning and evaluation that Professors Gilbert and Sawyer sought to fill with their first edition.

With this edition, Gilbert and Sawyer have updated their evidence-based presentation of strategies and methods. They have added more case vignettes to illustrate their concepts and methods in practical contexts. They have addressed the current issues involved in the increasing application of information technology to health education and have accordingly built a World Wide Web site to link the chapter content to late-breaking developments in the field. They also have updated and expanded the applications of their approach to special populations with a new chapter addressing minority health.

The second edition retains the down-to-earth practicality of the first edition, with its emphasis on skills required in practice, as delineated by the entry-level competencies put forth by the National Task Force on Preparation and Practice of Health Education. Among the foundational skills for this book's approach to selecting methods is the grounding of such selection in a process of needs assessment, problem diagnosis, priority setting, and the writing of concrete objectives.

The authors continue to walk that tightrope between the fuzzy philosophical precepts of health education and the precision of the "best practices" approach that can so easily be misapplied. By laying the question of pedagogy and the selection of instructional methods squarely in a diagnostic-planning framework, they avoid suggesting that some methods are inherently superior to others. Rather, the diagnostic-planning approach mandates that the "best" methods be considered those sensitive to a given context and population.

Unlike many other areas of education, health education must prove its contribution to behavioral changes if it is to earn the support necessary to continue. This means the support of public health, disease-prevention, and health-promotion programs and agencies. This book helps health education students and practitioners get beyond the gadgetry and puffery of new techniques that have only their novelty to recommend them. It recognizes the need to match methods with the characteristics and circumstances of the learners, the health goals to be achieved, and the forces beyond the individuals that will influence their ability to develop and change. These things in the final analysis are more important than how entertained the learners might be by multimedia mania, or how impressed they might be with pedantic pedagogy.

Lawrence W. Green
Director, WHO Collaborating Center on Tobacco and Health
Office on Smoking and Health
National Center for Chronic Disease
Prevention and Health Promotion

Preface

The philosophy presented in this text is based in the premise that the core of health education is the *process* of health education. There are many other tools for health educators, such as epidemiology, statistics, and program planning, but what is truly unique about a health educator is the focus on the "doing." To be an effective health educator means that you are skilled in conducting health education. As educators we may have access to the best knowledge available, but unless we are skilled and effective deliverers of this information, the usefulness of our work is clearly compromised.

Health Education is dedicated to the proposition that we must be good at the doing. Further, it is our belief that health educators need a much more systematic approach to the selection of methods of intervention. This text is intended to assist the health educator in reducing the possibility of a poor performance by encouraging the systematic development of sound, effective, and appropriate presentation methods.

This text is designed for any health educator or would-be health educator who wishes to become proficient in conducting health education programs. The authors strongly believe that the skills necessary to plan successfully for, and deliver, effective health education programs are fundamentally the same, regardless of where they are practiced—in a classroom, a workplace, a hospital, or a community setting. The principles of sound methodology remain constant. Therefore, this text is designed for multiple settings. It addresses the needs of the so-called "generic" health educator, and provides the tools for making appropriate programming decisions based on the needs of the clients and the educational settings.

A variety of learning aids are incorporated into the book. Each chapter contains health educator competencies, case studies, objectives, questions, and exercises. Also included are a glossary, a professional resource list, and up-to-date references.

This second edition demonstrates the evolving state of health education. The text includes a separate chapter on *Minority Health* and a new chapter that exemplifies the technology explosion, *Personal Computers and the Internet*. All other chapters have been updated and include Internet references. The unwieldy Resources section that so quickly becomes outdated has been removed in favor of Internet sources that can be constantly updated. Using the Jones and Bartlett web site (www.jbpub.com/healtheducation) will increase the rewards for using this text.

On the web site instructors will find PowerPoint presentations, essay questions, teaching tips, and worksheets. Students will find additional content information on the web site as indicated by the web icon in the margin of this text.

Responding to user request, the responses to the important case studies have been relocated to the end of each chapter and appear as *Case Studies Revisited*. This affords the reader the opportunity to critically consider the case at hand before reading the authors' responses. A new feature in this edition, called "Noteworthy," includes interesting and relevant features related to the chapter content.

We know that a good text is a book that fulfills the user's needs. We seek to constantly improve the book and look forward to hearing from students, instructors, and professionals who may have a comment, an idea, or a suggestion regarding the text.

Glen G. Gilbert
East Carolina University

Robin G. Sawyer
University of Maryland, College Park

Acknowledgments

The authors wish to give special thanks to the reviewers of the first and second editions.

First Edition: Jill Black, Springfield College; Loren Bensley, Central Michigan University; Gerald S. Fain and Karen Liller, University of South Florida; Onie Grosshans, University of Utah; Barbara J. Richards and B.E. Pruitt, Texas A&M University.

Second Edition: Lynn Bloomberg, Worcester State College; Michael Cleary, Slippery Rock University; Lyndall Ellingson, California State University—Chico; John Janowiak, Appalachian State University; and Katina Sayers, West Virginia University.

We would also like to thank Carol Jackson, Sandy Walter, Robert Gold, Lawrence Green, Gail Jacobs, Fran Gover, Bev Monis, Rosemarie Taylor, Jennifer Morrone-Joseph, Susan Karchmer, and Judy Patek.

We thank our many students over the years at the University of Maryland, East Carolina University, University of Virginia, Portland State University, University of North Carolina at Greensboro, South Eugene High School, Colin Kelly Junior High School, Penge High School, London and Calverton School, and the many other schools where we have conducted workshops and classes.

The authors would like to thank Marjorie Scaffa for her contribution to Chapter 3. They would also like to thank Judy Patek, an assistant principal, and Susan Karchmer and Jennifer Morrone-Joseph from Gallaudet University for their advice and expertise in writing Chapter 9. Their collective suggestions proved invaluable.

And finally thanks to the staff at Jones and Bartlett including Amy Austin, Associate Editor and Lianne Ames, Senior Production Editor.

About the Authors

Glen Gilbert   Glen is currently Professor and Dean of the School of Health and Human Performance at East Carolina University. He has taught university-level methods of instruction courses for over 15 years and has conducted in-service and consulting programs throughout the United States. He went on leave from his university post for two years to serve as Director of the School Health Initiative for the U.S. Department of Health and Human Services and worked with most states and with most federal agencies. As a former secondary school teacher and community health educator, he can relate to the real-world needs of health educators. He has authored over 70 professional publications and has taught at East Carolina University, the University of Maryland, Portland State University, the University of North Carolina at Greensboro, and the Ohio State University. He has been a health educator for over 25 years.

Robin Sawyer   Robin is currently an Associate Professor at the University of Maryland at College Park, where he has achieved popular distinction as an outstanding lecturer, teacher, and health educator. A native of Great Britain, Robin has worked in health education for many years on both sides of the Atlantic and has taught at the middle and high school levels in both countries. Known for his innovative instruction, he teaches courses in human sexuality, children's health, methods of instruction, and also teaches in the professional preparation program. Robin regularly presents on sexuality issues at the national level, and has had great success writing and producing award-winning films in the area of human sexuality. He is currently the coordinator of curriculum and instruction in the Department of Health Education.

Introduction

- Pat is conducting a mandatory inservice on HIV prevention for new correction personnel at the local jail.
- Michael is conducting a five-part workshop on health and safety for 45 physical plant employees at a local factory.
- Maria is performing a one-time presentation on the pap and pelvic examination for a group of 15 Hispanic women in a local community center.
- Natalie is conducting an individual birth control session for a sophomore student at a university health center.
- William is teaching a 10-part unit on family life to a class of 25 ninth-grade high school students.
- Tanya is performing a patient education session for two hypertensive middle-aged males at a local hospital.
- Dwayne is lecturing to 500 college students about sexually transmitted diseases and safer sex, as part of a series on contemporary sexual issues.
- Delores is speaking to a congressional panel on the importance of comprehensive health education.

Although these **health educators** are dealing with very different audiences—from very large groups to individuals, from high school students to elected national officials, from young to old, from the workplace to the school, from the community to the House of Representatives—they all share one crucial factor that will invariably determine success from failure . . . how well they actually educate. The philosophy presented in this text is based in the premise that the core of **health education** is the **health education process**. This means that what is most important is how well and effectively we perform the function of educating people and motivating them to make good health decisions.

There are many tools available to health educators, such as epidemiology, statistics, and program planning, but the essence of being a health educator is the actual "doing" of health education–that is, the conveyance of clear, appropriate **health information** to clients. As educators we may have access to the best knowledge available, but unless we are skilled and effective deliverers of this information, the usefulness of our work is clearly compromised.

This text is dedicated to the proposition that we must be good at the doing . . . the health education. Our goal is to favorably influence the health decision making of our clients. Further, it is our belief that health educators need a systematic approach to the selection of methods of intervention. Anyone who has sat through a poorly prepared, often boring and uninspired presentation/class should question the thought processes that resulted in such a negative experience. This text is intended to assist the health educator or would-be health educator in developing sound, effective, and appropriate presentation methods.

Our goal is to favorably influence the voluntary health decision making of our clients.

The authors of this text strongly believe that the skills necessary to plan for, and deliver, effective health education programs are fundamentally the same, regardless of where they are practiced—in a classroom, workplace, hospital, or community setting. Therefore, this text is designed for multiple settings and will address the needs of the so-called "generic" health educator. Case studies will provide opportunities to apply the principles found in each chapter to specific situations. The reader should consider the specific case study and determine the appropriate course of action. A discussion of each case study can be found at the end of each chapter (under "Case Studies Revisited"). Following is an example of such a case study and its evaluation.

Example of Case Study

The government authorizes $3 million to evaluate a large clinical trial aimed at influencing the health behaviors of Americans. A group of volunteers provides pamphlets and educational counseling at a large shopping mall, and each volunteer spends about an hour with over 5,000 people. The research design for evaluating the program is solid. Proper comparison groups are in place, and the instrumentation for assessing change is of high quality. We know what the behaviors, attitudes, and knowledge were before, during, and after the intervention (treatment), and we are certain threats to internal and external validity of the study have been controlled. The outcome measures are well matched with the objectives of the health education program. According to all measures, however, the intervention does not change anything.

Example of Case Study Revisited

There are, of course, many possibilities for the no-change results, but here are three questions that we want you to consider in particular:

1. Were the methods selected for the intervention appropriate and properly implemented?
2. Was adequate time provided for the intervention to achieve the objectives?
3. Were the people conducting the intervention properly trained? Were they in fact health educators?

Also note the following points:

- Although we do not have the objectives before us, it seems clear that few behavioral objectives could be reached by an intervention consisting solely of pamphlets and educational counseling by volunteers.

- An hour is not enough time to change most behaviors unless you have a very highly motivated clientele.
- Volunteers can play important and sometimes powerful roles but do not qualify as health educators.

This only moderately exaggerated example shows why health educators must work to improve the art and science of health education. Becoming a high-quality health educator requires hard work and dedication. A top-quality health educator is always working to develop communication skills, increase current knowledge of the subject matter, and remain a motivator. It is hoped that this text will provide some of the tools needed to accomplish the goals and objectives of health educators.

Process of Health Education

It is important to remember that health education is, as the name implies, education about health. Health education has its roots in education and public health. It draws on many disciplines including psychology, sociology, education, public health, and epidemiology. It is a unique discipline in many ways. One of the challenges for the health educator is that while the principal tool is education, the sought outcomes are often behavioral. Other disciplines in education focus almost exclusively on knowledge. Health education is called upon to alter people's drug-taking behavior, lower cholesterol, and improve fitness, to name only a few of the many complicated expectations. Other education disciplines are not held to such lofty goals.

Remember always to be grateful for the millions of people everywhere whose despicable habits make health education necessary.
—Mohan Singh

Health educators must learn to set meaningful, appropriate, and achievable goals and objectives. After setting clear, high-quality objectives the health educator must seek to meet those objectives through appropriate ethical methods.

History of Health Education

Health education has been offered in some form since the beginning of time. Humanity has always sought to lead a longer and healthier life. Means's classic text *A History of Health Education in the United States* reviews early health education activities in the United States. It is interesting to note Harvard College required hygiene in 1818 of all seniors (Means, 1962, p. 36). The American Public Health Association was formed in 1872, and the National Education Association started a Department of Child Safety in 1894 (Means, 1962, pp. 46–48). The American School Health Association was formed in 1927 as the then American Association of School Physicians. The American Association for Health Education began as part of what is now titled the Alliance for Health, Physical Education, Recreation, and Dance when it began as the American Association for Health and Physical Education in 1937.

Education about health became more common in the 1800s and early 1900s with numerous reports and advocates. Some noted advocates include Horace Mann, Thomas Denison Wood, the American Academy of Medicine, the Metropolitan Life Insurance Company, the U.S. Public Health Service, and the U.S. Office of Education. The first reported academic department of health education was located at Georgia State College for Women around 1917. The first known recipient of a health education degree was Cecile Oertel Humphrey, who, after additional course work at Harvard during the summers of his program at Georgia State College, received a bachelor of science in health education. A thesis was required, and his was entitled "The Inferiority Complex—Its Relation to Mental Hygiene." No report is available on what has become of Mr. Humphrey (Means, 1962, p. 144). Teachers College, Columbia University, began an undergraduate degree in 1920 and was one of the early granters of graduate degrees in health education.

Health education has functioned as a separate discipline for approximately the last 30 to 60 years. As a relatively new discipline, it has always struggled for a strong sense of identity. One illustration of this is the large number of health education professional organizations, each with overlapping goals. Another is the odd fact that health education degrees are sometimes offered at higher-education institutions with few, or in some extreme cases, no health educators on the faculty. Despite these problems, health education continues to evolve into an important discipline with a unique orientation to addressing the health education needs of the world.

Throughout the history of health education, numerous agencies have recognized its potential to address health problems. Federal agencies have supported many studies and projects designed to improve the quality and impact of health education. An important effort was the Role Delineation Project begun in 1978 (funded by the then U.S. Bureau of Health Manpower and carried out by the National Center for Health Education), which examined the role of the entry-level health educator and generated a defined role. This defined role was based on surveys of practicing health educators in 1978. The end product was a defined role for the entry-level health educator. Although obviously in need of continual updating, the definition of the role was a significant step in the evolution of health education as a discipline. An important finding suggested that the health educator's role was essentially the same regardless of the health education setting. The result was the definition of the **generic health educator,** a concept very important for the training of health educators. It states that health educators should all possess certain common skills. These skills were later more fully defined as *competencies for entry-level health educators* by a panel of experts meeting at Ball State University. Still later these competencies became the basis for a test by the National Commission for Health Education Credentialing (NCHEC) to certify health education specialists. The competencies are also used by the National Council for the Accreditation of Teacher Education (NCATE) as part of the teacher-training accreditation review process.

This *generic health educator* concept has important ramifications for the training of health educators because it puts more emphasis on the acquisition of skills than on health content. Health educators practice in a variety of settings, including school health education, community health education, worksite health education, and patient health education, and it is clear that some skills would be used more in some settings than in others. Yet, the basic skills are generic to all settings. Health educators need to acquire these basic skills. It is ludicrous, for example, for an individual to believe he or she can function well as a health educator without training in educational principles. This text is organized and presented to facilitate the acquisition of many of these basic skills.

Goals of the Text

After reading and synthesizing this text, the health educator will be able to

- Plan properly for health education instruction.
- Develop quality lesson/presentation plans and unit plans.
- Plan for the special needs of target populations.
- Select appropriate methods through a systematic approach.
- Use methods of intervention properly.

Health Education Competencies

Entry-Level The entry-level health education competencies were first developed during the early 1980s and published in 1985. Now that the competencies have existed for several years, the health education profession is working to reverify them through the Competencies Update Project (CUP) initiated in 1998 by the National Commission for Health Education Credentialing (NCHEC). To facilitate this project, two phases of research that directly concern competency development will be conducted, first to examine how other professions distinguish among levels of practice, and second to monitor health education position announcements for additional specification of entry-level competencies. The timeline for the possible dissemination of report findings is projected to be the latter part of the year 2000.

Advanced-Level or Graduate-Level Competencies The document "Standards for the Preparation of Graduate-Level Health Educators," first published in 1997, addressed appropriate competencies for the more advanced-level health educator. A more recent document, published in 1999, "A Competency-Based Framework for Graduate-Level Health Educators," expanded on the earlier document, adding three new areas of graduate responsibility. These competencies are intended to provide a sense of what is expected of a more advanced health educator and allow professional preparation programs to adapt their curricula to ever-changing educational and societal needs.

Use of Competencies in Text
Each chapter begins with the relevant entry-level competencies and sub-competencies and any appropriate new graduate-level competencies. In some instances the entry-level and graduate-level competencies are the same, and in these cases this similarity is noted.

A complete listing of the entry-level competencies and subcompetencies and graduate level competencies can be found in Appendix A.

Format of the Text

- Each chapter begins with a listing of the generic entry-level and/or graduate-level competencies developed for the National Task Force on the Preparation and Practice of Health Educators, Inc. A complete listing of the competencies can be found in the appendix.
- Each chapter also begins with a graphic (Figure 1-1) that illustrates the components of proper method selection addressed in the chapter. As the caption explains, the heavy-bordered boxes identify the components addressed in this text. One or more of these boxes will be shaded to indicate the subject or subjects of a chapter.
- Each chapter states the objectives to be achieved by the reader.
- Case studies are used throughout the text and are revisited at the end of each chapter.
- Each chapter ends with a summary, a series of exercises, and a list of references.
- A glossary can be found at the end of the text.
- Scattered throughout the text can be found health education proverbs from "Mohan Singh," the pseudonym of Horace G. "Hod" Ogden. Before his death in 1998, Mohan Singh directed many programs for the institution now known as the Centers for Disease Control and Prevention (CDC) during his more than 20 years with the U.S. Public Health Ser-

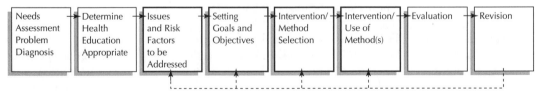

Figure 1-1 Method Selection in Health Education

vice. He always felt it was important to keep life in perspective and that having a good laugh was one way to do that. We are certain he must be laughing about the continuing life of his sayings, often constructed on napkins in Atlanta and D.C. beverage houses. We are pleased to continue spreading these timeless messages for health educators willing to listen.

Method Selection Components

Many public health and health education texts deal with program planning and evaluation. This text focuses on the *conduct* of health education—the pedagogy. **Pedagogy** is the art or profession of teaching. Pedagogy is what health education practice is about.

1. **Needs assessment and problem diagnosis.** This text begins with the assumption that some type of needs assessment has been done and it has been determined that health education is a viable alternative.

2. **Determination of whether health education is the appropriate intervention.** This text also begins with the assumption that it has been determined that health education is the appropriate intervention. As health education can be very complicated, expensive, and difficult, this is an important assumption. Often other methods of health promotion may be more appropriate. Altering the environment, for example, might make better use of resources: if students are eating unhealthy lunches, it may be easier to ensure they eat lunch at school where they will be offered only healthy choices. Such tactics can lead to much better behavior at relatively low cost. However, the long-term behavior may not be altered with only a change in the physical environment.

3. **Issues and risk factors to be addressed.** This text will consider some of the issues and risk factors to be taken into account when making decisions. See Chapters 2, 3, 9, and 10.

4. **Setting goals and objectives.** Goals and objectives are an important component of pedagogy and are addressed in Chapters 2 and 3.

5. **Intervention/method selection.** Selection of the appropriate intervention or method for health education is the major issue addressed in this text. See Chapters 4 through 10 and the appendix.

6. **Evaluation.** *The issue of evaluation is so major that it cannot be sufficiently addressed in this text.* The importance of this area cannot be overestimated. Entire books and courses are dedicated to evaluation, as is fitting for such important and lengthy material. Therefore, although there are many references to evaluation here, no chapter is dedicated to the issue. Instead, the reader is referred to books that can treat the subject in detail.

7. **Revision.** Good, practical evaluation will lead to revision of any intervention. Revision is an important tool that should be part of any program. However, since it should be based on evaluation, revision is not addressed in this text.

SUMMARY

1. A major goal of the text is a systematic approach to the selection of methods of intervention.

2. Education about health has been part of general education since antiquity. Health education as a formal discipline, however, is relatively new.

3. Successful health education interventions and presentations require the development of realistic and meaningful goals and objectives.

REFERENCES

Means, R. K. (1962). *A History of Health Education in the United States.* Philadelphia: Lea and Febiger.

National Task Force on the Preparation and Practice of Health Educators, Inc. (1983). *A Guide for the Development of Competency-Based Curricula for Entry Level Health Educators.* New York.

National Task Force on the Preparation and Practice of Health Educators, Inc. (1985). *A Framework for the Development of Competency-Based Curricula for Entry Level Health Educators.* New York.

U.S. Department of Health and Human Services (1981). National Conference for Institutions Preparing Health Educators: Proceedings, Birmingham, AL, 1981. DHHS Publication 81-50171.

2
CHAPTER

Planning for Instruction

Entry-Level and Graduate-Level Health Educator Competencies Addressed In This Chapter

Responsibility I: Assessing Individual and Community Needs for Health Education
   Competency A: Obtain health-related data about social and cultural environments, growth and development factors, needs, and interests.
   Competency C: Infer needs for health education on the basis of obtained data.

Responsibility II: Planning Effective Health Education Programs
   Competency B: Develop a logical scope and sequence plan for a health education program.
   Competency C: Formulate appropriate and measurable program objectives.
   Competency D: Design education programs consistent with specified program objectives.
   Competency E: Develop health education programs using social marketing principles.

Responsibility III: Implementing Health Education Programs
   Competency A: Exhibit competence in carrying out planned educational programs.
   Competency B: Infer enabling objectives as needed to implement instructional program in specified settings.

> Note: The competencies listed above, which are addressed in this chapter, are considered to be both entry-level and graduate-level competencies by the National Commission for Health Education Credentialing, Inc. They are taken from *A Framework for the Development of Competency Based Curricula for Entry Level Health Educators* by the National Task Force for the Preparation and Practice of Health Education, 1985; and *A Competency-based Framework for Graduate Level Health Educators* by the National Task Force for the Preparation and Practice of Health Education, 1999.

Method Selection in Health Education

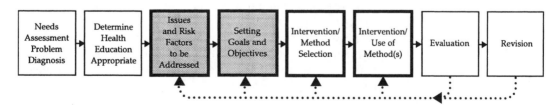

Heavy-bordered boxes indicate subjects addressed in this text; shaded boxes indicate subject(s) of current chapter.

After studying the chapter the reader should be able to

- Conduct an appropriate needs assessment for a given community setting.
- List the major considerations that should be made before selecting an educational objective.
- Write behavioral objectives in the cognitive, affective, and psychomotor domains for a given concept or contact area.
- List the most common mistakes in objective selection.

KEY ISSUES

Program planning	Outcome objectives
Conducting a needs assessment	Writing goals and objectives
Relationship of objectives and evaluation	Selecting verbs
Selecting objectives	Common mistakes
Objective domains	Ethics as part of planning
Process objectives	Seating arrangements
	The learning environment

Program Planning

Method selection is only one element of program planning. Program planning has issues that are beyond the scope of, and therefore not addressed by, this text. Many other books are devoted to those issues. We begin with the assumption that the "problem" has been identified and health education has been determined to be part of the needed solution. This is, of course, a major assumption. It is usually valid for school settings, where the **curriculum** framework for health education is already in place, and for health educators working for a categorical agency that has decided to focus on one or two elements of health education. If the decision for health education has not been made, then the reader should turn to planning models and conduct a thorough diagnosis of the problem before turning to health education and this text. Figure 2-1 shows the full range of method selection, with shaded boxes indicating the subjects that are the focus of this text.

Case Study: Pat Pat has set the elimination of drug use by all adolescents in her community as her objective for a community-wide drug education program. She plans to work cooperatively with several local agencies including the schools and later to apply for federal funding to support the program. Following two years of this approach, she gets a small local grant to evaluate her program. Preliminary reports show that drugs are used by about 15 percent of adolescents in the community. (See Case Studies Revisited page 42.)

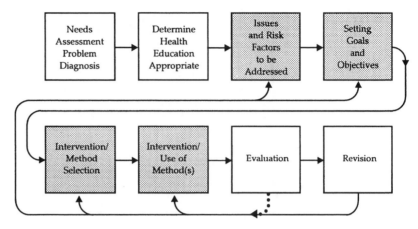

Figure 2-1
Method Selection in
Health Education

Shaded boxes indicate subjects included in this text.

Needs Assessment

Although program **goals** and **objectives** are often set for the health educator by some other group, a **needs assessment** (step one of Figure 2-1) is always appropriate. Outside agencies will often develop excellent objectives, but may still fail to account for special characteristics found at the local level. When goals and objectives are established for health educators, it reduces the complexity of their needs assessment, but generally, they should still play a significant role in objective establishment, by interpretation if not by setting the objectives directly.

The needs assessment, as the term implies, seeks to determine the needs of a targeted population. Before health educators set out to do something, it is important for them to know how this **target population** perceives its needs.[1] Generally, the better we know the target population, the more we should be able to accomplish. The amount of time and resources we devote to the needs assessment will depend on issues such as the duration, priority, and prior work experience with the group. If we have worked with the group recently, we may need to spend little time, but if this is a new group it may require considerable time and effort. We must review what we know of this target population. A simple needs assessment survey is depicted in Figure 2-2.

Case Study: Joe Joe has been asked to make a needs assessment report for a planned health education program targeting the local community. The total budget for the

---

[1]Green and Kreuter use the term *diagnosis* to describe this phase of health promotion planning. They describe this phase in detail in their classic text *Health Promotion and Planning an Educational and Environmental Approach.* It is also sometimes referred to as *reconnaissance.*

WORKSHOP NEEDS ASSESSMENT

Please answer the following questions as completely and honestly as you can. The information collected will be used in determining the content of the health education workshop.

1. What do you hope to get from this workshop/class?

_____
_____
_____

2. Why are you here?

_____
_____
_____

3. One thing you hope will be covered.

_____
_____
_____

4. One issue that has been covered too much and would be a waste of time for this workshop is?

_____
_____
_____

Other comments?

_____
_____
_____
_____
_____
_____

Figure 2-2
Simple Needs Assessment Survey

three-month intervention is $2,000 plus 20 to 30 hours of Joe's time. The planned components of the needs assessment include the following:

1. Local health statistics
2. Planned survey of target audience
3. Knowledge testing as a pretest
4. Focus group of neighborhood residents

(See Case Studies Revisited page 42.)

Target Population

The two types of information that need to be obtained regarding a target population are **demographics** and statistics:

Demographics   Developmental characteristics
Interest surveys
Knowledge levels

Attitudes held
Health skills
Expert opinion

Statistics   National or international trends
Regional
Local

Many sources of information about the needs and interests of a target population exist including

1. National and regional vital statistics
2. National or regional health surveys
3. State reports on health status
4. School- or community-based surveys.
5. Self-constructed surveys.

It is important that health educators assess this information to minimize unneeded work while taking into account the desires of the target group. Conducting a needs assessment puts a group on notice that you recognize its importance and value its opinions. These are necessary ingredients for success.

Prior to a program we should collect demographic information such as age, ethnicity, gender, and other characteristics that may impact objectives and method selection. If we are working with young people, we may turn to information on the developmental characteristics of this age group. Surveys may exist that will tell us something about the knowledge or interests of this age group. If such surveys do not exist, we may be able to conduct such surveys. This data collection, sometimes referred to as **baseline data,** provides information that helps us determine how to conduct our program and serves as a basis of comparison. Any major program must include such baseline data, since there will always be interest in what benefits have been accrued for the dollars invested.

We should also consider what statistical information may be available. International, national, regional, or local reports can provide vital information on needs. Such reports can also be used to demonstrate the importance of a topic. When they don't, it may be important to conduct our own needs assessment specific to our target population. Collecting such information also demonstrates an interest in tailoring the program to the needs of the local target group and may serve as part of the intervention program by pointing out individual needs. Identification of personal needs often leads to some attempt at behavior change. People who know they are at higher than average risk for some loss of health will sometimes try to reduce that risk. How serious they perceive the risk to be will often determine how they respond. As will be discussed later, such information is often very important in selling the program to funding agencies, gathering local support, and encouraging participants to cooperate in the program.

Focus Groups

He who lives by bread alone needs sex education.
—Mohan Singh

There are a number of ways to design and use focus groups as a needs assessment and planning tool. Basically a representative group of the target population or a very similar group is assembled for a focused discussion. Sometimes an incentive is necessary to secure participation, such as a meal or a twenty dollar bill. Prior to the meeting, questions are developed to gather the sought after information, typically including the demographics, beliefs, and health practices of the community, as well as the names of respected leaders. Often the meeting is taped for later transcription. The leader is responsible for ensuring that useful information is collected through both preassembled questions and careful follow-up of cues from the comments of the group. Often unanticipated information is collected that can alter the methods selected for the intervention.

The focus group is a very useful tool. A professional focus group facilitator can be employed, or a member of the planning team may become a good facilitator with practice. Most good community health educators do at least a very brief version of a focus group before starting any program in a new community.

See Chapter 3 for a discussion of models and theories. Health educators need to consider very real and practical motivators for the people they are addressing with their programs.

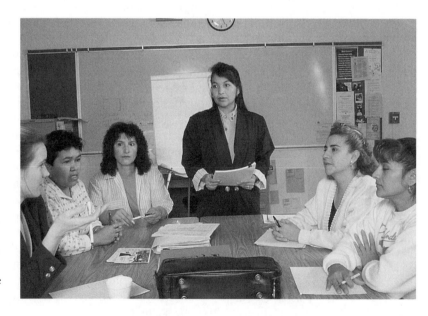

Focus groups are a useful needs assessment and planning tool. The organizer should concentrate on creating the right mix of people.

The Links Among Goals, Objectives, and Evaluation

Alice "Would you tell me please, which way I ought to walk from here?"
"That depends a good deal on where you want to get to," said the Cat.
"I don't much care where," said Alice.
"Then it doesn't matter which way you walk," said the Cat.
"—so long as I get somewhere," Alice added as an explanation.
"Oh, you're sure to do that," said the Cat, "if you only walk long enough!"
—Lewis Carroll,
Alice in Wonderland and Through the Looking Glass

You may have heard the statement, "If you do not know where you want to go it is usually impossible to get there." These words of wisdom apply well to all health education endeavors. We often see health educators trying to get somewhere without being clear about where that somewhere might be. Even more interesting, we often see them trying to evaluate what they have done trying to get there. Obviously, this is not a prudent practice. Health educators must state clearly where they want to go. Not only is this vital for evaluation, it is essential for good planning in selecting an intervention. There are clear links among goals, objectives, method/intervention selection, and evaluation.

Let us examine some examples (with discussion) of how inappropriate conclusions can be reached when we have no clear-cut objectives.

1. "My program went well because we distributed 750 pamphlets on drug abuse."

    If the program objective was to distribute pamphlets, then the objective was met but it was a very poor objective. Distribution numbers or numbers of people that visit a booth in a shopping mall are examples of very limited measures that tell us nothing about changes in knowledge attitudes or behaviors.

2. "My program went well because the 40 people attending the lecture on drug abuse seemed very interested and asked many questions."

    Looking interested tells us nothing about what is being learned. It does tell us something about the methods employed (process evaluation). It may indicate that people find the topic or method of presentation interesting, but it tells us nothing about what has been learned.

3. "My program went well because, after the five antidrug television spots were aired, the state drug use numbers went down."

    Although this is a positive trend, it does not tell us if that trend is related to our program. It may have nothing to do with our activities, and it would be inappropriate for us to assume so without further information.

4. "My program went poorly because, after our intensive intervention with all county high school students, the state drug use numbers went up."

    Again, we do not know if this trend had any connection to our program. The number for our students might be much better due to our program, but without clear objectives we cannot adequately measure our outcomes.

5. "My STD prevention program went poorly because, after our intensive intervention throughout the county, our STD statistics showed an increase."

    Again, we do not know if this trend had any connection to our program. The statistics for STDs commonly go up for a period of time following an intensive campaign because people seek treatment. If we set objectives to lower incidence rates in a short period of time we would be setting up our program for failure.

It is difficult to evaluate these statements without knowing the objectives, but all suggest that the evaluation measures have not been well thought out.

Case Study: Jerry   Jerry was extremely enthusiastic about beginning a sex education program in his high school. The principal had been skeptical about the potential controversy and had put Jerry off for two years. Finally, the principal gave Jerry the administrative and financial support to begin a program, provided he furnish the principal with a course outline and specific objectives. In his haste to consummate the agreement, Jerry quickly prepared an outline, including objectives that promised a substantial decrease in unintended pregnancy and sexually transmitted infection rates. One year later, with budget reductions looming, Jerry is asked to justify the continued support of his sex education program. Much to Jerry's chagrin, the principal points to a higher number of pregnancies than last year, and no available data whatsoever of any sexually transmitted infection rates. What fundamental errors did Jerry make? (See Case Studies Revisited page 42.)

Why Use Objectives?

Objectives serve many useful functions. They provide the health educator with a clear notion of what is to be accomplished. Consequently, it becomes much easier to select methods and to focus all efforts. This focus is vital if we are to develop comprehensive, coordinated approaches to influencing health knowledge and behaviors. Therefore, it is important to begin with the question, what is the target? (See Figure 2-3.) Then we must define the target as specifically as we can.

Objectives reveal to us whether we have selected an inappropriate target, in which case it may be impossible to hit (see Figure 2-4).

Objectives also make evaluation efforts possible. Without objectives it is impossible to measure the achievement of change in knowledge, attitudes, or behavior. You cannot evaluate any type of change unless you first clearly state exactly what you intend to change.

Objectives, moreover, make it easier to convey our instructional intent to others. Learners in any setting do better when it is clear what is to be learned. This is true of participants in workshops as well as students in more formal educational settings. Plus, reviewing well-stated objectives allows learners to assess if a program is the correct program for them.

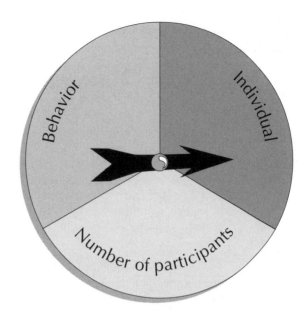

Figure 2-3
Determining a Target

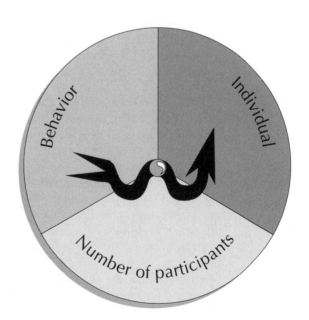

Figure 2-4
Importance of
Appropriate Target

Issues in Setting Objectives and Selecting Interventions/Methods

Some issues to be considered in setting objectives and selecting interventions or methods are as follows:

1. Maturity level of the learner
2. Content to be covered
3. Environment
4. Materials and equipment available
5. Time allotment
6. Group size
7. Time of day

When we set our objectives it is important to make them realistic given our resources. Of course, our objectives are often set by someone else, but the principles are the same. What can we accomplish in the time available with the resources at our disposal?

We must take into account the *maturity level of the learner.* Is the information pitched at the correct level for the learner? If it is too high, comprehension will be a problem; if it is too low, boredom and distraction will occur. Are the selected activities sufficiently varied to stimulate audience attention? This is an important concern when working with young people.

What type of *content* do you intend to cover? Large amounts of complex, didactic information may need to be broken down into smaller more understandable units, again depending on the level of the learner. Varying strategies might also alleviate the boredom factor and result in more effective learning.

What is the physical *environment* like? Can you, for example, lay out four "Annie" CPR mannequins on the floor of a very confined space to conduct important certification classes? Can you successfully perform group facilitation which might include sensitive issues in a space with little privacy? The available environment cannot be underestimated when considering objectives.

Can you obtain the *materials and equipment* you would like to include in a program? For example, is a certain video you would like to use available or affordable? Do you have access to a projector or VCR? Before you include activities in program outlines and strategy selection, check to make sure that the resources are available. How much *time* do you have with specific groups, and how often will you meet? Is it worth spending 20 minutes incorporating an icebreaker exercise with a group that will only meet one time for two hours? The answer to this question depends on the specific objectives that you construct. Should you construct objectives that include behavior

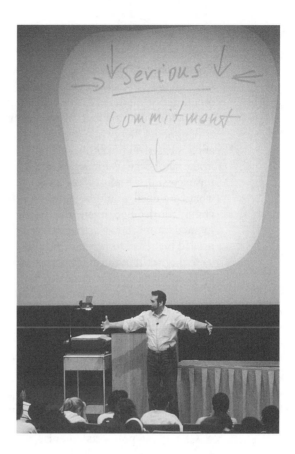

The success of your presentation depends on the correct environment and access to appropriate presentation tools.

change when you will only meet with a group for a total of two hours? You must be realistic about which activities can be utilized and what objectives can be achieved within certain time constraints.

Group size will certainly drive your method selection. Presenting to a large group of 250 individuals will definitely require a different strategy than group process for a small number of people. Consider what might be the most effective ways to communicate with individuals and groups when considering group size.

Anyone who has had early morning classes or dozed during an after-lunch or dinner speech will appreciate the importance of *time of day*. Will you need to wake up the group, quiet them down, struggle to keep their interest, or what? Early morning or postlunch groups might require a wake-up activity, so always consider this issue when developing strategy selection.

Often we must also determine if we can hope to achieve and perhaps measure outcome/impact objectives, or if we should focus on process objectives. Time and resources permitting, we should consider both.

Process Objectives

Process objectives are concerned with what we hope to do along the path to our outcome objectives. This includes a look at how well we are implementing our methods. Are we maintaining interest, and are we providing high-quality information? Most curriculum packages are not implemented as designed. Often when programs are evaluated, the outcome of the evaluation is based on the faulty assumption that all users implement the program in the same way. Whether we are totally successful, partially successful, or unsuccessful, we must have a clear picture of what was done and not just what we hoped would be done in order to evaluate our results. Often programs are deemed ineffective when in fact the program was not implemented or only a few activities or methods from that program were actually used. This refers to program **fidelity.** How faithful to the planned program were the health educators? A lack of fidelity points to the need for training and marketing the total program to the intended user.

Some process objectives might include the following:

- Getting people to participate
- Recognition of need
- Quality of workshop presentations
- Needs assessment
- Peer review
- Fidelity
- Self-assessment
- Changes in policy statements
- Quality control standards

Writing Outcome/Impact Objectives

Beware, lest the fragile lotus of health education be trampled by the elephants of reality.
—Mohan Singh

Outcome/impact objectives are concerned with what we are seeking to change in knowledge, attitudes, and behaviors. How will the participants be different as a result of our educational intervention? These outcomes can be assessed after a short-duration program or long-term program. Obviously, what we can expect must be based on the contact time, motivation, and intensity of our program. For a short-term program it may be realistic to expect gains in knowledge but not attitude or behavior change.

Some outcome/impact objectives might include the following:

- Changes in knowledge
- Changes in attitudes
- Changes in skills
- Changes in behavior
- Cost effectiveness

Writing General Goals

Goal: *A broad statement of direction used to present the overall intent of a program or course.*

Different authors and authorities use a variety of terms and definitions regarding goals and objectives. We will use the term *goal* to mean a broad statement of direction used to present the overall intent of a program or course. A goal does not need to be stated in measurable terms, since it is a broad statement. *Objectives* should always be stated in measurable terms and should complement and more fully explain the intent of a goal. A goal gives us a general sense of the intent of the program or class.

Some goals might include the following:

1. Participants will be able to prepare healthy meals.
2. The use of nonprescription drugs will be reduced.
3. Participants will develop good parenting skills.
4. Unwanted pregnancies will be reduced.
5. Students will understand the digestion process.
6. Participants will show appreciation for the environment.

Goals for Healthy People

The classic document *Healthy People: The Surgeon General's Report on Health Promotion and Disease Prevention* (1979) contains the following goals:

1. To continue to improve infant health and, by 1990, to reduce infant mortality by at least 35 percent, to fewer than 9 deaths per 1,000 live births.
2. To improve child health, foster optimal childhood development, and, by 1990, reduce deaths among children ages 1 to 14 years by at least 20 percent, to fewer than 34 per 100,000.
3. To improve the health and health habits of adolescents and young adults and, by 1990, to reduce deaths among people ages 15 to 24 by at least 20 percent, to fewer than 93 per 100,000.
4. To improve the health of adults and, by 1990, to reduce deaths among people ages 25 to 64 by at least 25 percent, to fewer than 400 per 100,000.
5. To improve the health and quality of life for older adults and, by 1990, to reduce the average annual number of days of restricted activity due to acute and chronic conditions by 20 percent, to fewer than 39 days per year for people aged 65 and older.

Since these are national goals they have been written so they are measurable. As explained earlier, this is not always the case with goals. Most are written as broad statements and are not measurable.

Narrowing Goals to Measurable Objectives

Goals provide a sense of where we want to go, but they usually do not provide clear, precise statements of our destination. We must break these broad

---

SAMPLE PROGRAM PLANNING WORKSHEET

_____

1. What needs to be done? List issue(s) or program(s):

_____
_____
_____
_____
_____

2. State the general goal:

_____
_____

3. State the objective(s) to be evaluated as clearly as you can:

_____
_____
_____
_____
_____
_____

4. Can this objective be broken down further? Break it down to the smallest unit. It must be clear what specifically you hope to see documented or changed knowledge, attitudes, or a behavior.

_____
_____
_____
_____
_____

5. Can each objective be evaluated? If not restate it.

_____

Figure 2-5
Program Planning
Worksheet for Narrow-
ing Goals to Objectives

statements into measurable objectives. One method for doing this is to use a worksheet to guide us to our objectives. After examining our problem, we set general goals. Next we break the problem down as far as we can go. We state our objectives as clearly and precisely as we can. See Figure 2-5 for a sample program planning worksheet.

Writing Self-Contained Outcome/Impact Objectives

Objectives must be much more specific than goals. They must be measurable and clearly indicate what will be different after implementation of the health education program. There are many educational experts knowledgeable in the writing of educational objectives. Most health agencies and organizations will have their own method for stating objectives. Most such methods will be far less specific than what is recommended here and therefore easier to write. We have taken the components from other systems and have constructed a system called _self-contained objectives_. That means, of course, that all the elements are contained within the objective statement. The objective can "stand on its own" and make sense. Each objective makes clear what is expected, according to what source of information, and is stated in such a way that the achievement is measurable. The authors present this method first because it is a format that forces the user to examine important issues in the object process. Most agencies use some abreviated version of this format. Objectives need not always be measured, but they must be measurable. In the real world there are not always sufficient funds, time, personnel, or the need to measure all objectives, but if measurement is not possible, then the objective is not clearly stated.

The steps in writing self-contained objectives are as follows.

1. Begin with the phrase, "The _____ (student/participant/parent) will be able to . . ."
2. Select an action verb.
    a. The participant will be able to *list* seven common depressant drugs . . .
    b. The student will be able to *match* drugs with the appropriate classification . . .
    c. The student will be able to *demonstrate* mouth-to-mouth resuscitation . . .
    d. The participant *will show a willingness to take personal action* against drug use in the neighborhood . . .
3. Provide indication of what constitutes evidence of success.
    a. The participant will be able to list seven common depressant drugs *according to the handouts provided.*
    b. The student will be able to match drugs with the appropriate classification *found in the course textbook.*
    c. The student will be able to demonstrate mouth-to-mouth resuscitation *according to the American Red Cross.*
    d. The participant will show a willingness to take personal action against drug use in the neighborhood by *volunteering* to be part of night patrols in the neighborhood or conducting a door-to-door recruitment.
4. Consider if you have selected objectives appropriate to your needs and domains. For example,
    a. Cognitive/knowledge objective requiring recall of information.
    b. Cognitive/knowledge objective requiring some synthesis or recall.
    c. Psychomotor/"doing" objective requiring performance of a skill.
    d. Affective/"attitude" objective seeking willingness to take action.

Sample Objectives

1. Participants will be able to list and describe the four local agencies available to provide child abuse prevention support as presented during the workshop.

2. Participants will report improved self-efficacy in communication with family members according to the guidelines presented during the workshop.
3. Students will show a willingness to take personal action to improve the environment by voluntarily participating in community-organized cleanups or by voluntarily taking personal action to reduce waste in their community.

Other Objective-Writing Formats

There are many styles of writing objectives, and the health educator may be forced to adapt to the style adopted by the agency or school. Self-contained objectives are suitable for most purposes, and we recommend their use. Further, once you can author self-contained objectives, it becomes relatively easy to master other methods. However, there are advantages to other styles. Some formats make it easier to use objectives over and over again with little change and may be used for different content areas.

1. General instructional objectives (learning outcomes).
    a. Write each objective as an *intended learning outcome*.
    b. Use a verb that is general enough to encompass a domain of student performance. Omit the lead-in phrase, "The student will be able to. . . ." Use verbs such as *knows, understands, applies.*
    c. Include only one learning outcome for each general objective.
    d. Keep these objectives free of subject matter so that they can be used with various units.
    e. State each general objective so that it is definable by a set of specific learning outcomes. (For short units, two to four general objectives will usually suffice.)
2. Specific instructional objectives (learning outcomes).
    a. Place the specific instructional objectives under the general learning objectives. Be certain they are relevant to the general learning outcome under which they are placed.
    b. Use a verb to begin each specific learning outcome. This verb should specify definite, observable student performance. Avoid using verbs such as *sees* and *realizes,* which are vague and not observable.
    c. Under each general learning outcome, list a representative sample of specific learning outcomes to describe the performance of those students who have achieved the objective. (It is impossible to list all learning outcomes.)
3. Examples
    a. Drugs (high school/college level).
        (1) Knows systems of classification.
            (a) Lists various systems of classification.
            (b) Explains the advantages and disadvantages of each system.
            (c) Designs an original system.

     b. Stress control (high school/college level).
       (1) Understands breathing techniques.
         (a) Discusses uses of these.
         (b) Demonstrates them.
         (c) Expresses willingness to use technique.
     c. First aid—choking (junior high/elementary level).
       (1) Knows correct procedures.
         (a) Explains when and when not to use the techniques.
         (b) Recites the steps.
         (c) Performs the procedures.

Suggested Recipe for Writing Health Education Outcome/Impact Objectives

1. Make a rough outline of what you hope to accomplish in this educational setting. Jot down key elements of what you hope to achieve.
2. Ask yourself the following: When they finish with this lesson, workshop, or unit, how will the participants feel or act or what new knowledge or skills will they possess that were not present before this event?
3. Try to state each specific item of information, feeling, and skill as a behavioral objective.
4. Ask yourself if each objective is something the targeted population has gained or could gain from your instruction? If the answer is no, it is not a good objective.
5. Check your verb to see that it is specific (see Table 2-1).
6. Can you measure your objective? Remember you do not have to follow through on measuring each objective, but it must be possible to do so, or it is not a true behavioral objective. Assessment of affective objectives is controversial because many people do not believe they can be measured. Generally, affective assessment is based on a measurable action that a "reasonable person" would assume represents a held attitude or feeling.
7. Psychomotor objectives represent skills that can be performed (i.e., mouth-to-mouth resuscitation). The focus must be the physical performance. Mouth-to-mouth resuscitation requires cognition, but the focus is on the performance of the skill. Visiting an agency is not a psychomotor objective, because walking to the agency is not really the focus and because it would generally be an assignment. Assignments are not objectives. Assignments help us to achieve objectives.

After writing your objectives, double-check each one with the following questions:

1. Have you avoided "fuzzy" verbs? (See Table 2-1 for suggested verbs.)
2. Can you measure the outcome of your objective?

Table 2-1
Suggested Verbs for
Health Education Goals
and Objectives

Goals	
Analyze	Apply
Appreciate	Commit
Conceptualize	Create
Demonstrate	Know
Perform	Plan
Synthesize	Use

Objectives		
Arrange	Categorize	Choose
Clean	Classify	Conduct
Construct	Compute	Describe
Design	Define	Discuss
Drink	Diagram	Feature
Itemize	Eat	Identify
Mark	Lead	List
Operate	Match	Name
Position	Perform	Pick
Sort	Report	Show a willingness
Volunteer	Specify	Underline

3. Is the standard by which achievement will be measured clearly stated?
4. Is each objective something that is really worth achieving?
5. Is there a sufficient number of objectives to cover your true intention of instruction?
6. Are you guilty of not stating your true intentions just because you find it difficult?

Objective-Writing Exercises

Read the following scenarios, take a few moments to consider appropriate outcomes for each situation, and then write down what you would consider to be appropriate behavioral objectives. What are the most needed skills, beliefs, or knowledge? Obviously, you will have to give some consideration to the actual content you would potentially cover in each situation and how you would divide up your time. Remember to consider such basic principles as size of group, setting, time, number of objectives, domain of objectives, and so on.

1. You are a middle school health education teacher. You are about to teach your *first* lesson on heart health to a class of 20 seventh-grade students of mixed academic ability. This particular unit consists of five class periods, and each period is 50 minutes long.

2. You are a community health educator facilitating a program on smoking cessation for 10 middle-aged adults. The program consists of 10 two-hour weekly workshops and you are planning to conduct the *first* workshop.

3. You have been invited to a local high school to deliver a one-hour informational presentation on AIDS to a special assembly consisting of 400 ninth-grade students.

4. You are teaching a two-hour workshop on CPR to 15 Safeway employees in the employee lounge. Your goal is CPR certification of the group.

5. You are a middle school health education teacher beginning the third of five 50-minute class periods on the topic of alcohol. For this period you have decided that the goals should focus on attitudes about the negative aspects of alcohol use. One strategy you have selected is the development of posters by the students depicting alcohol messages. There are 30 students in the class.

6. You are a community health educator who has been asked to facilitate a 90-minute workshop for approximately 25 Hispanic women on the importance of pelvic examinations. Levels of fluency in English are poor.

7. You are a college health educator who has been asked to conduct a one-hour workshop on safer sex for approximately 20 students in a residence hall.

8. Two students in a campus residence hall have recently experienced date rape. As the campus health educator you have been requested by that residence hall's resident assistant (RA) to conduct a one-hour presentation on date rape. The RA expects about 50 students to attend the presentation scheduled to be held in the first-floor lounge.

9. You have been facilitating a weekly six-week course on childbirth. The class meets for 90 minutes and consists of six couples in various stages of pregnancy, from 36 to 41 weeks. This is the last of the six sessions, and you are planning objectives that will allow you to wrap up the course.

10. You are a high school health educator teaching in a very progressive and enlightened school district. You are teaching human sexuality and are about to begin a two-day, 50-minute-period unit on homosexuality. You are planning objectives for this first class.

Common Mistakes in Objective Selection

Beware of the following common mistakes in setting objectives:

1. Selecting an objective that is not achievable.
2. Using verbs that are not specific.
3. Selecting objectives that do not truly represent what you wish to achieve.
4. Selecting objectives that are not realistic given the resources available.
5. Stating an activity and not an objective.

Examples of Goal and Objective Setting

The National Health Objectives When the 1990 Health Objectives were released, they received little attention outside the Public Health Service. They soon became an important force driving agendas and setting funding priorities for all sectors of government. Having clear, specific objectives has forever changed the U.S. Public Health Service. The process in setting the Year 2000 Objectives became much more politicized because public and private groups were aware of their influence. The objectives have become powerful tools in setting government and private policy. The 2010 objectives have grown in number and complexity and have been the subject of much debate.

The U.S. Public Health Service Office of Disease Prevention and Health Promotion was established as a coordinating and policy development unit of the Office of the Assistant Secretary of Health. Since the early days the office has reported to Dr. J. Michael McGinnis, who was charged with coordinating the development of the Surgeon General's reports and the health objectives for the nation. In 1979 the first Surgeon General's report on health promotion was released ("Healthy People: The Surgeon General's Report on Health Promotion and Disease Prevention"), which reviewed the gains made in health promotion. In addition, the report established broad national goals according to life stages and focused on reduction of mortality.

During the same period a process was put in place to develop national health objectives. This took over a year, with first drafts developed by 167 invited experts serving on panels centered around 15 subject areas held and sponsored by the Centers for Disease Control (CDC) in Atlanta. Members were drawn from a variety of backgrounds. The purpose was to develop national, not federal, objectives. It was felt that by establishing clear targets, agencies would focus on meeting those objectives—a common practice for business for many years but a new concept for much of government. Available research was used to determine appropriate targets, and the compilation of information pointed to the need for additional data (needs assessment). A major effort was made, but the task became even more complicated when the process was repeated for the year 2000 objectives. By this time people knew that influential people, including virtually all federal funding sources, were paying careful attention to the objectives. As a result, major lobbying efforts became part of the process of setting the objectives.

Some of the original drafts of the year 2000 objectives differ significantly from the final product. The Office of Disease Prevention and Health Promotion and the CDC are to be commended for pulling together the various factions and completing the target objectives. This is an important example of what needs to be done for any health education program. Clear objectives must be established at the outset if the project is to be successful and to make measurement possible. The national health objectives have resulted in significant changes in the way the U.S. government, and especially the U.S. Public Health Service, does business.

Sample Year 1990 Objectives

By 1990 every junior and senior high school student in the United States should receive accurate, timely education about sexually transmitted infections. (Currently, 70 percent of school systems provide some information about sexually transmitted infections, but the quality and timing of the communication varies greatly.)

By 1990 the proportion of adults who smoke should be reduced to below 25 percent. (In 1979, the proportion of the U.S. population that smoked was 33 percent.)

By 1990 all states should include nutrition education as part of required comprehensive school health education at elementary and secondary levels. (In 1979, only 10 states mandated nutrition as a core content area in school health education.)

By 1990 the proportion of children and adolescents ages 10 to 17 participating in daily school physical education programs should be greater than 60 percent. (In 1974–75, the share was 33 percent.)

By 1990 the proportion of employees of companies and institutions with more than 500 employees offering employer-sponsored fitness programs should be greater than 25 percent. (In 1979 about 2.5 percent of companies had formally organized fitness programs.)

By 1990 no public elementary or secondary school (and no medical facility) should offer highly carcinogenic foods or snacks in vending machines or in school breakfast or lunch programs.

Sample Year 2000 Objectives

4.13 Provide to children in all school districts and private schools primary and secondary educational programs on alcohol and other drugs, preferably as part of quality school health education. (Baseline: 63 percent provided some instruction, 39 percent provided counseling, and 23 percent referred students for clinical assessments in 1987.)

5.4 Reduce the proportion of adolescents who have engaged in sexual intercourse to no more than 15 percent by age 15 and no more than 40 percent by age 17. (Baseline: 27 percent of girls and 33 percent of boys by age 15; 50 percent of girls and 66 percent of boys by age 17; reported in 1988.)

16.3 Reduce breast cancer deaths to no more than 20.6 per 100,000 women. (Age-adjusted baseline: 22.9 per 100,000 in 1987.)

17.13 Increase to at least 30 percent the proportion of people aged 6 and older who engage regularly, preferably daily, in light to moderate physical activity for at least 30 minutes per day. (Baseline: 22 percent of people aged 18 and older were active for at least 30 minutes five or more times per week and 12 percent were active seven or more times per week in 1985.)

18.9 Increase to at least 75 percent the proportion of primary care and mental health care providers who provide age-appropriate counseling on the prevention of HIV and other sexually transmitted infections. (Baseline: 10 percent of physicians reported that they regularly assessed the sexual behaviors of their patients in 1987.)

19.12 Include instruction in sexually transmitted infection transmission prevention in the curricula of all middle and secondary schools, preferably as part of quality school health education. (Baseline: 95 percent of schools reported offering at least one class on sexually transmitted infections as part of their standard curricula in 1988.)

Note: Strategies to achieve this objective must be undertaken sensitively to avoid indirectly encouraging or condoning sexual activity among teens who are not yet sexually active.

Preliminary Sample Year 2010 Objectives

4 (formerly 19.5) Reduce the number of new cases of herpes simplex virus type 2 (HSV-2) infection so that the prevalence in persons 20 to 29 years of age is no greater than 15 percent. (Baseline: 17.2 percent of this age group had HSV-2 during the period 1988 to 1994.)

Select Populations	1988–94
African American	33.6%
Asian/Pacific Islander	Not available
Hispanic	Not available
Mexican American	14.8%
White, non-Hispanic	14.7%
Total	17.2%

1 (formerly 19.2) Reduce the prevalence of *Chlamydia trachomatis* infections among young persons (15 to 24 years old) to no more than 3.0 percent. (Baseline: see following table.)

		1997	
Select Populations	Female (family planning)	Female (STD clinic)	Male (STD clinic)
African American, non-Hispanic	11.1	15.3	18.1
American Indian/ Alaska Native	6.3	13.1	12.6
Asian/Pacific Islander	4.7	12.0	16.6
Hispanic	5.2	14.0	18.5
White, non-Hispanic	3.1	9.2	11.5
Other	4.4	9.6	10.7
Total	4.7	12.3	15.7

6c Reduce to 5.8 percent the proportion of youth reporting use of any drugs during the past 30 days. (Baseline: 9 percent of youth reported drug use in 1996.) (See Chapter 8 for objective on past-month use of tobacco.)

Select Populations	1996
African American	8.6%
American Indian/Alaska Native	Not available
Asian/Pacific Islander	Not available
Hispanic	9.2%
White	9.2%
Male	Not available
Female	Not available

3 Reduce drug-related deaths to 1.3 per 100,000. (Age-adjusted baseline: drug-related deaths occurred in persons per 100,000 in 1996.)

Select Populations	1996
African American	8.5
American Indian/Alaska Native	5.0
Asian/Pacific Islander	1.4
Hispanic	6.0
White	4.8
Male	7.3
Female	3.0

9 (developmental)   Increase the proportion of the nation's public and private elementary, middle/junior high, and senior high schools that require daily physical education for all students.

9 (developmental/formerly 8.12)   Increase to _____ percent the proportion of managed care organizations and hospitals that provide community disease prevention and health promotion activities that address the priority health needs identified by their communities.

Select Populations	
African American	Not available
American Indian/Alaska Native	Not available
Asian/Pacific Islander	Not available
Hispanic	Not available
White	Not available
Male	Not available
Female	Not available

13 (formerly 1.10) Increase to 85 percent the proportion of worksites offering employer-sponsored physical activity and fitness programs.

Worksite Size	1992
<50 employees	Not available
50–99 employees	33%
100–249 employees	47%
250–749 employees	66%
750 employees	83%

Target Setting Method: 2 percent better than the best.

6 Increase to at least 85 percent the proportion of young people in grades 9 through 12 who engage in vigorous physical activity that promotes the development and maintenance of cardiorespiratory fitness three or more days per week for 20 or more minutes per occasion. (Baseline: 64 percent of students in grades 9–12 participated in such activity in 1995; 80 percent of students age 8–16 did so in 1988–94.)

Select Populations	1995
Boys	
9th grade students	80%
10th grade students	79
11th grade students	72
12th grade students	67
Girls	
9th grade students	62
10th grade students	59
11th grade students	47
12th grade students	42

Note: Examples of vigorous physical activities include basketball, jogging, swimming laps, and tennis.

Sample Community Standards   The CDC have produced model standards for communities (Healthy Communities 2000: Model Standards) that formulate model objectives for community adoption. The user simply fills in the blanks. Of course, agreement is the more difficult phase, but having model objectives that have been formulated by a respected element of the U.S. Public Health Service is very helpful.

By _____ (2000) reduce homicides to no more than (7.2) per 100,000 people. (Age-adjusted baseline: 8.5 per 100,000 in 1987.)

By _____ (2000) reduce weapon-related violent deaths to no more than (12.6) per 100,000 people from major causes. (Age-adjusted baseline: 12.9 per 100,000 by firearms, 1.9 per 100,000 by knives, in 1987.)

By _____ (2000) reduce suicides to no more than (10.5) per 100,000 people. (Age-adjusted baseline: 11.7 per 100,000 in 1987.)

By _____ (2000) increase the high school graduation rate to at least (90) percent, thereby reducing risks for multiple problem behaviors and poor mental and physical health. (Baseline: 79 percent of people aged 20 through 21 had graduated from high school with a regular diploma in 1989.)

By _____ all community prevention programs will have an identifiable strategy for the use of health education including at a minimum the following:

a. Specification of population clusters with identifiable health problems or risks
b. Assessment of behavior related to those problems
c. Statement of educational objectives
d. Educational methods to be employed with each target group
e. Timelines for implementation
f. Periodic evaluation of educational effectiveness

By _____ programs to promote and distribute condoms including but not limited to television, radio, and print advertising and outreach to those engaged in high-risk behavior should be part of organized community health education.

Reduce the proportion of adolescents who have engaged in sexual intercourse to no more than 15 percent by age 15 and no more than 40 percent by age 17. (Baseline: 27 percent of girls and 33 percent of boys by age 15; 50 percent of girls and 66 percent of boys by age 17; reported in 1988.)

Ethics as Part of Planning

Many ethical issues are involved in health education intervention. We are attempting to change people in some way. Will these changes and methods of change be ethical? To ensure that the answer is yes, certain steps should be taken to protect people's rights. Until recently, the most widely adopted code of ethics was the SOPHE code. A brief version of the SOPHE code is given in Figure 2-6. This code stated that a health educator should influence people without coercion and that changes of behavior should be voluntary. A more recent code of ethics has been developed by the Coalition of National Health Education Organizations and has superseded the SOPHE code (see appendix).

SOPHE's Code of Ethics (Brief Edition)

To guide professional behaviors of its members toward highest standards, SOPHE adopted a Code of Ethics in 1976 and acknowledged the need for periodic review and improvement of the Code.

- I will accurately represent my capability, education, training, and experience, and will act within the boundaries of my professional competence.

- I will maintain my competence at the highest level through continuing study, training, and research.

- I will report research findings and practice activities honestly and without distortion.

- I will not discriminate because of race, color, national origin, religion, age or socioeconomic status in rendering service, employing, training, or promoting others.

- I value the privacy, dignity, and worth of the individual, and will use skills consistent with these values.

- I will observe the principle of informed consent with respect to individuals and groups served.

- I will support change by choice, not by coercion.

- I will foster an educational environment that nurtures individual growth and development.

- If I become aware of unethical practices, I am accountable for taking appropriate action concerning these practices.

Figure 2-6
SOPHE's Code of
Ethics (Brief Edition)

Human Subjects Review

When we design programs and select intervention methods, it is important we keep ethical considerations in mind. For example, if we are conducting any data collection, we must go through a formal review process to protect the rights of human subjects in research. These *institutional review boards* (IRBs) are a requirement for any programs that receive federal funding. They are established by government, colleges, universities, and other agencies to review ongoing research projects. They have formal guidelines to protect the rights of subjects, including the right to know what will happen, the right to privacy, and the right to be free from harm.

Ethical Obligations to Employer

We are responsible to our employer, which means we are obligated to give full effort to our job. If we have been hired to work a 40-hour week, we must ethically devote 40 hours to the work as defined by our employer. It is not ethical for us to define what our work is unless we are self-employed. If we believe our employer is asking us to do something that is unethical, it is our obligation to discuss it with him or her. If it is then clear we are being asked to do something improper, we should report it to the next-higher authority,

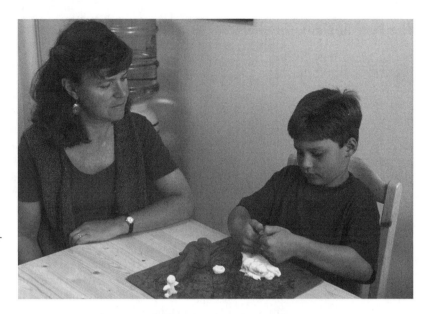

Institutional review boards use formal guidelines to monitor ongoing research projects that involve human subjects.

Quality health education is not easy, and it is not accidental.

resign, or do both. If we are asked to teach something we do not believe in due to religious or other conflicts, we are obligated to discuss this with our employer. Perhaps someone else can teach that topic or other accommodation can be made, but it is not ethical for us unilaterally to change the curriculum or lesson to fit our personal beliefs. We must work through channels to either get it changed, teach it, or allow someone else to teach it.

We also have the obligation to keep up to date and to employ the best methods. We often hear of the shortcomings of health education programs. After reading this text, you will probably recognize that we do have the tools to be successful, but many practitioners are not applying what we know. This is an ethical issue. Quality health education is not easy, and it is not accidental—it takes hard, dedicated work.

Case Study: Nathaniel

Nathaniel has been assigned to teach a personal health course at a local community college. The outline calls for two days of coverage of HIV-AIDS issues. Nathaniel is not very conversant in these issues so he substitutes two additional days in the nutrition area, which he enjoys. Several students and student reporters go to the dean to urge the dean to be certain AIDS is covered in personal health courses. The dean says that it is part of all personal health courses. Several students have just completed Nathaniel's course and state emphatically that it is not. The dean is very angry when she discovers that Nathaniel has not covered the prescribed material. Can Nathaniel defend his position? (See Case Studies Revisited page 42.)

The Learning Environment

The mental/emotional environment can be influenced by the physical environment in which we conduct our classes or workshops. We must do what we can to make the total environment as pleasant as possible. If we have control over the space, we should strive to develop a cheerful positive appearance that is more conducive to learning. It is common sense that a room that is warm and cheerful is important for good learning. Select warm colors and organize the space to be inviting. Adding colorful paper and posters also sets a positive mood. Be certain to change the colors and posters on a regular basis. Often in community settings we have limited control over the physical setting.

Case Study: Susan

Susan inherits a classroom that is run down and gloomy in appearance. Many years ago it was painted a battleship gray, which has now faded. The bulletin boards are old and worn. She believes that this is contributing to a negative atmosphere and wants to do something about it. She has requested through her principal that it be repaired. She discusses the problem with her students, who organize a fund-raising drive that results in $85 for paint and paper. Over the break students volunteer to help scrub and paint the room. The transformation is dramatic. The three days of vacation time spent painting result in a major change in the total environment. Susan notices a significant change in the classroom climate. (See Case Studies Revisited page 43.)

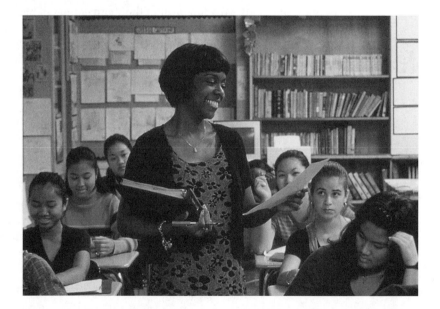

Rooms that are decorated cheerfully with warm colors offer an inviting learning environment.

Noise Levels Noise can be a major distraction in the learning environment. Select a site free of distractions as much as possible. Soft background music can sometimes overcome some noise from the outside. Other noise can come from participants and can also be a distraction or could simply indicate a high degree of interest. Noise must be assessed in terms of what helps achieve learning. Many classrooms are so quiet that learning is unlikely to be taking place. Participants need opportunities to show enthusiasm and ask questions. The reason for the noise is an important consideration. All participants should have an opportunity to hear and be heard.

Seating Arrangements The way you organize your seating is very important. Most situations allow for some change. Determine what would be the best seating arrangement for the objectives you hope to achieve. If you want interaction, a circle might be best. If you feel you need most interaction to be between you and the group, a semicircle might be best. If it is a large group, you might consider multiple rows with your position elevated. If you want small-group work, you might consider small clusters. Figures 2-7 through 2-12 depict various seating arrangements.

It is important to plan ahead and not let seating happen simply by accident. Arrive early for workshops and plan your environment. Arrange the

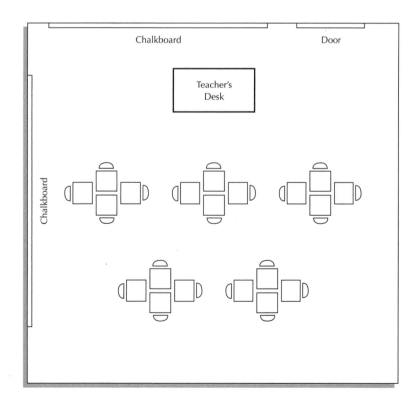

Figure 2-7
Classroom Seating
Objective: Interaction
and Small-Group Work

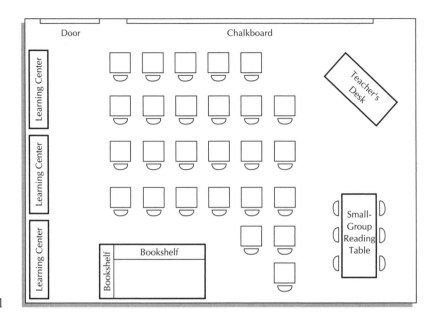

Figure 2-8
Classroom Objective:
Flexibility with Control

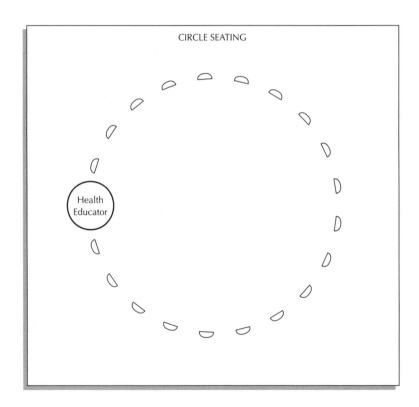

Figure 2-9
Community or School
Objective: Interaction

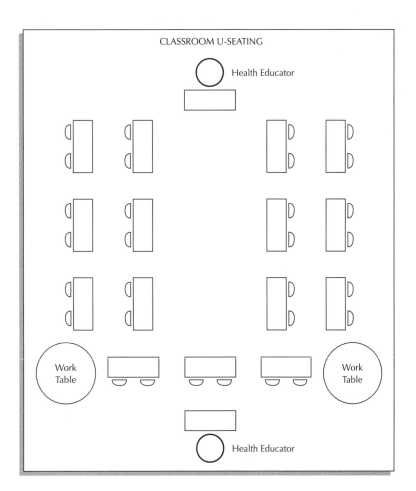

Figure 2-10
Classroom Objective: Flexibility with Emphasis on Interaction

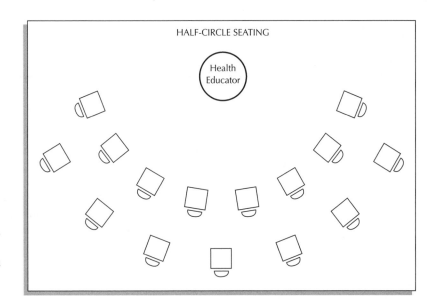

Figure 2-11
Classroom or Community Objective: Controlled Interaction with Health Educator in Controlling Position

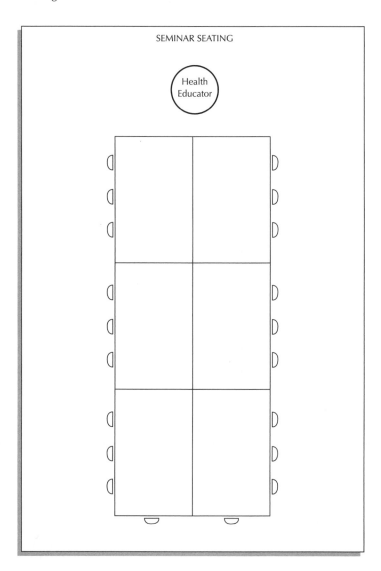

Figure 2-12
Community or School
Objective: Controlled
Interaction

seating and let people know it is not okay to change it. If you do not want people sitting in the back, then do not place seats in the back. If you are in the classroom, do not let students pick where they sit until you know them well. Certain students or participants should never sit together. Be certain to also consider any special needs students have such as hearing or sight limitations. Putting someone in an incorrect seat can produce a behavioral problem. For example, a participant who cannot hear may become very disruptive simply because he or she cannot participate.

Using the Total Environment

In the past many health education programs have assumed that the few contact hours of the program could lead to major changes in the target population without giving consideration to the total environment in which individual members exist. It is important that we give consideration to the total physical and mental climate in which these people live.

While we may not have the capability to significantly alter this environment, we can probably provide the knowledge or skills to alter perceptions of the environment. That is, we might help participants overcome feelings of lack of control or helplessness or we might provide information on where to get help to change the environment.

Case Study: Maria Maria has conducted a community workshop on the need for prenatal care. The major objective was to increase knowledge regarding the reasons to seek such care and increase compliance. The workshop was well attended, and the information seemed to be received with interest. Post-workshop assessment shows knowledge was significantly increased. However, a six-month follow-up shows no increase in compliance. (See Case Studies Revisited page 43.)

For more information and tools related to this chapter visit
www.jbpub.com/healtheducation.

EXERCISES

1. You have been asked to develop a sexuality unit for ninth grade high school students. What do you think would be appropriate goals for such a unit? Also, write three sample objectives you feel would be reasonable, being sure to include at least one from the *affective* domain.

2. Select a health topic and target population. Now, in thinking of how to justify the development of your program, list specific resources or agencies from which you could obtain supportive data. (These must be *real* sources.) You will need to conduct some research and then cite addresses or Internet information related to the agencies or other sources you would use to support your proposal.

3. What are the three major reasons for developing objectives?

4. Describe four important factors to consider when developing objectives or selecting methods.

5. What are the major differences between goals and objectives?

6. Describe how could you utilize national health objectives like Healthy People 2000 or 2010 to develop your own local program objectives. Illustrate your answer by selecting any specific health topic.

CASE STUDIES REVISITED

Case Study Revisited: Pat

Since Pat's only stated objective was to end drug use, she has failed by her own standards. Pat has not set realistic objectives in measurable terms for her program, and because of this mistake the program was virtually certain to fail. Further, Pat has not determined through a needs assessment what the current status of the community is in terms of its needs and interests and the prevalence of drug use. If, for example, Pat had discovered that drugs were being used by 35 percent of adolescents in the community, she could structure her objectives to reflect a modest but realistic behavior or attitude change. Pat has failed to plan carefully for instruction. (See page 10.)

Case Study Revisited: Joe

The strengths of this plan are that Joe has collected local statistics and is planning to survey the community and hold a focus group. The knowledge testing will provide a baseline, but is knowledge all that is sought as an outcome?

Cost estimates in time and money are not provided, but this program could be too expensive given the total budget. Needs assessment plans need to be realistic. (See page 11.)

Case Study Revisited: Jerry

Through his haste and poorly conceived, unrealistic objectives, Jerry has placed the entire sexuality program in jeopardy. He made the same two fundamental errors in planning, as Pat did in the earlier case study. First, Jerry did not conduct a thorough needs assessment before designing program goals and objectives. If Jerry promises a reduction in sexually transmitted infections, he will need to obtain data as to their existing prevalence in order to make a subsequent comparison. The likelihood of even being allowed to collect such sensitive data in a public school is at best marginal. Second, in constructing his objectives Jerry was extremely unrealistic as to what any single program could accomplish. Constructing program *goals* related to reducing rates of unintended pregnancy and sexually transmitted infections would be appropriate, but specific behavioral *objectives* that need to be measurable should be much more modest and reasonable in scope. As discussed in Chapter 10, setting such unattainable objectives in a controversial area such as human sexuality can do irreparable and sometimes fatal damage to a program that may be constantly under scrutiny. (See page 16.)

Case Study Revisited: Nathaniel

Nathaniel's actions were poorly thought out and based on selfish motives. If Nathaniel was supposed to teach to an already existing syllabus, then he should have prepared sufficiently to be able to cover all topics. Alternately, Nathaniel could have used a more knowledgeable guest speaker or colleague to cover a particular topic. Nathaniel has certainly not helped himself professionally by angering his dean, and his actions would be difficult to defend. (See page 35.)

Case Study Revisited: Susan Susan has demonstrated an understanding of the effects that the environment can have on learning, and she has shown a great deal of initiative in enhancing her own particular environment. The atmosphere in Susan's classes may not change overnight, but she has optimized the possibility for change. Health educators should not underestimate the effects that the physical environment can have on learning, and in some cases how easily the environment can be improved. (See page 36.)

Case Study Revisited: Maria Maria has conducted a useful workshop that obviously provided some needed factual information. However, in preparing for her presentation, Maria failed to consider the total environment of her target population, and just what compliance would necessitate. Maria provided no information on the accessibility of the clinic, how to get there, and failed to emphasize the very low costs involved. She gave no real thought to the total environment of this group or the potential barriers to effecting a positive behavior change. (See page 41.)

SUMMARY

Selecting or writing the appropriate educational goals and objectives is important for any health education program.

1. The selection of an objective should always consider the resources available to achieve that objective.

2. A needs assessment is an important step before selecting or writing objectives or selecting methods.

3. Goals may be general, but objectives must be specific and measurable.

4. In writing objectives, the educational purposes (process or outcome) must be considered.

5. All domains should be considered if adequate time and resources are available.

6. Methods should be selected with proper ethics in mind.

7. The total environment must be considered when planning for instruction.

REFERENCES

Bloom, B. (1956). *Taxonomy of Educational Objectives: The Classification of Educational Goals Handbook I: Cognitive Domain.* New York: David McKay.

Gilmore, G. D. (1977). Needs assessment process for community health education. *International Journal of Health Education, 20,* 164–173.

Green, L. W., & Kreuter, M. W. (1991). *Health Promotion and Planning: An Educational and Environmental Approach.* Mountain View: Mayfield.

Green, L. W., Levine, D. M., & Deeds, S. G. (1975). Clinical trials of health education for hypertensive outpatients: Design and baseline data. *Preventive Medicine, 4,* 417–425.

Green, L. W., Levine, D. M., Wolle, J., & Deeds, S. G. (1979). Development of randomized patient education experiments with urban poor hypertensives. *Patient Counseling and Health Education, 1,* 106–111.

Krathwohl, D., et al. (1956). *Taxonomy of Educational Objectives: The Classification of Educational Goals Handbook II: Affective Domain.* New York: David McKay.

Morisky, D. E., DeMuth, N. E., Field-Fass, M., et al. (1985). Evaluation of family health education to build social support for long-term control of high blood pressure. *Health Education Quarterly, 12,* 35–50.

Morisky, D. E., Levine, L., Green, L. W., et al. (1983). Five-year blood pressure control and mortality following health education for hypertensive patients. *American Journal of Public Health,* 73, 153–162.

Popham, J., & Baber, E. (1970). *Establishing Instructional Goals.* Englewood Cliffs, NJ: Prentice-Hall.

Ross, H., & Mico, P. (1980). *Theory and Practice in Health Education.* Palo Alto: Mayfield.

Taba, H. (1962). *Curriculum Development.* New York: Harcourt, Brace and World.

Toohey, J. V., & Shireffs, J. H. (1980). *Health Education, 11,* 15–17.

U.S. Department of Health and Human Services. (1980). *Promoting Health/Preventing Disease: Objectives for the Nation.* Washington, D.C.: Government Printing Office.

U.S. Department of Health and Human Services. (1992). *Healthy Communities 2000: Model Standards.* Washington, D.C.: Government Printing Office.

U.S. Department of Health and Human Services. (1992). *Healthy People 2000: National Health Promotion Objectives: Full Report, with Commentary.* Boston: Jones and Bartlett.

Selecting an Intervention/ Method

Co-authored by
Marjorie E. Scaffa
University of South Alabama

Entry Level and Graduate Level Health Educator Competencies Addressed In This Chapter

Responsibility I: Assessing Individual and Community Needs for Health Education
   Competency A: Obtain health related data about social and cultural environments, growth and development factors, needs, and interests.
   Competency C: Infer needs for health education on the basis of obtained data.

Responsibility II: Planning Effective Health Education Programs
   Competency B: Develop a logical scope and sequence plan for a health education program.

Responsibility IV: Evaluating Effectiveness of Health Education Programs
   Competency A: Develop plans to assess achievement of program objectives.

Responsibility VII: Communicating Health and Health Education Needs, Concerns, and Resources
   Competency A: Interpret concepts, purposes, and theories of health education.
   Competency B: Predict the impact of societal value systems on health education programs.

Method Selection in Health Education

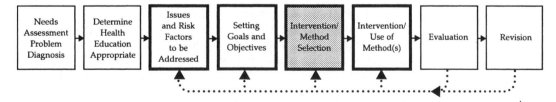

Heavy-bordered boxes indicate subjects addressed in this text; shaded boxes indicate subject(s) of current chapter.

Publisher's Note: This chapter includes copyrighted material from Marjorie E. Scaffa's doctoral dissertation entitled "The Development of Comprehensive Theory in Health Education: a Feasibility Study" and is used with permission. The publisher and authors gratefully acknowledge Dr. Scaffa's contribution.

Note: The competencies listed on page 45, which are addressed in this chapter, are considered to be both entry-level and graduate-level competencies by the National Commission for Health Education Credentialing, Inc. They are taken from A Framework for the Development of Competency Based Curricula for Entry Level Health Educators by the National Task Force for the Preparation and Practice of Health Education, 1985; and A Competency-based Framework for Graduate Level Health Educators by the National Task Force for the Preparation and Practice of Health Education, 1999.

OBJECTIVES   After studying the chapter the reader should be able to

- List the major considerations in selecting an educational intervention/method.
- Employ appropriate theories and models in method selection.
- Present a rationale for proper selection of a method.
- List the most common mistakes in method selection.

KEY ISSUES

Objectives	Budget
Educational principles	Resources/site/environment
Theory and model application	Characteristics of the
Educational domains	educational provider
Characteristics of the learner	Cultural appropriateness
and the community	Using a variety of methods
Group size	Packaging the total
Contact time	intervention strategy

Objectives as Drivers of Selection

Selecting the appropriate educational intervention is vital to achieving your objectives. Therefore, the objectives should drive the selection of all educational interventions and methods. In other words, the methods selected must be appropriate for the objectives sought. The previous chapter has described the components of setting goals and objectives. This chapter emphasizes the importance of reviewing objectives before selecting methods. Such a review is always the first step in selection. Interventions and methods must be linked with the objectives they are likely to achieve.

We use the term **intervention** to describe the total overall strategy to achieve our objectives. A **method** refers to one component of the intervention such as an educational game or a health fair. Each is only one of perhaps many methods we could employ to achieve our objectives. All educators have the selection process in common, but the health educator must also consider how the chosen strategies might influence clients' attitudes that influence health and directly influencing health behaviors. Further, the health educator must often work with very modest amounts of time and limited resources. Given that health educators may be asked to help clients modify complex and deeply rooted practices, selecting the correct methods is indeed a challenge. Nevertheless, we do have an arsenal of methods and a knowledge base to help us with these decisions. This chapter will review the issues to be considered when selecting an intervention strategy (method).

| **Case Study: John** | John is offering a workshop for low-income expectant mothers as part of his work for the March of Dimes. He personally likes role playing as a method, so he has written up several role plays about life after the delivery. The site for the two-hour workshop is a nice upscale hotel, and he has mailed approximately 100 invitations. This is a very culturally diverse community with many Asians, Salvadorians, and Mexican Americans. John is surprised at the low participant turnout and very indignant when the few mothers-to-be in attendance walk out rather than participate in role plays. (See Case Studies Revisited page 74.) |

Educational Principles

You should also review basic educational principles when determining which methods to employ. Have you applied as many educational principles as possible, such as reinforcement, repetition, and practice? Reviewing these principles will often trigger new ideas about which methods to use or not to use.

In order to address health issues through health education, it is important that we draw on the vast knowledge base that education has developed to tell us how to educate learners. The following principles, adapted from Gilbert's text (1981), are of enormous importance to health education.

Principles Related to Motivation Teaching is effective only when clients are motivated to learn. Some principles of motivation follow:

- Learning is more effective when the learner is motivated by results intrinsic to the experience.
- Individuals tend to repeat behaviors that are rewarded (reinforced).
- Immediate reinforcement is more effective than delayed reinforcement.
- Fear and punishment have uncertain effects upon learning. They may facilitate or hinder learning.
- An individual learns best when he or she believes the learning is important.
- Learners can be helped to understand a concept, principle, or generalization by showing them how varied experiences relate to it and then how it can be applied to a new situation.

Principles Related to Needs and Abilities

Clients can learn only to the extent of their abilities, and they are usually motivated to learn only that which they perceive as necessary. Therefore, educators must determine the needs and abilities of their client base. Principles related to this task follow:

- Behaviors sought should be within the range of possibility for the learner involved.
- Generally, the higher the educational level of any given group, the greater is the willingness to use the printed word.
- The lower the educational level, the greater is the need for oral or picture media.
- There are marked individual differences in any given group of learners.
- Individuals usually slant persuasive communications to fit their own biases. It is important to protect learners from your biases.
- Creative individuals show a preference for the complex and the novel.
- When problems or issues are a common concern, group thinking is an effective approach to learning.

Principles Related to General Nature of Learning

Health educators, like any other educators, should be familiar with the following principles of the functions of learning:

- In order for learning to occur, repetition is usually required.
- Learning should be an active process that involves the dynamic interaction of the learner with that which is to be learned.
- Other things being equal, recent experiences are more vivid than earlier ones.
- Learning generally proceeds from the general to the specific, then to the general (whole–part–whole).
- **Transfer learning** is not automatic. We must teach for transfer.
- Behaviors or skills sought must be practiced.
- Learning generally progresses from the known to the unknown, from the concrete to the abstract, and from the simple to the complex.
- Periods of practice interrupted by periods of rest result in more efficient learning than do longer periods of practice with few or no interruptions.
- Time spent recalling and discussing what has been read facilitates learning more than mere rereading.

Theory and Model Application

Health educators and researchers from many disciplines have developed numerous theories and models to try to explain human behavior with regard to health practices and ways we might intervene as health educators. These models and theories have important applications in method selection. If we wish to test a model or theory, we should be careful to select a method compatible with that model or theory. If we have theoretical notions, we should draw on the available theories and models and related research to improve on our ideas. For example, we should ask how models and theories such as the health belief model or social learning theory apply to our strategy, and how we can utilize these ideas to improve and focus our total intervention and individual methods.

Ideas can be classified in many ways. Cornish (1980) suggests they be classified in two categories: concepts and theories. He defines a **concept** as a generalized notion, a mental map, or an image of some phenomenon and a **theory** as a description of two or more concepts and the relationship among them (Cornish, 1980). Thought involves the manipulation of concepts and theories and provides us with models of how the world functions. A **model** can be defined as a semantic or diagrammatic representation of concepts and their interrelationships that allows for operationalization, experimental assessment, and application of a theory (Parcel, 1984). Not all theories have corresponding models, and not all models are founded on specific, well-defined theories.

Current Status of Theory in Health Education

One of the fundamental characteristics of a true profession is that it has a theoretical base underlying its practice, within which parameters the profession operates (Shireffs, 1984). As an interdisciplinary field, health education draws its body of knowledge from a variety of sources. Health education relies on the biological sciences for much of its content; the behavioral sciences for much of its philosophy, program development, and implementation strategies; and education for much of its methodology (Rubinson and Alles, 1984).

Due, in part, to its broad interdisciplinary nature, some argue health education lacks a clearly defined, readily identifiable body of knowledge. Since the body of knowledge is growing, it is sometimes diffuse and hard to identify, particularly because of the lack of consensus on what is the core of health education. As stated earlier, this text is based on the idea that the core of the discipline of health education is the *process* of health education. This means that what is most important is how well and effectively we perform the function of educating people about health decisions. This process of health education, then, is the crucial focus for a health educator. There are many other tools available to health educators, but what is unique about health education as a discipline is that health educators are trained to perform the process of health education. Various models and theories are available as tools to facilitate the basic task.

Typically, in the development of the sciences, theory precedes application. However, health education has been traditionally, and continues to be, very practice oriented. The field has evolved without having a well-developed, unique theoretical base (Creswell, 1984; Dwore and Matarazzo, 1981; Frazer, Kukulka, and Richardson, 1988). A premise that has predominated in health education for many years is that knowledge and a positive attitude will lead to health-enhancing behavior change (Shireffs, 1984). This assumption has been demonstrated to be simplistic, ill founded, and ineffective, yet much of the field continues to practice health education and conduct research utilizing this principle (Shireffs, 1984; Frazer, Kukulka, and Richardson, 1988).

Health education has borrowed well-defined theoretical frameworks from other disciplines, most notably social learning theory, problem-behavior theory, theory of reasoned action, communications theory, and behavioral theory (Parcel, 1984). Although these models from the behavioral sciences are valuable, it must be recognized that they are not health behavior specific and have been shown to be of limited usefulness in the treatment and prevention of disease and dysfunction (Dwore and Matarazzo, 1981). Indeed, few of the theories have been developed by individuals who would call themselves health educators.

A well-developed theoretical base in health education is helpful for a variety of reasons. Theory can provide the foundation and context for basic and applied research and program design, implementation, and evaluation. Following is a description of some the popular constructs or concepts, theories, and models found in the professional health education literature and a critique of their appropriateness for health education practice and research. This is not meant to be an exhaustive account of relevant theoretical approaches, but rather a sampling in order to illustrate the current state of theory as they are applied health education.

Constructs

Of all of the sociopsychological variables that may affect health-related behavior, three appear to receive the most attention in health education literature: locus of control, self-efficacy, and behavioral intent. These constructs can aid us in method selection or evaluation.

Health Locus of Control

The **health locus of control** construct was first described by Wallston et al. (1976). It was developed as a health-specific adaptation of the internal-external locus of control concept postulated by Rotter in 1954 as one component of social learning theory (discussed shortly). Locus of control was considered a means of predicting behavior based on an individual's expectations of reinforcement. Reinforcement was believed to be either under the control of the individual (**internal locus**) or under the control of outside forces (**external locus**). Externality has been associated with feelings of powerlessness, and internality with self-motivated behaviors (Wallston and Wallston, 1978).

Health locus of control, it was suggested, could be used to predict a variety of health behaviors, including information seeking, compliance with medication regimens, smoking cessation, and appointment keeping (Wallston and Wallston, 1978). Levenson (1974) expanded the health locus of control construct to include two dimensions of externality: belief that reinforcement is due to fate or chance and belief in control by powerful others. If an individual perceives that an event is contingent upon his or her own actions, then the person is considered to have an internal locus of control. If, on the other hand, an individual perceives that an event is contingent upon the actions of powerful others or occurs as a result of luck or chance, then he or she is considered to have an external locus of control (Parcel, Nader, and Rogers, 1980). It is readily apparent that if we have this information about a group it would influence our selection of intervention (Casey, Kingery, Bouder and Corbbett, 1993).

Currently, several health-specific locus of control scales exist. These include the original health locus of control scale by Wallston et al. (1976), the multidimensional health locus of control scale by Wallston, Wallston, and DeVillis (1978), and the children's health locus of control scale by Parcel and Meyer (1978).

Case Study: Marcel

Marcel is working with a community group on a series of workshops designed to improve general levels of health, particularly related to nutrition and heart health. As he begins his introductory statements on the benefits of good food, Marcel notices several cynical looks and some careless whispering. Putting aside his carefully prepared notes, Marcel stops the workshop to query the participants' reactions. After several minutes of discussion, what becomes clear to Marcel is that many of the participants feel that they cannot influence their own health behavior. Instead of continuing on with the planned presentation, Marcel decides to employ a health locus of control instrument and finds over 50 percent of the group feel external forces control their health status. Marcel then decides to modify his programming by designing an intervention that not only includes factual information related to heart health, but also strategies to address the issue of locus of control, such as having physicians help in directing participants behavior. (See Case Studies Revisited page 74.)

Self-Efficacy

Self-efficacy is defined as the individual's perception that he or she will be able to perform a specific behavior successfully (Bandura, 1977). A belief in one's own competence to execute a task is required to produce a desired outcome. Self-efficacy expectations are derived from several sources of information: previous performance accomplishments, vicarious experiences **(modeling),** verbal persuasion, and emotional arousal (Bandura, 1977).

Successful performance increases expectations of mastery whereas repeated failures diminish them. The effects of failure, however, are partially dependent on the timing and the pattern of the negative experiences. Watching others who are similar to oneself overcoming obstacles by determined effort increases self-efficacy. Modeling by a variety of personally significant individuals is more effective than repeated modeling by a single person. Self-efficacy is increased if the modeled behavior has clear and observable outcomes. Verbal persuasion is an effective adjunct to performance accomplishments and modeling, but it rarely increases self-efficacy when used by itself.

Increased levels of anxiety usually interfere with performance and lower efficacy expectations. Behavioral control of these anxiety levels and cogni-

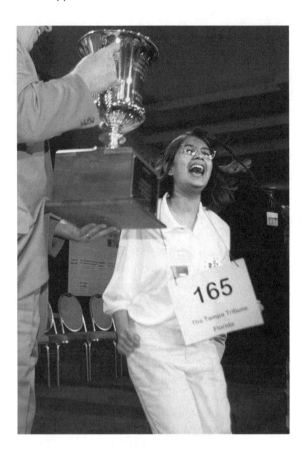

Self-efficacy, the belief that one will perform a behavior successfully, probably aided Nupur Lala as she spelled her way to victory.

tive reappraisal of related physiological and emotional states can increase self-efficacy (Bandura, 1977).

It is hypothesized that efficacy expectations influence what behaviors will be initiated, the degree of effort that will be expended, and the persistence of the behavior over time. Perceived self-efficacy has a direct influence on an individual's choice of activities and settings (Bandura, 1977). Expectation of successful performance alone will not produce the desired behavior; necessary skill capabilities and incentives are also required. The reader can readily see the relationship of these models and concepts to educational principles.

Efficacy expectations change over time and vary on several dimensions, including magnitude, generality, and strength (Bandura, 1977). *Magnitude* refers to the level of difficulty with which an individual experiences a sense of competence. *Generality* refers to an ability to extend one's sense of efficacy beyond a situation. *Strength* refers to the degree to which the expectation can be extinguished by disconfirming experiences. Weak expectations are easily abandoned, whereas strong expectations may persist in spite of some negative experiences (Bandura, 1977).

It has been suggested that simple self-efficacy measures may be helpful as a starting point in interventions focused on exercise, stress, diet and medicine use (Clark and Dodge, 1999).

Case Study: Nancy

Nancy is working with a group of senior smokers. Although Nancy is an ex-smoker herself, the group, being much older, does not see her as a role model. Instead of simply moving ahead and ignoring this issue, Nancy decides to bring in a panel of older ex-smokers to review the skills needed to stop smoking. The individuals on the panel discuss in depth their experiences with stopping smoking, and the group seems to relate well to the session. Nancy finds a pronounced difference in group response following this panel. Self-efficacy has clearly improved. Nancy is pleased that she was able to incorporate a strategy that seemed to facilitate learning but is somewhat disappointed at herself for not anticipating this problem before it arose. (See Case Studies Revisited, page 74.)

Behavioral Intent

Behavioral intent, according to Ajzen and Fishbein (1973), is the immediate antecedent of overt behavior. It is an individual's resolution (intent) to perform a specific act with respect to a given stimulus in a given situation. It is the attitude about a specific behavior that is relevant, not attitudes toward objects, people, or situations.

Behavioral intent is thought to be a function of two basic factors. One is personal in nature and the other is reflective of social influences. The *personal factor* is the individual's attitude, positive or negative, toward performing a specific behavior—that is, whether or not he or she is in favor of or against engaging in this behavior. The *social factor* is the individual's perception of the social pressures to act or not to act in a specific manner. This factor is often referred to as the **subjective norm.** Neither of these two factors in isolation are thought to be sufficient to determine behavioral intent. Ajzen and Fishbein (1973) state that the personal factor plus the subjective norm is necessary to create behavioral intent.

Behavioral intent can be an excellent needs assessment and evaluation method before and after intervention. Measuring this trait is particularly useful when efforts to evaluate actual behavior change may be too costly or time-consuming to be practical. We must, of course, have realistic expectations for our health education program.

Case Study: Don

Don is involved in teaching CPR to a group of metal shop employees. He has little time or resources to carry out an extensive evaluation but is concerned that in previous training workshops participants appeared to have little confidence and seemed unlikely to use the skills covered. Don considers his options and decides to utilize simulation mannequins, which will help participants gauge their skills, and use a pretest/posttest questionnaire to measure any changes in levels of behavioral intent. He employs questions regarding self-assessed skill level and the likelihood of using CPR if faced with a real situation. He is elated to see a marked increase in scores after his 10-hour inservice. (See Case Studies Revisited page 75.)

Among the many theories referred to in health education literature, two are cited more frequently than others: social learning theory and theory of reasoned action. Again, theories can provide a basis for method selection. Much needs to be done to test these theories and link them to appropriate health education interventions.

Social Learning (Cognitive) Theory

In *Social Learning and Clinical Psychology,* Rotter (1954) established the foundation for **social learning theory,** which has since been renamed **social cognitive theory** (Bandura, 1986). He postulated that it was an individual's expectations of the consequences of a particular action that determined whether or not that behavior was performed.

Bandura (1977) expanded on Rotter's work and developed the concept of self-efficacy as an integral component of social learning theory. As previously explained, self-efficacy is defined as the individual's perception that he or she will be able to successfully perform a specific behavior (Bandura, 1977). It is the belief in one's own competence to execute an action that will generally achieve the desired outcome. The most basic postulate of social learning theory is that individuals perform behaviors that result in certain outcomes. However, both the behaviors and the outcomes are mediated by expectancies. An **expectancy** is the value an individual places on a particular outcome (Bandura, 1977).

Efficacy expectations—whether or not an individual believes in his or her ability to perform a given behavior—are derived from personal performance attainments, vicarious experience, verbal persuasion, and emotional arousal. Successful accomplishment of a behavior enhances one's expectation for future endeavors. The more similar the current task to ones performed successfully in the past, the greater are the efficacy expectations. Observation of others who are perceived as being similar to oneself engaging in activities and achieving the desired outcome can also increase one's expectations for accomplishment. Verbal encouragement and permission to try a specific behavior and a perceived physiological and emotional state conducive to successful execution of the task will also enhance an individual's confidence and self-efficacy relative to that behavior, according to the theory. A recent study with school health education teachers reveals a low rating of self-efficacy for recognition of students at risk for suicide (Price, Telljohann, and Wahl, 1999). Schools that offered inservice programs on suicide and crisis intervention demonstrated higher student scores on self-efficacy.

Outcome expectations are the individual's belief that a given behavior will lead to specific outcomes (Bandura, 1977). The locus of control construct is considered an element of outcome expectations by Bandura (1977) and others (Rosenstock, Strecher, and Becker, 1988; Wodarski, 1987; DiBlasio, 1986; Eiser, 1985). The interaction of the constructs of self-efficacy and locus of control forms the foundation for social learning theory and is the basis on which behavior can be predicted (Bandura, 1977). It is expected, according to the theory, that individuals who have high levels of self-efficacy and an internal locus of control will be more likely to attempt to execute a particular behavior than those with low levels of self-efficacy and an external locus of control. These individuals would have a high level of confidence in their ability to successfully accomplish the task and would tend to believe that performance of the behavior would directly affect the outcome (Rosenstock, Strecher, and Becker, 1988). Individuals with low levels of self-efficacy and an external locus of control would be less likely to attempt a given behavior, as they have low levels of confidence in their ability to perform the behavior and tend to believe that their actions would not produce the desired outcome anyway (Rosenstock, Strecher, and Becker, 1988).

Of course, it has been suggested that if we have large numbers of people with high levels of self confidence (self-efficacy) and high locus of control, they probably don't need much health education. Perhaps we should focus on improving both elements in certain populations before we focus too much on health content.

Behavior change, in the social learning theory paradigm, can be achieved directly by reinforcement of particular behaviors; indirectly, through social modeling or observing someone else being reinforced for the behavior; and, as a third option, through self management, in which the individual monitors and rewards himself or herself (Parcel and Baranowski, 1981). According to Rosenstock, Strecher, and Becker (1988), lifestyle changes will occur if the individual believes that

1. The current behaviors pose a threat to a personally valued outcome, for example, health or appearance (environmental cue).
2. The specific behavior change will be likely to reduce these threats (outcome efficacy).
3. He or she is personally competent to perform the desired behavior (efficacy expectation).

Applications of Social Learning Theory in Health Education

Several studies have utilized the social learning theory (SLT) approach in examining health behaviors. DiBlasio (1986) investigated the drinking and driving behavior of students in grades 10 through 12. Five SLT constructs were operationalized and measured through self-report. These constructs included exposure to and identification with various groups, modeling, differential reinforcement, personal attitudes and beliefs, and positive or negative social rewards or consequences. The theory was supported, as all of the constructs significantly contributed to the adolescents' decisions to drive under the influence or ride with someone who was intoxicated. The greatest predictor of all of the constructs was exposure to or identification with specific groups. DiBlasio's (1986) recommendation, based on these results, was to

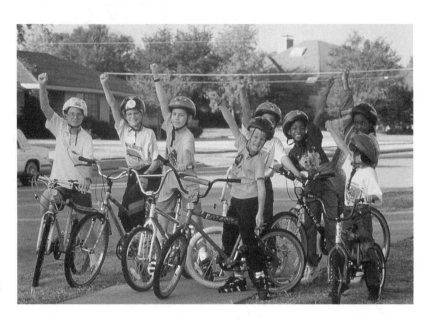

Identification with specific groups can greatly influence the behavior of children and adolescents.

include parents and peers in the planning of prevention programs regarding driving under the influence. Knowledge of such findings is very important for method selection and determining how we utilize contact time.

Wodarski (1987) evaluated the usefulness of SLT in the development and implementation of an educational intervention for adolescents on drinking and driving. A teams/games/tournament approach was designed to enhance self-efficacy and to provide positive social outcomes for the desired behaviors. The results indicated that, when compared to a control group, the intervention students demonstrated a significant decrease in self-reported alcohol consumption and a significant increase in knowledge and self-efficacy related to drinking behavior. Such studies may point to the need for physical education and recreation programs for youth beyond the fitness values.

Parcel and Baranowski (1981) described the application of SLT as it relates to phases in the behavior change process. They concluded that the various constructs of SLT were relevant at different stages in the process of behavior change. Baranowski's four phases of behavior change include pretraining, training, initial self-testing, and continued performance.

In the *pretraining* phase expectancies are the key constructs. What a person believes about a given health problem, what anxieties are associated with these beliefs, and the perception of changeability are all relevant issues during this phase.

In the *training* phase the focus is on developing the capability to perform the desired behaviors and on learning to cope with problems associated with the change process itself. The construct of **behavioral capability** states that if an individual is to engage in a specific behavior, he or she must have *knowledge* of the parameters of the behavior and the *skill* to carry it out successfully. According to SLT, behavioral capability can be acquired through the observation of others engaged in the behavior or social modeling, as well as direct skill training (Parcel and Baranowski, 1981).

In the *self-testing* phase the construct of self-efficacy appears to be the most influential. Confidence in one's ability is essential if the skills learned in the training phase are to be implemented. The technique of successive approximations is particularly useful in the development of self-efficacy.

In the final phase, *continued performance*, the construct of self-control is the most salient. In order for a behavior to be maintained over time, an individual must be able to resist the temptation to discontinue the behavior and to delay gratification. Contracting and self-monitoring are methods of enhancing self-control (Parcel and Baranowski, 1981).

In general, social learning theory provides a unique perspective for health education practice. The constructs of self-efficacy, outcome expectancy, behavioral capability, modeling, and self-control appear to be particularly relevant for the development of health education interventions.

Case Study: Jessica

Jessica is working with a group of young people at the YMCA with the hope of increasing their resistance skills to offers of drugs. After reading about various models and theories of health behavior, Jessica plans to cover ways of saying "no thanks." She makes a determined effort to have each person practice saying "no" in a role play in front of the other group members. Each session is critiqued by the other members, and other suggestions for strategies are fully discussed. Even though this is a time-consuming methodology, each person has three such sessions of saying "no." The self-confidence of the group members regarding the possession of needed skills and the feeling that they can and will use the skills is greatly enhanced. (See Case Studies Revisited page 75.)

Theory of Reasoned Action

Attitude theory serves as the basis for the work of Fishbein and Ajzen and their **theory of reasoned action.** This theory postulates that an individual's attitude toward an object is a function of his or her beliefs about the object. **Attitudes** are defined as learned predispositions to consistently respond to objects in favorable or unfavorable ways (Fishbein, 1973).

The theory of reasoned action is based on two assumptions. One assumption is that human beings are usually very rational and make systematic decisions based on available information. It dismisses the notion that unconscious motives can influence behavior and insists that individuals carefully consider the implications of their behavior before engaging in specific activities (Ajzen and Fishbein, 1980).

A second assumption is that most behavior is under volitional control and that in a specific situation an individual forms an intent to act that subsequently influences overt behavior (Ajzen and Fishbein, 1973). This behavioral intent is viewed as the most immediately relevant predictor of behavior. According to the theory, behavioral intent is determined by the individual's attitude toward the behavior, normative beliefs regarding the behavior, and motivation to comply with the norms (Ajzen and Fishbein, 1973).

Attitude toward the behavior, in this context, is defined as the individual's positive or negative evaluation of performing the behavior. **Normative belief,** or subjective norm (mentioned earlier), refers to the individual's perception of the social pressures to perform or not to perform the behavior in question. Conflict between an individual's attitude toward the behavior and the subjective norm is not uncommon. Assigning relative weights to these two determinants greatly enhances the predictive value of the behavioral intent construct and the explanatory value of the theory (Ajzen and Fishbein, 1980).

According to Ajzen and Fishbein (1973), the central equation of the theory is that behavior is determined by behavioral intent that is equal to the individual's attitude toward the act plus the individual's normative belief multiplied by his or her motivation to comply with the norm.

The theory of reasoned action has several limitations. Although it makes reference to attitudes toward behavior, it does not include attitudes toward objects, people, or institutions. These attitudes may also have an impact on behavioral intent. In addition, other factors that may influence behavior, such as personality variables and demographic characteristics, are not considered. Ajzen and Fishbein (1980) contend that it is unnecessary to attempt to link these external variables to behavioral phenomena, as the intervening factors, that is, behavioral intent, can account for these effects.

Another possible limitation is the degree of specificity necessary for the theory to accurately predict behavior. The relationship between attitude, behavioral intent, and behavior is not consistently supported in the literature. Behavioral intent appears to be a relatively good predictor under many conditions. The more abstract or generalized the measure of intention, the less is its predictive capability. A measure of behavioral intent such as "I intend to exercise" is much less predictive than the statement "I intend to walk two miles, three times a week for the next three months." The longer the time interval between the measure of intent and the observation of the behavior, the less likely the behavior is to occur. Behavioral intent appears to be unstable and variable over time, which limits its usefulness as a predictor of behavior.

Other Selected Theories Relevant to Health Education

Problem-Behavior Theory

Three other theories applicable to health education are problem-behavior theory, communications theory, and behavioral theory.

Jessor and Jessor (1977) developed **problem-behavior theory,** which has its conceptual roots in social psychology. It is an attempt to develop a profile of vulnerability or predisposition toward health-threatening behaviors such as alcohol consumption, drug use, smoking, and risky sexual behavior. This theoretical framework is based on the interrelationships and interactions among three major explanatory concepts: personality, perceived environment, and behavior. Each concept has specific variables that have implications for the incidence of problem behaviors. A major contribution of this theory is its application in the explanation of risk-taking behavior of adolescents in the normal developmental process.

Communications theory is not a single theory but rather many approaches designed to change people's attitudes and behavior through persuasive techniques (Parcel, 1984). One eclectic approach is known as the **information-processing paradigm** (McGuire, 1981). In this model the communication-persuasion process occurs in six phases and consists of five components. The components of communication are described as source, message, channel, receiver, and destination. The phases, or behavioral steps, in the process of persuasion are presentation, attention, comprehension, yielding, retention, and overt behavior (McGuire, 1981). Communications theory has been used effectively in health education in the design and conduct of a public health campaign (McGuire, 1981). It may also be useful in an attempt to inoculate children against persuasion in the media and peer pressure (Parcel, 1984).

Behavioral theories are multiple and are variations derived from Watson and Skinner's notions of behaviorism. **Behavior modification** is a technique, based on behavioral theory, designed to develop new behaviors or alter existing behaviors (Stainbrook and Green, 1982). Basically, the presupposition of behavioral theory is that behavior is a function of reinforcement conditions. If a behavior is reinforced, then it will increase in frequency. Reinforcement may be positive, as in the administration of some pleasurable consequence, or negative, as in the removal of some pleasant condition.

In its most radical form, behaviorism focuses on the study and control of external environmental variables. Internal constructs such as attitudes and mental processes are dismissed as unimportant at best, and irrelevant at worst (Stainbrook and Green, 1982). Behavioral strategies have proved effective in the treatment of habit disorders, behavior or conduct problems, and in skill acquisition and development.

Models

Clearly, two models relevant to health education are very popular in the literature. One, the **health belief model,** is a model of the precursors of health behavior; the other, the **PRECEDE-PROCEED model,** is a program planning and evaluation tool. A third, lesser known model is called the **transtheoretical model** or **stages of change model.**

Cummings, Becker, and Maile (1980), in a review of 14 models used in health education research, concluded that there is considerable overlap in the constructs or variables that make up these frameworks. These investigators attempted to develop a unified framework for explaining health behavior by involving the authors of the various models in categorizing over 100 variables derived from the models. Six factors emerged from the multidimensional scaling analysis: (1) access to health care services; (2) attitudes toward health care; (3) perception of threat of illness; (4) characteristics of the social network, interactions, norms, and structure; (5) knowledge about disease; and (6) demographic characteristics (Cummings, Becker, and Maile, 1980).

Health Belief Model

Of all of the models studied by Cummings, Becker, and Maile (1980), the health belief model was by far the most extensively utilized. This model was originally developed by Hochbaum, Kegeles, Leventhal, and Rosenstock to explain preventive health behaviors, and the lack of such behavior, but was quickly adapted to study sick roles and illness behavior (Becker, 1974; Kirscht, 1974). The model is based on theories from social psychology, most notably, Lewin's *aspiration theory* (Maiman and Becker, 1974). Two underlying premises of the model are the phenomenological orientation and the historical perspective. The *phenomenological orientation* states that it is the individual's perceptions that determine behavior, not the environment. A *historical perspective* mandates a focus on the current dynamics affecting an individual's behavior, not on past history or prior experiences (Rosenstock, 1974).

The health belief model describes the relationships between people's beliefs about health and their health-specific behaviors. The beliefs that mediate health behavior are, according to the model, perceived susceptibility, severity, benefits, and barriers (Figure 3-1). *Perceived susceptibility* is the individual's subjective impression of the risk of contracting a disease or illness. *Perceived severity* refers to the convictions a person holds regarding the de-

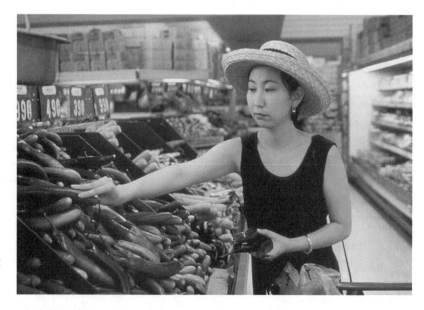

Choosing healthy foods because you know that they are good for you is an example of the health belief model. Your choice illustrates the relationship between your beliefs about health and your health-specific behaviors.

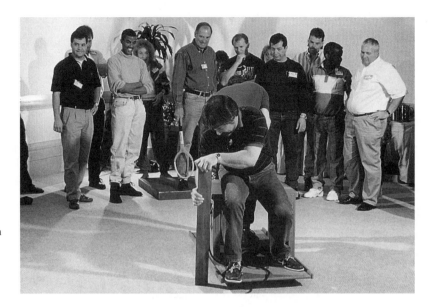

Icebreaker activities can be a helpful way to begin a workshop or class with a positive tone.

3. Set the ground rules for participant interaction.
4. Can truly energize participants.
5. Can put participants at ease.

Disadvantages are that they

1. Can be time-consuming, reducing time for more important needs.
2. Can make participants uncomfortable.

Notice that these activities have the potential to make participants either comfortable or uncomfortable. Choose them wisely, considering participant characteristics.

Example 1: The Name Game

1. Sit in a circle so that all faces can be seen.
2. Reviewing the rules: You cannot write names down; All will participate; associate names with faces, since we will change places later.
3. First person says his or her own name (generally only first name).
4. Second person says first person's name and then his or her own.
5. Procedure is repeated until final person says all names plus his or her own.
6. Reverse directions and have first person say all names in reverse order.
7. After several persons have completed game in reverse, change places and pick several people to say names.
8. Repeat until all are comfortable saying all names.

*Example 2: Get It
Off My Back*

Purpose   1. To introduce a new area of instruction.
2. To get a group better acquainted.
3. To review.
4. To determine the knowledge of the group.

Background   The facilitator must do background work on the topic to be covered and identify key vocabulary words. Examples include drug names, nutrients, diseases, and pollutants.

Player Objective   To identify the word on your back.

Materials   Three-by-five-inch cards and masking tape.

Rules of Play   1. After reviewing all rules, a three-by-five-inch card with a word on it is placed on the back of each participant. It is important that no one sees the card placed on his or her own back.
2. You can ask only yes-and-no questions.
3. You can ask each person only one question. If you have asked a question of all participants, you may repeat the process.
4. You must get at least three yes answers to your questions before you can make a guess at the word on your back.
5. The first person to guess correctly is the winner. Continue the game until at least half of the group has been successful.
6. Instruct participants to answer "I don't know or I am not certain" rather than taking a chance on giving the wrong yes or no answer, as wrong answers will ruin the game. If no one is certain of the correct answer, the facilitator should give the answer.
7. Repeat the game if there is time.
8. Debrief by discussing the logic followed in discovering the words being guessed at.

*Example 3: Special
Name Tags*   Construct special name tags to include information that will open up common ground and put the group at ease. Figure 5-1 shows an example.

After completing the answers to the questions posed on the name tag, each person should pair up with another and ask clarifying questions. Participants can decline to answer any question but generally find these questions nonthreatening. This is a good beginning activity to promote some safe self-disclosure that contributes to a positive atmosphere.

Other Examples   Two other examples of getting-acquainted activities follow:

1. Pair up participants and give them two minutes to interview each other before introducing their partner to the group.
2. Ask each participant to reveal a personal trait of which they are proud.

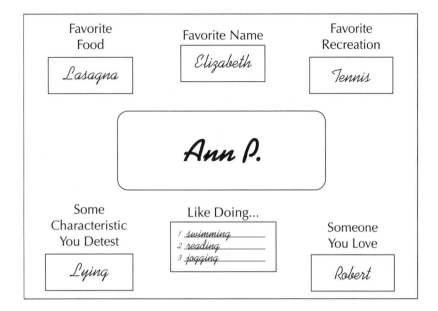

Figure 5-1
Name Tag Serving as
Icebreaker

Method/Intervention 2: Audiotapes

Audiotapes can be used in many creative ways and are often combined with other methods. You can **simulate** situations or play real voices.

Advantages and Disadvantages

Advantages of audiotapes are that they

1. Are low in cost.
2. Provide a structured and controlled experience.
3. Are easy to use.
4. Can provide excellent feedback.

Disadvantages are that they

1. Appeal to only one sense.
2. Require equipment.
3. Require special equipment for large groups.
4. Material can be boring.

Example 1: Interviews with Experts

Interviews with experts on the subject involved can be played back for the group. Try to select charismatic leaders or voices.

Example 2: Self-Interview

Invite participants to have a conversation with themselves. The tape asks questions for each to answer. For example, propose a conversation with a crystal ball. The participant controls the on-and-off button and asks the crystal ball about his or her future if certain unhealthy behaviors are followed. (See also Chapter 7.)

Method/Intervention 3: Audiovisual Materials

Audiovisual materials include videotapes, films, overhead transparencies, DVDs, presentation software, and filmstrips. The use of audiovisual equipment will be discussed in detail in Chapter 7. Here we will just summarize the advantages and disadvantages and provide some brief examples of use.

Advantages and Disadvantages

Advantages of audiovisuals are that they

1. Provide potential for variety.
2. Serve as an attention-getter.
3. Are often relatively cheap and easy to use (as in the case of blank videotapes and overhead transparencies).
4. Can serve as a class or individual project (as in the case of making a video).
5. Are inexpensive.

Disadvantages are that they

1. Are unpredictable in outcome.
2. Require equipment that may be expensive (such as interactive videodiscs).
3. Can create a situation in which some are unwilling to participate and allow others to do all the work.

(See also Chapter 10.)

Examples   Following are some examples of how to use audiovisual materials.

1. As a supplement to lecture, provide real-life examples and experts.
2. Make tapes (audio or video) as a group. For example, a videotape could be made of community problems, using the approach of an investigative reporter.
3. Use videotapes to monitor behaviors such as drug transactions. This practice can become a deterrent to such behavior.
4. Record by audiotape or videotape a confrontational situation, such as parents and child arguing over the use of a drug of interest to the group. Use actors to portray the wrong way and a better way of engaging in such a confrontation.

Method/Intervention 4: Brainstorming

Brainstorming is a method of eliciting ideas and information from a group. It can be used to define a problem or to consider possible solutions to a problem. It can be very effective in developing a positive group attitude since it recognizes the importance of each group member. It often provides a sense of group empowerment. Basically, it is a free-thinking forum with the facilitator working to elicit as many possible solutions to a problem as possible. This is followed by grouping and reorganizing ideas until they are well understood and all are considered.

Rules Rules for brainstorming are as follows:

1. There are no bad ideas. Do not make negative remarks about ideas as this will stifle creativity.
2. All ideas/solutions will be considered (listed).
3. Go around the group in a circle and list ideas that are possible solutions to the problem or issue at hand. If possible, use large sheets of paper and hang them on the walls. Alternatively, use a chalkboard or transparencies.
4. Individuals can pass on their turn if they feel they have no new idea to contribute.
5. Continue the process until people run low on new ideas. Make certain not to stop before all new ideas are presented.
6. The process can end here or can move to a second step.
7. The second step is to consolidate common themes and ideas. This must be done with the full consent of the group. It may be possible to consolidate the list to a more manageable list without losing the essence of the ideas presented.
8. The third step is to prioritize the ideas. This step may not be necessary, but if needed it should be done with ample time for discussion. If consensus cannot be reached, some form of voting may be necessary. Consider the group dynamics before deciding on an oral or secret ballot.

Advantages and Disadvantages Advantages of brainstorming are that it

1. Provides an opportunity for all to be important contributors.
2. Requires little equipment.
3. Builds a cooperative environment.

Disadvantages are that it

1. Is unpredictable in outcome.
2. Can make some individuals uncomfortable, feeling forced to contribute.
3. Can be time-consuming if taken through all steps.
4. Can fail if people refuse to participate.

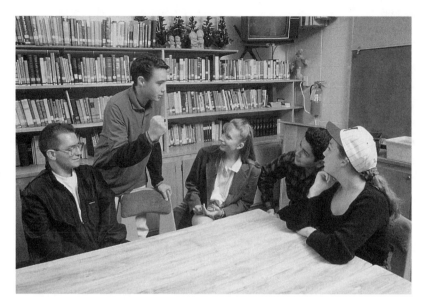

Solutions to many problems can be generated in brainstorming activities if the activity is conducted correctly. It is important to remember that no ideas are bad and to include everyone.

Examples   Use brainstorming to generate ideas on how to address such problems as

1. School littering
2. Access to local services
3. Using condoms
4. Teenage pregnancy
5. Poor food selection
6. Drug sales in the neighborhood

Sample Operational Procedures   Following is an example of operational procedures in brainstorming:

1. Brainstorm objectives using large wall charts.
2. After creating an exhaustive list, quickly review the intentions/wording of each stated objective.
3. Establish priority objectives.
4. Assign suggested implementation responsibility.

Assumptions   Effective brainstorming rests on certain assumptions that should be clarified for the group before beginning the operational procedures previously mentioned.

1. All contributions are welcomed and should be considered.
2. All suggested objectives will be reported unless withdrawn by the person making the suggestion.

3. It is permissible, in fact encouraged, to overlap with other groups.
4. Rotation input will be used, but anyone can decline to make suggestions.

Method/Intervention 5: Case Studies

A powerful tool for health educators is the **case study,** which presents situations for the sake of problem diagnosis and solution. The situations can be real and based on historical events, or they can be based on hypothetical events, structured to fit any content area. This book is replete with case studies on a variety of issues. Entire textbooks in public health are written around collections of case studies (Kreuter, Lezin, and Green, 1998).

Advantages and Disadvantages

Advantages of case studies are that they

1. Generally require little equipment.
2. Are able to address difficult topics in a controlled manner.
3. Allow for good control over content.
4. Can be structured to appear realistic.
5. Provide an excellent opportunity to learn in a practical fashion.

Disadvantages are that they

1. Can be time-consuming.
2. Can result in pooling of ignorance.

Example I: Case Study of Diabetes Prevention Program in Charlotte, NC

Your agency has received a large grant (100K) to develop a diabetes prevention program in a predominantly **Hispanic** community (approximately 50 percent of inhabitants are of Mexican ancestry). You have been assigned the task of determining the components of the program. Consider how you would go about determining which intervention methods and teaching strategies to use. Ask yourself how you can be certain you are being sensitive to the needs of the community.

- What steps would you follow?
- Where would you physically locate the program?
- What specific teaching or other intervention methods might be productive, and why?

Example 2: Case Study of Problem Pregnancy Prevention Program in Raleigh, NC

Your agency has received a large grant (100K) to develop a problem pregnancy prevention program in a predominantly Chinese-American community. The community comprises approximately 2,000 girls/young women age 12–19. The pregnancy rate has been approximately 10 percent per year. Approximately 13 percent speak very little English. You have been assigned the task of determining the components of the program. Consider how you would go about determining which intervention methods and teaching strategies to use. Ask yourself how you can be certain you are being sensitive to the needs of the community.

- What steps would you follow?
- Where would you physically locate the program?
- What specific teaching or other intervention methods might be productive, and why?

Example 3: Case Study of AIDS Prevention Program in Washington D.C.

Your agency has received a large grant (100K) to develop an AIDS prevention program for the deaf in your community. It is estimated you have approximately 2,000 **deaf** and **hard-of-hearing** adults age 18–40 living in the community. Most live in the northwest and northeast part of the city. There is a large cluster near Gallaudet University. Approximately 40 percent are African-American and approximately 15% are Hispanic. You have been assigned the task of determining the components of the program. Consider how you would go about determining which intervention methods and teaching strategies to use. Ask yourself how you can be certain you are being sensitive to the needs of this community.

- What steps would you follow?
- Where would you physically locate the program?
- What specific teaching or other intervention methods might be productive, and why?

Method/Intervention 6: Computer-Assisted Instruction

Computer-assisted instruction is best combined with other teaching techniques. The main issue is to find the software that meets your objectives and a setting that has the hardware to implement the program. The possibilities are exciting, but the costs can be high. The use of such technology is currently much more common in school settings but could be used in community settings. Many people have computer and Internet access at home, and if the program can be shared, this can be a major way to reach large numbers of people.

Health education software has been slow to develop because it is often difficult to make a profit on software that can be very high in developmental costs. The market is often small, and unfortunately much of the software has been the object of software pirating.

Other possible approaches to gain access to adequate hardware are to use local community colleges or to purchase portable machines. Libraries generally have computers for public use and often lend public domain software. Public domain software can also be obtained over networks and public systems via the Internet. In the future such applications will probably be even more feasible.

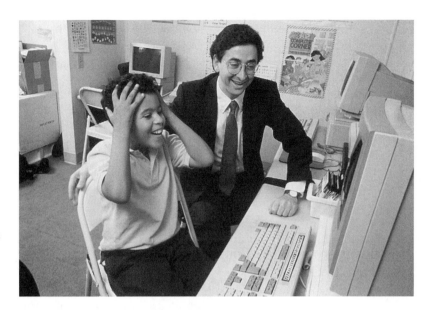

Computer use in health education can provide an element of fun and variety to a lesson or workshop.

Portable projection systems are now available, making use of a large screen. This means one computer can be used to reach a large audience. Changes can be made on the spot, and new technology permits on-screen movement and sound. Custom lessons/presentations can be developed that are very professional attention-getters. (See also Chapter 6.)

Advantages and Disadvantages

Advantages of computer-assisted instruction are that it

1. Can provide an element of fun.
2. Is considered **innovative.**
3. Provides variety.
4. Can involve participants actively in the learning process.
5. Provides almost immediate feedback.
6. Makes self-pacing exercises possible.
7. In some applications, such as simulations, requires higher-level thinking.
8. Can provide individualized programs.
9. Can be used to reinforce other lessons.

Disadvantages are that it

1. Can be expensive.
2. Requires special equipment.
3. Requires special software.
4. Requires special training in computer use.
5. Can be frightening to someone new to computers.

Examples   Following are some examples of applications of computer-assisted instruction.

1. Dietary analysis programs.
2. Health risk appraisals.
3. Health games.
4. Monitoring compliance, such as with medications.
5. Simulations.
6. Expert system applications.
7. Using computers to plot trends such as birth rates or violent acts.
8. Automatically sending reminder notices using computer voice messaging.

(See also Chapter 6.)

Method/Intervention 7: Cooperative Learning and Group Work

Cooperative learning is a broad category of learning experiences that center on learning from fellow participants. Generally participants are working toward a common goal. It includes group work such as brainstorming but can be as straightforward as permission to share personal experiences. It has the potential to enhance group spirit and can be very important in group situations.

When to Use   Working in small groups can be an effective **strategy** in both the school and community settings. The health educator must first establish some very clear behavioral objectives before deciding whether or not small-group work is even appropriate. There are many reasons for incorporating group work into the learning process. Group work can facilitate cooperative learning, problem solving, the sharing of ideas, brainstorming, or be nothing more than a device to allow the members of the group to get to know one another. The ability to use group work may be driven by the overall number of participants, their willingness to participate, facilities that allow for small-group setup, and the health educator's aptitude for running small-group exercises.

Advantages and Disadvantages   Advantages of cooperative or group learning are that it

1. Can provide an element of fun.
2. Potentially creates an atmosphere of cooperation.
3. Utilizes multiple thinkers and therefore can create high-quality, innovative answers.
4. Allows participants to learn in a more active and involved manner, therefore decreasing the potential for boredom.
5. Encourages cooperation and collaboration that a large group setting might inhibit.

6. Stimulates innovation in thought, which again might not be encouraged in a large group.
7. Allows participants to quickly become acquainted with each other. This is particularly useful in making people feel at ease in a new situation.
8. Exposes individuals to a variety of viewpoints and ideas that might not surface in a large group setting.
9. Can foster an acceptance of differences in heritage, socioeconomic status, **disabilities,** and so forth.

Disadvantages are that it

1. Is unpredictable in outcome.
2. Has the potential for being very disruptive in the school setting. **School health educators** must be very clear about their expectations regarding behavior and noise levels and be prepared to end an activity prematurely should the students get out of control.
3. Can sometimes be dominated by overassertive individuals. In both school and community settings, facilitators need to circulate among the groups to minimize the effects of such behavior. In the school setting, if there are tasks to be performed within groups (such as recorder or reporter), the health educator should appoint these individuals before the groups begin work to avoid disruptive arguments.
4. Has the potential to wander off the track of the activity, particularly in the school setting. Again, the health educator can minimize this problem by regularly checking in with individual groups and bringing them back on task.

Examples Examples of cooperative learning or group work follow:

1. Brainstorming on how to prevent drug sales on certain street corners.
2. Share personal experiences.
3. Make individual presentations assigned by instructor. Instructor reviews format prior to presentation and ensures that quality experience will be provided.
4. Plan an environmental day such as Earth Day.
5. Design an antismoking ad poster or 30-second videotape.
6. Form dyads or triads for problem-solving tasks.
7. Prepare and practice delivery of a report (small-group practice and critique).

Method/Intervention 8: Debates

Debates are the organized discussion of differing points of view. By providing structure we hope to achieve better understanding of multiple points of view and perhaps some wisdom. Debates also can potentially develop skills in oral persuasion.

Advantages and Disadvantages

Advantages of debates are that they

1. Can provide an element of fun.
2. Can develop many skills.
3. Provide variety.
4. Can expose group to many diverse opinions.

Disadvantages are that they

1. Require careful controls.
2. May reinforce current positions.
3. May develop into controversy.
4. Can make some people uncomfortable.
5. Can fail if people refuse to participate.

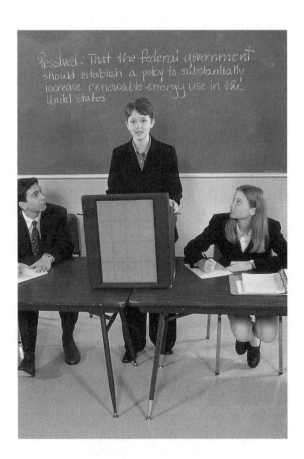

Debates help students practice oral skills and look at issues from alternative viewpoints.

Debates can be inspirational events or the dull sharing and reinforcement of opinions. What happens is a result of organization and planning. First, you must review your objectives and determine if a debate will be helpful in achieving them. Do you wish to bring in outside debaters, use a debate team, or plan a notable debate and invite the community? What would be useful? If you wish to use your group or class, it is important to structure the debate so you can be certain to achieve your objectives. Since you are not teaching debate, remember that debate skills are an important secondary benefit but not the primary objective. The primary objective is usually the knowledge gained from preparation and observation of the debate or considering an issue from an alternative viewpoint.

Case Study: Pat   Pat Thomas, a school health educator, decides to have a debate on the issue of abortion. She asks for volunteers for the debate from the class. They select their position, and the debate follows in one week. The students provide excellent arguments on both sides of the issue. Pat feels good about the experience until she notices hostility among the students following the debate. Upon questioning the class she learns almost no one changed his or her position in any way, and many feel upset that others will not change their position given the righteousness of their cause. What happened? What could improve the chances that learning will take place and students consider both sides? (See Case Studies Revisited page 172.)

Some common debate characteristics follow:

1. Keep participants from knowing which side—pro or con—they will present until the last minute. This forces them to consider and prepare for both sides of an issue.
2. Set a structured time frame in advance—for example, three minutes for each side's opening arguments followed by three minutes rebuttal and three minutes closing.
3. Have the order of arguments drawn at random.
4. Consider ascertaining the participants' position on an issue and assigning them to debate the opposite side.

Examples   Examples of debate issues in health education follow:

1. Should helmet laws be mandatory?
2. Should condoms be provided to minors on demand?
3. Should parents be notified of all medical procedures (STD treatment, abortion, etc.)?
4. Should abortion be legal?

5. Should free needles and sterilization kits be provided to drug users?
6. Who is responsible for the problem of pollution, violence, poverty, etc.?

Method/Intervention 9: Displays and Bulletin Boards

Displays and bulletin boards are graphics and text combined in formats to attract attention. They can provide a positive educational environment and reinforce important points. They can also reach groups not attending any formal presentation or course.

Advantages and Disadvantages

Advantages of displays and bulletin boards are that they

1. Can set a positive environment.
2. Can be an ongoing educational tool.
3. Can reach special populations such as "walk-bys."
4. Provide variety.

Disadvantages are that they

1. Can be expensive.
2. Require special materials.
3. Can be time-consuming.
4. Can raise the concern of vandalism.

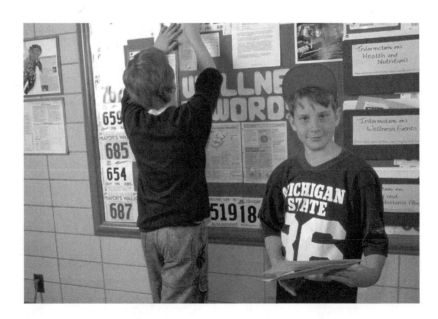

A well-organized bulletin board can add to a positive classroom environment.

Good bulletin board planning begins by analyzing its various elements: the title materials to be used, their arrangement, lettering, and color choices. Interest will be aroused by attention-getters such as puns, riddles, exaggeration, associations, comic strip figures, and other familiar figures. Elements to be used should be considered in terms of the following variables:

1. *Topic selection.* Focus attention on single theme or subject. Message should be short and to the point.
2. *Materials (background).* The best materials will vary with the theme or subject. Once you have a rough sketch, take time to decide which materials will create the desired effect. You can use construction paper, white newspaper print, burlap, wallpaper, newspaper, gift-wrapping paper, or corrugated paper.
3. *Display materials.* Use actual objects and three-dimensional objects whenever possible. You can also use drawings, next best to real objects, cartoon and stick figures, pictures, or cotton roving (this can be used to tie the board together, indicate direction, or add decorative touch).
4. *Arrangement.* A formal arrangement with two sides balanced allows all items to be quickly seen but may tend to be boring. It is best suited for complicated arrangements. An informal, or unbalanced, arrangement is more interesting and eye-catching. Key elements should dominate. With either arrangement, use captions employing the left-to-right principle. Place these at the bottom only if the bulletin board is at eye level. Frames give an appearance of completeness. Use construction paper corners or paper strip corners for final touch.
5. *Lettering.* A bold, even stroke of about $\frac{1}{6}$ of a letter is the most legible lettering. It must balance yet not overshadow the rest of the board. Capital letters, manuscript letters, fancy or textured can be used. Use felt-tip pens, rope, paint, cutouts, ribbon or yarn, spray paint, stencils, twigs, popsicle sticks, and so on.
6. *Color.* Attention, force, and meaning are obtained through skillful contrasting of color. Choose colors that catch attention and not those that blend into the background. You can pick colors for shock effect. Red, green, and blue are good at all times, but dark and light tones add dramatic and pleasing effect. *Contrast makes the difference!*

Method/Intervention 10: Educational Games

Educational games are activities that utilize an element of fun and of competition. They differ from other games in that the educational objectives are clear and are the main focus of the activity. Games are generally competitive activities, and the user should consider the effects on all participants of using such a format.

Advantages and Disadvantages   Advantages of educational games are that they

1. Provide an element of fun.
2. Provide competition that can be motivating.
3. Provide variety.
4. Provide opportunities for repetition of important information.
5. Can be excellent introduction activities or good reviews.
6. Can encourage and enhance teamwork.

Disadvantages are that they

1. Tend to focus on cognitive information for the most part.
2. Can be embarrassing for individuals who know little of the topic.
3. Can place too much emphasis on competition.
4. Can become disruptive if enthusiasm gets out of control.
5. Can fail if winning becomes more important than learning.

Often participants can design their own games and rules. Utilizing existing frame games is a good way to develop interest. Use the format followed in current popular TV game shows.

Example 1: Football Game   The Football Game can be adapted to baseball, basketball, etc.

Purpose
1. To review (could be used as a means of oral evaluation).
2. To start a card file collection of good testing items for future tests, reviews, and oral evaluations.

Background   Facilitator must make up a large number of appropriate questions.

Rules of Play
1. Divide into two teams.
2. Flip a coin to see which team will be on offense first.
3. First offense begins from the team's own 40-yard line.
4. Questions are asked in rotating order. If the answer is correct, the team advances 10 yards.
5. If the first person fails to answer the question, the next member is permitted to answer the question but a down is lost. If the first question was a true-false question, a new one is asked.
6. If the question is missed by the fourth person, the ball is lost on downs.
7. Questions are asked from pile 1 down to the 30-yard line.
8. Questions are asked from pile 2 between the 30-yard line and the 10-yard line.
9. Pile 3 contains the touchdown questions when the team reaches the 10-yard line.
10. Pile 4 contains the point after touchdown conversion.
11. From the 20- or 10-yard lines, a field goal may be attempted from pile 5.

12. After a touchdown and conversion attempt, the team scored on starts a new offensive from its own 40-yard line.
13. If a field goal attempt is successful, the team that kicked starts a new offensive from its own 40-yard line. If unsuccessful, the defense takes over on its own 20-yard line.
14. A five-minute halftime is taken in the middle of the period for consultation with team members and references on questions missed during the first half. Change possession of ball for second half.
15. In case of a tie score, the team with the most first downs (in this case the most correct answers) shall be the winner.

Materials Needed
1. A series of questions on three-by-five-inch cards or cards that look like footballs, separated into piles.
2. Place cards showing numbers of piles.
3. Representative football field—could be a model or magnetic board, or you could draw one on a blackboard, showing line divisions.
4. Blackboard or scoreboard display of team scores and first downs.
5. Method of showing progress of ball. Three possibilities are
   a. Mark the blackboard with chalk (use colored chalk if you have it).
   b. Use a model, moving a small indicator of some kind back and forth on top of it.
   c. Use a magnetic board.

Example 2:
Baseball Game

The Baseball Game is another sports oriented educational game.

Rules of Play
1. Allow three outs to a side (three misses).
2. Limit singles to a maximum of three per inning. This will keep one team from dominating time.
3. Score by force-in only. This will prevent arguments. Be certain to explain.
4. Play as many innings as time permits (not more than nine).
5. If question is correctly answered, runner advances the corresponding bases.
6. Singles are easy questions, doubles harder, and so on.
7. If game ends in a tie, decide winner by total number of correct answers.

Alternate Rules of Play
1. Divide into two teams.
2. Make up series of questions: true-false for singles, easy questions for doubles, harder questions for triples and home runs.
3. Runner must be forced in to score.
4. Limit three singles and three doubles per inning.
5. Talking by team at bat results in an out; talking by team on defense results in an out for the next inning.
6. Winner scores most runs.
7. Add third-inning stretch for study.
8. Missed questions may be used again later.

Example 3:
Hollywood Squares

Hollywood squares is a cognitive (knowledge) oriented game. It is especially suitable as an introductory game or as a review activity. The basic design (frame) is taken from the television game of the same name, and questions may be based on any desired content area. The instructor can make up questions or have students develop them as an assignment. Consider using another more current TV game show format.

Setting

1. Select nine people to act as celebrities, and ask them to leave the room. They might be selected earlier and come prepared.
2. Arrange chairs in the front of the class.
   a. Put three chairs in a straight row facing away from the blackboard toward the rest of the class. Allow room for three persons to stand behind and three to sit on the floor in front.
   b. Put lectern at back of class as shown in Figure 5-2, with two captains.
3. Prepare a scoreboard to one side of the blackboard in case there is time for more than one game.
4. Divide remainder of class in half alternately.
   a. Advise (name: _____) that she is captain of team X and seat her.
   b. Advise (name: _____) that he is captain of team O and seat him.
   c. Be sure to seat X on right of lectern, O on left.

Celebrities Briefing

Celebrities wear tags and take on the role of famous people, or they can just be themselves.

1. Questions will be directed to you; answer independently.
2. If you do not have a good answer, alibi or bluff—but make up your mind quickly, because there will be a time limit.
3. When you come back into the room, situate yourselves in the front of the room as I direct you.

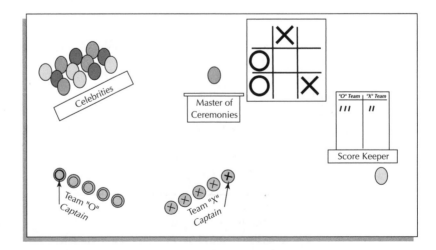

Figure 5-2
Room Setup for Hollywood Squares Game

4. Please, no conversation, except to answer or bluff.
5. Do not be afraid to ask for a question to be repeated.
6. Any questions?

Return to Class
1. Celebrities are seated.
2. Check to see that teams are situated.
3. Brief class on the game.
   a. The object of the game is to get three squares in a row either up and down, across, or diagonally. To do this, the team must decide whether or not a celebrity is giving the right answer or making one up.
   b. Each completed game is worth 250 points. The team with the most points at the end of class will win a fabulous prize. The winning team will be given some prize, perhaps be allowed to leave early. If used with a community group, provide gold stars or prizes.
   c. Since we are deviating from the original format of "Hollywood Squares" in as much as teams will compete instead of single contestants, it is necessary to set a time limit of 30 seconds on deliberation between captain and team. Final decisions on how to answer each question will be left to the captain of each team. Please answer as quickly as possible.
   d. The facilitator will be the final judge of whether an answer is correct.
4. Are there any questions?

Begin
1. X, you start by choosing a square.
2. Question 1.

Questions Questions should be based on important concepts and stated objectives. They should also be asked in such way that they lend themselves to bluffing.

Materials Needed Nine large cards with "X" on one side and "O" on the other side are needed. Two cards are used to designate teams; one "O" card and one "X" card.

***Example 4:*
*Health Bingo*** The Health Bingo Game uses a card like that shown in Figure 5-3.

Purpose
1. To review information.
2. To introduce information.
3. To evaluate workshop or class.

Background Facilitator must make up a list of questions suitable for the game. Each round requires 24 questions.

Player Objective To achieve "bingo" by getting five correct answers in a row or column or diagonal line.

Health B I N G O				
22	2	11	5	13
1	17	20	9	7
4	8	Free Space	3	14
24	10	6	19	21
18	15	23	16	12

Figure 5-3
Health Bingo Card

Materials   Bingo cards and pencils.

Rules of Play
1. Each person randomly assigns numbers (1-24) to the small corner boxes of their bingo cards.
2. Facilitator begins game by drawing or otherwise randomly selecting the first number and reads a question.
3. Players locate square and write the correct answer (if they know it).
4. The process is repeated until someone calls "bingo."
5. The facilitator then checks the card to ensure there are five correct answers. If one or more is incorrect, play resumes; otherwise the person is named the winner.
6. At this point the facilitator reviews the questions and answers.

Example 5: The room setup for the Educational Relay is shown in Figure 5-4.
Educational Relay

Purpose
1. To introduce a new area of instruction.
2. To get people up and active.
3. To review material.

Background The facilitator must prepare a set of cards for each team (usually there are three teams with 15 to 20 cards each). Each set of cards should be the same except for a mark identifying each team. Three different-colored sets of cards could be used, for example. Cards each have a word appropriate to the topic being covered. Each container is labeled with the name of the category. An example would be containers labeled with food groups and cards with names of foods.

Player Objective To get the cards in the correct container, and also to complete the task first.

Materials
1. Three sets of three-by-five-inch cards.
2. Three containers (large brown bags work fine).

Rules of Play
1. Teams are selected, and the room is cleared to allow running a relay.
2. Each member must start behind a line, pick up a card, run and place it in the correct container, and return to tag the next person in line. The next person repeats until all cards are used.
3. The winning team (first team to deposit all cards) receives 5 points for best speed; the second team receives 3 points; the third team receives 1 point.
4. The facilitator moves to the containers and removes the cards, checking with the group for correct answers. Each *correct* answer is worth 1 point.

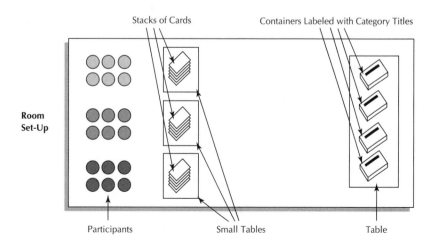

Figure 5-4
Room Setup for
Educational Relay

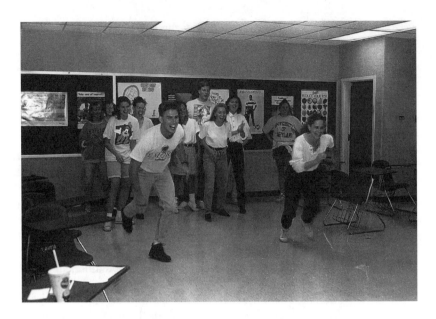

Active participation promotes learning.

5. The team with the highest point total is the winner.
6. Be extra careful with safety. Make certain the room is safe for a relay. Encourage people to walk if appropriate.

Method/Intervention 11: Experiments and Demonstrations

Experiments and demonstrations can serve as important tools for the health educator. Providing a factual demonstration is important for presenting information, reinforcing information, and enhancing recall. Demonstrations can be used in community settings with careful planning. They are often remembered for a long time.

Advantages and Disadvantages

Advantages of experiments and demonstrations are that they

1. Are visual and often hands-on.
2. Can serve to teach the scientific method.
3. Usually have a high interest level.
4. Reinforce theoretical aspects of a topic.

What I hear, I forget.
What I see, I remember.
What I do, I learn.
—Chinese proverb, author unknown

Disadvantages are that they

1. Can be costly.
2. Require time-consuming setup.
3. Require special equipment.

4. Are unpredictable in outcome.
5. Without proper controls and setup, can be dangerous.

Example 1: Fish Tank Ecology Demonstration

The Fish Tank Ecology Demonstration requires clearance and may evoke emotional responses. You must be prepared to deal with these issues from animal rights groups and others. Be certain this activity is appropriate for the age group involved.

Materials Required

1. Fish.
2. Fish tank.
3. Small fishnet.
4. Litter, assorted sizes.
5. Appropriate story.
6. Clearance of agency or school to conduct activity (human subjects clearance may be required).

Description

One medium-sized fish tank is set up in plain view of the audience. Inside the tank is a goldfish. Next to this tank is a smaller tank or large jar with clean water. A fishnet is evident and in plain view.

Procedures

1. The facilitator sets up the demonstration without explanation but makes certain the audience sees all components, especially the fishnet.
2. The facilitator introduces someone to present a story. An excellent choice would be the Dr. Seuss story, *The Lorax*. The story is then read to the group.
3. Every so often the facilitator adds a piece of litter to the fish tank. This is done in full view of the audience. Hold up the litter item and examine the label before placing it in the tank.
4. As the story goes on, the litter becomes increasingly toxic. Progress from solid objects such as cans to soap products and oil.

Discovery is learning.
—Francis Bacon

5. If someone says to stop littering, ignore that person, but if someone takes action, allow that person to put the fish in the clean tank.
6. The activity ends when the story is over and the tank is thoroughly polluted or someone saves the fish.
7. The story reader usually leaves after reading the story.
8. Debrief the group as follows:

   Question: What happened?
   The usual response is, "You killed the fish."
   Question: Who killed the fish?
   Response: You all the killed the fish. You all knew what was happening but did nothing to save the fish. That is exactly what is happening to our environment. We talk a lot but do nothing. Every one of you could have saved this fish but you all made excuses and did nothing.

   If someone saves the fish, present the fish to that person and commend him or her for taking action.

Example 2: Smoking Experiment (Accumulation of Tar 1)

This Smoking Experiment is the first of two showing accumulation of tar, both taken from a Public Health Service book by G.G. Gilbert and M. Ziady (1986). Figure 5-5 illustrates the experiment.

Purpose To show the accumulation of tar in water by change of color and smell.

Appropriate Age Group Middle through secondary school.

Materials
1. Gallon jar with a two-holed stopper.
2. Cigarettes and matches.
3. Delivery tubes (glass, plastic, or rubber hose).
4. Cigarette holder.
5. Hand squeeze pump or vacuum pump.

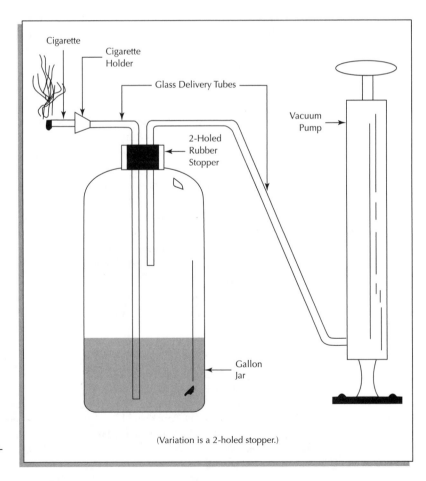

Figure 5-5
First Smoking Experiment Showing Accumulation of Tar

Procedure
1. Assemble cigarette tar separating apparatus as shown in the diagram.
2. Fill the gallon jar half full with water.
3. Place cigarette in intake and light.
4. Using vacuum pump, draw smoke from cigarette into gallon jar and water.
5. Pump until cigarette is burned completely. Replace with additional cigarettes until tars can be seen in water.
6. Examine color and smell of water.

Key Points for Discussion
1. What happens to your lungs when you smoke?
2. What are the similarities between this experiment and what happens to your lungs?
3. What chemicals are in the water?
4. Where can we find out more about the effects of smoking?
5. How does your body rid itself of these tars?

Example 3: Smoking Experiment (Accumulation of Tar 2)

This Smoking Experiment is the second of two showing accumulation of tar, both taken from a Public Health Service article by G.G. Gilbert and M. Ziady (1986). Figure 5-6 illustrates the experiment.

Purpose
To show the accumulation of tar in cotton balls.

Appropriate Age Group
Primary school.

Materials
1. Plastic window cleaner container or other empty plastic container, transparent if possible.
2. Ballpoint pen barrel or other tubing approximately the size of a cigarette.
3. Cotton.
4. Cigarettes and matches.
5. Ashtray or other item to catch ashes.

Procedure
You may wish to conduct the experiment outside or with the windows open to avoid side-stream smoke.

1. Rinse the container thoroughly.
2. Make an opening in the cap of the container to fit the tubing into the cap.
3. Place the tubing in the opening and seal tight with cement or clay if needed.
4. Insert loosely packed cotton ball into tubing.
5. Insert cigarette into open end of tubing.
6. Press firmly on the plastic container to force air out, light the cigarette, and then proceed with slow and regular pumping action.

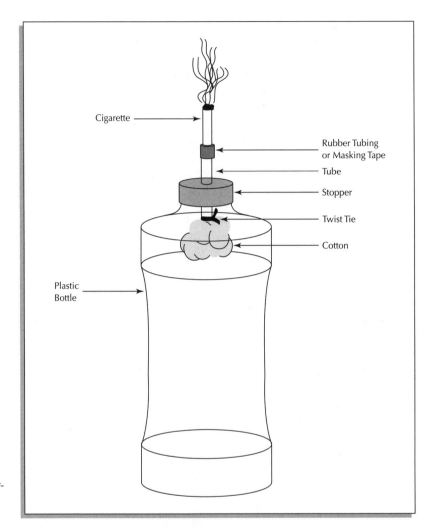

Figure 5-6
Second Smoking Experiment Showing Accumulation of Tar

7. Withdraw cotton from tubing to show accumulation of tar.
8. Pass container around for individuals to smell and to observe that smoke continues to be expelled for a period of time.

Variation   1. Divide into groups and conduct several experiments, keeping a close watch for safety.
2. Try same experiment with filter cigarette.
3. Compare filter and nonfilter cigarettes.

Key Points for Discussion   1. What happens to your lungs when you smoke?
2. Is this experiment similar to what happens to your lungs?
3. Consider this effect multiplied by 20 or 30 times per day for 5, 10, or 20 years.

Other Examples   Three other examples of experiments follow:

1. Put powder on a doorknob that is visible only under a black light. Use the black light experiment to discuss transmission of disease.
2. Test local streams for contaminates.
3. Test wall paints for the presence of lead.

Method/Intervention 12: Field Trips

Field trips are visits with individuals, to sites of interest, or both. Such visits provide special opportunities to put people or activities in the context of the environment. Such activities are common in many schools but should also be considered in community health programs. If you expect individuals to use services, for example, it would be a good idea to visit the site and get acquainted with the personnel. Chances are much greater that these services will be utilized.

When to Use   It is appropriate to use field trips when you believe the trip will actually help meet your objectives. Being on site affords special opportunities not found elsewhere, and visiting a site can often have a demystifying effect. If you want to ensure that your group is more comfortable in using a facility, for example, a field trip would be a good idea. Knowing how to get there can be an important issue. Which bus to take or where to park can be important considerations. These issues have been shown time and again to be major barriers for action.

You may gain access to special expertise or equipment that is important to reaching your objectives only through field trips. Prior planning is most important if you want to ensure a successful trip. You should always personally visit the site first before taking a group. Take only those groups that you are certain you can handle. This is especially important with any group that will be in a potentially dangerous area. One method often used is to establish a list of questions to be answered by each visitor and collect the responses following the trip. Always conduct a debriefing session after the visit.

Advantages and   Advantages of field trips are that they
Disadvantages

1. Can be structured to address difficult objectives.
2. Are often very entertaining and enjoyable.
3. Put people in the context of their environment.
4. Often have models and materials not available elsewhere.

Disadvantages are that they

1. Usually require transportation and can be costly.
2. Can be very time-consuming.

3. Are unpredictable in outcome because of uncertainty of interaction.
4. Often raise the concern of liability coverage.

Case Study: Meshah   Meshah took a group of high school students to a comprehensive community health clinic to meet with the staff. The agenda was so full the students had little opportunity to ask questions. On the bus home Meshah engaged the students in discussion about the football season. Unknown to Meshah, the students still had many questions about privacy issues, access to care, and the qualifications and training of staff. Many students left with incorrect assumptions because of the lack of follow-up. How could Meshah have structured this visit more effectively? (See Case Studies Revisited page 172.)

Health Museums or Health Education Centers   Several centers around the country specialize in health education activities. These are very exciting places that have a wealth of materials on display. Most are hands-on places that schedule group visits. Generally, they have

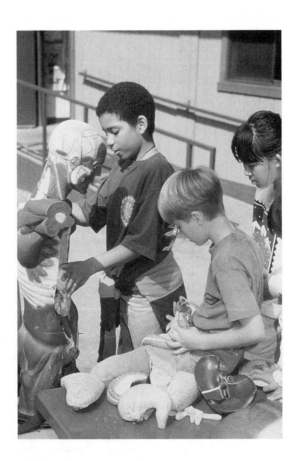

Health education centers are entertaining places to bring students for a hands on learning experience.

specially trained staff who will lead tailormade sessions. Examples of such centers include:

1. Center for Health Education in Indianapolis
2. Poe Center for Health Education in Raleigh, North Carolina
3. National Health Museum at Walter Reed Hospital in Washington, DC
4. Denver Museum of Natural History: Hall of Life Health Education Center.

Examples   Four examples of field trips follow:

1. Visit an emergency room.
2. Visit a public health clinic and take on the role of a client.
3. Ride with a police officer for an evening.
4. Interview individuals who have experienced a health problem of special interest.

Method/Intervention 13: Guest Speakers

Guest speakers can be a tremendous resource in both the school and community settings. Many individuals have knowledge or experiences that make them uniquely qualified to add a great deal to health-related topics. Individuals who have experienced or are experiencing health problems can help bring alive and personalize what might be viewed as dull and irrelevant health information. Other speakers might be experts in a field who can bring up-to-date information about topical health issues.

One caution must be made, however. Health educators must think carefully about what they are trying to achieve before using guest speakers (see the information on constructing behavioral objectives in Chapter 2). For example, all too often school and college health educators, in an attempt to increase the students' awareness of their own susceptibility to HIV, will bring in a guest speaker who is HIV positive. The speaker is a middle-aged man who discusses how he contracted the virus through homosexual sex. The students usually feel moved by the tragedy of the situation and the courage of the individual, but leave the presentation with their stereotypical view strongly reinforced, that HIV is still really a gay disease. Objectives must be clearly defined before utilizing a speaker, and the health educator should avoid the trap of using someone simply because "it seemed like the right thing to do!"

Advantages and   Advantages of guest speakers are that they
Disadvantages

1. Allow groups access to experts in the field and the opportunity to obtain up-to-the-minute information.

2. Enable participants to personalize, or put a face to, a health issue that up to this point might have seemed abstract.
3. Give participants a "break" from the regular presenter or teacher.
4. Allow participants to meet individuals who might be influential at the local, state, or even national levels. This opportunity can facilitate networking.

Disadvantages are that they

1. Can be ineffective if the speaker is poor. Many individuals have some good information to share, but because their speaking skills are so poor, their presentations are boring and thus ineffectual. Every effort should be made to hear a speaker before extending an invitation.
2. Can present an unbalanced picture of an issue. The single guest speaker tends to bring one viewpoint to an educational setting, which, of course, is not always a bad thing. However, care must be taken to at least consider this factor, and, when discussing controversial issues in particular, make an effort to present the opposing viewpoint.
3. In a school setting, will require notification and permission from the administration. It is of particular importance to obtain such permission when "sensitive" issues such as human sexuality or drug education are being addressed.
4. May not be the kind of person to whom participants can relate. Issues such as the speaker's race, gender, age, and national origin are all important factors to consider when bringing in a guest speaker to a community. Close consultation with community leaders is an effective way to facilitate the choice of speaker.
5. May charge a speaking fee. Although many speakers will not charge any type of fee, those individuals who have a particular expertise, who are regular speakers, and who have a good reputation will invariably charge a speaking fee. This can range from a few hundred to a thousand or more dollars per engagement. Always be sure to ask about a fee before arranging a presentation!

Example: Eating Disorders Unit   Assume that you have been asked to teach a small unit on eating disorders to college students. You have covered the "theory" of the issue, but it is clear to you that despite the statistics you have given related to the prevalence of this problem, the students are having a difficult time understanding how individuals become involved with eating disorders. After a little research on your part, you discover that the campus has an eating disorder support group which provides students who are willing to share their stories with other students. A student from the group attends your class, and suddenly eating disorders has a face and a personality . . . and because the face and personality probably look very similar to those of the regular class members, the effects of using such a guest speaker can be profound.

Method/Intervention 14: Guided Imagery

Guided imagery as a method involves experiencing through a guided sensory journey some health-enhancing behavior or potential outcome. It generally involves closing of the eyes and being guided through some experience. It is commonly used in stress management and sports psychology.

When to Use
It is appropriate to use guided imagery when you believe the experience will actually help meet your objectives.

Advantages and Disadvantages
Advantages of guided imagery are that it

1. Can positively influence attitudes and values such as efficacy.
2. Can be entertaining and enjoyable.
3. Is low in cost.
4. Can be motivational.

Disadvantages are that it

1. Requires some training and practice.
2. Can be time-consuming.

Examples
Three examples of guided imagery follow:

1. *Pain control*—see Table 5-2 for a description of this exercise.
2. *Stress education*—soft music such as sea sounds is accompanied by directions to imagine walking on a beach.
3. *Weight control*—the participants are directed to imagine themselves at their ideal weight and how good it feels and looks.

Method/Intervention 15: Humor

Humor can be used as an attraction or a reinforcing activity. It is an important tool for health educators. It can liven up a meeting and help to establish rapport with an audience. However, it is important to note that people differ in what they find humorous. Be certain to avoid humor that may offend. For example, the bumper sticker proclaiming, "Support Mental Health or I Will Kill You" is funny to many but upsetting to others. Likewise, "How in the Health Are You?" may offend some people. Also, it is important to keep humor focused on objectives.

Table 5-2 A Basic Experience for Pain Control

Now relax, close your eyes, take a deep breath, and repeat mentally to yourself each sentence after I say it:

My arms and legs are heavy and warm (six times).
My heartbeat is calm and regular (six times).
My body breathes itself (six times).
My abdomen is warm (six times).
My forehead is cool (six times).
My mind is quiet and still (three times).
My mind is quiet and happy (three times).
I am at peace.
I feel my feet expanding lightly and pleasantly by 1 inch (two times).
My feet are now expanding lightly and pleasantly by 12 inches (two times).
The pleasant 12-inch expansion is spreading throughout all the parts of my legs (two times).
My abdomen, buttocks, and back are expanding 12 inches lightly and pleasantly (two times).
My chest is expanding 12 inches pleasantly and lightly (two times).
My arms are expanding 12 inches lightly and pleasantly (two times).
My neck and head are joining in the 12 inches of expansion (two times).
My entire body is relaxed, expanded, and comfortable (six times).
My mind is quiet and happy (two times).
I withdraw my mind from my physical surroundings (two times).
I am free of pain and all other sensations (two times).
My body is safe and comfortable (six times).
My mind is quiet and happy (two times).
I am that I am (pause two minutes).
Each time I practice this exercise my body becomes more and more comfortable. And I carry this comfort with me to my normal awareness. As I prepare to return to my normal awareness, I will bring with me the ideal comfort which I have created in my focused concentration. As I open my eyes, I take a deep comfortable breath and a big comfortable stretch.

Source: *The Pain Game* by C. Normal Shealy, M.D. Copyright © 1976 by C. Norman Shealy, M.D. Used by permission of Celestial Arts, P.O. Box 7327, Berkeley, CA 94707.

William and Pauline Carlyon (1987) have some good suggestions for using humor:

- Remember, humor is not just a joke. It is one of a range of positive emotions you want to evoke.
- Do not assume that others share your sense of humor and its underlying social attitudes.
- Beware of satire and irony. They are easily misread as sarcasm or ridicule.
- Do not tell jokes, unless they are "on you." Save your standup comedy for your family and friends, who are familiar with your eccentricities.
- Avoid ethnic humor and dialect imitations particularly. You will almost always sound insulting.
- Do listen to your clients/patients/students and encourage their humor by participating in its enjoyment. Only they know the humor that's best for them.

Advantages and Disadvantages

Advantages of humor are that it

1. Provides an element of fun.
2. Is a good attention-getter.
3. Provides variety.
4. Can address affective information or issues in a palatable format.
5. Can provide new perspectives.

Disadvantages are that it

1. Is unpredictable in outcome since everyone has a different sense of humor.
2. Requires special setup.
3. May require permission to use.
4. May be viewed as a waste of time by some participants.

Examples

Some examples of how to use humor follow:

1. Ask the group to design cartoons that would influence a target group.
2. Use cartoons on a overhead projector with text removed and ask the group to write new text that would influence the target population.
3. Ask the group to write humorous health sayings.
4. Photocopy cartoons or humorous health sayings and make transparencies from them to spice up presentation.
5. Tell a funny story. This could be a story about yourself and the health issue.
6. Show a humorous commercial related to the topic.
7. Tell a joke related to issues.

Method/Intervention 16: Lecture

Lecturing is a primary tool of the health educator. It is often maligned as a method, but in fact it is the most common tool in health education although it is often poorly utilized. Good lecturing requires practice and organization. Most of us will not become world-class orators, but we can become competent speakers. We strongly urge you to enhance your speaking skills by reading some books on public speaking, taking a course, or joining a toastmasters club to improve your skills. You will constantly be called upon to make presentations as a health educator. Whether you are in school or community health education, you must develop skills in making presentations. Your presentations may be to small or large groups, but the basic principles are the same.

Any time you must lecture for over 20 minutes, utilize some of the other methods or prepare a truly stirring presentation. It is unlikely that you can keep the attention of your audience much beyond this time frame unless audience members are personally highly motivated (i.e., graduate students or victims of the disease you are discussing, who perceive you to clearly have information they want) or you are charismatic. Preparation is the key to a successful presentation. (See also Chapter 4.)

Advantages and Disadvantages

Advantages of the lecture style are that it

1. Allows you to cover large amounts of information in a short time.
2. Can be used with very large groups.
3. Requires little equipment, although a microphone is important for large groups.

Disadvantages are that it

1. Can be a difficult method for holding the attention of an audience.
2. Requires a very high level of expertise on the topic to do well without other aids.
3. Is not a good way to attract an audience unless the speaker is well known and respected.
4. Is generally effective only for short periods of time.

Prepresentation Tasks

Preparation for presentation, or *prepresentation* tasks, include the following:

1. Select or write objectives (see Chapter 2).
2. Analyze audience—needs assessment (see Chapter 2).
3. Develop appropriate content for lecture. Be careful not to cover too much material at one time. Consider providing a handout to reinforce important points.
4. Develop lecture notes as part of your lesson plan (see Chapter 4). This preparation should be done well before the presentation. Knowing you are prepared is a great confidence builder. Preparing the night before often gives you the jitters and is self-defeating.
5. Develop an alternate plan in case something does not work right. What do you do if the audiovisual equipment does not work or the participants do not ask questions when you want them to?
6. Practice making your presentation. If you have the time and resources, video- or audiotape it and play it back. Practice keeping your hands at your side. Do not hold your notes. It is okay to glance at them when needed, but do not be tied to them. If this is a topic you do not know well, use overheads or some other visual aid. This will ensure you do not miss any key points, and people will look at your visual aid a good part of the time, taking some of the pressure off you.

The Presentation

Guidelines for presentation follow:

1. Clarify what you will cover—what are your objectives? Students or clients will learn more if you make it clear what you want them to get out

of your presentation. Speak at an appropriate level, but do not be patronizing.

2. Present your information clearly, repeating important points.

3. Whenever possible check to be certain the audience is understanding your message. Always remember you are lecturing to reach your objectives. You are not there to only entertain. You are a health educator hoping to influence lives. Use humor if it helps achieve your objectives.

4. Review key points and prepare for the next step in your program. What do you want participants to do? What is the next step?

5. Finally, review these "Dos" and "Do Nots" of presentation:

The "Do Nots" of Presentation

Do not play with chalk like dice.

Do not put your hands in your pocket or use some other distraction with your hands.

Do not say "I don't know this area very well" or "I don't know why I was asked to cover this."

Do not get tied to a podium or your notes.

The "Dos" of Presentation

Do smile and move about.

Do reinforce key points.

Do let the audience know you are a credible speaker on the topic.

Do use visual aids as appropriate.

Do show an aura of confidence.

Do make eye contact.

Method/Intervention 17: Mass Media

The term **mass media** refers to the use of media to reach large audiences or the use of available mass media materials to educate a target group. These materials include television, newspapers, magazines, pamphlets, billboards, and radio. Be certain to consider local media such as ethnic publications and community-based publications. Developing your own mass media program is generally expensive and requires special skills. However, many publications will provide free access for worthy causes and may even make their professional staff available. Generally, we recommend the use of specialists for such work. These specialists need not be Park Avenue firms, but can be local businesses or local community college or university staff personnel.

Another way to use media is to utilize available media examples through videotaping or copying. Often formal permission can be granted for educational programs. Many of the **voluntary health agencies** such as the American Cancer Society have high-quality materials.

An important issue is often preparing groups to analyze media messages and to examine fallacies.

Advantages and Disadvantages

Advantages of the mass media are that they

1. Can reach a large number of individuals.
2. Can reinforce important ideas.
3. Can create a positive environment for change.

Disadvantages are that they

1. Are usually inadequate to change complex behaviors because of the brevity of the messages.
2. Can be very expensive.
3. May require special personnel.

Whom to Contact

Here are some guidelines on whom to contact:

1. For newspapers, contact the education or medical science editor if they have one, otherwise, the appropriate news editor.
2. For television, contact the public service director or the program director.
3. For radio, contact the public service director or the program director.

Example: Local Media Campaign

Conduct a mass media campaign for a health fair. Contact the local television station regarding what they need. They may wish to conduct live interviews for their public service programs or as part of local news segments. The key is to be cooperative and flexible about air time. Generally stations are very cooperative in providing some time. The following media kits can give you ideas about putting together a campaign to support school health education or other health topics.

1. American School Health Association, Marketing Kit—A Healthy Child: The Key to the Basics, available from ASHA, P.O. Box 708, Kent, OH 44240. 330-678-1601.
2. Health Education Advocacy Kit, available from American Association for Health Education, 1900 Association Dr., Reston, VA 22061. 703-476-3437.

Method/Intervention 18: Models

Models are useful visual aids for instruction. Examples of models include anatomical facsimiles, breast models for self-examination practice, model communities, car models, and any variety of materials to make a point or draw people visually into a discussion.

Advantages and Disadvantages

Advantages of models are that they

1. Can provide variety.
2. Can be used to provide "hands-on" experiences.

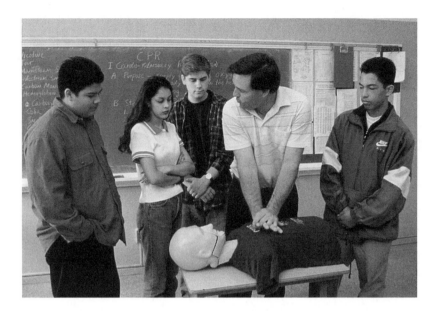

Models offer a much more interactive approach to learning than photos or illustrations can offer.

3. Are very attractive and good attention-getters.
4. Can be much more meaningful than a picture in a text.

Disadvantages are that they

1. Require equipment.
2. Can be expensive.
3. Require extra setup.

Examples   Some examples of how to use models follow:

1. Use mannequins to teach CPR.
2. Use a heart model for teaching heart attack prevention and care.
3. Use model breasts for teaching breast self-examination.
4. Use model testicles for teaching testicular self-examination.

Method/Intervention 19: Music

Music can be used in several ways to achieve objectives. It can be used as a method or as part of a method. Music is a powerful mood setter. Music can be used in the background as a way of setting the mood for a skit or role play. It can be used to draw attention to the message found in the lyrics. Students can make up their own lyrics. Music affects us all. We can select music to help us create a special mood or capture the interest of a group.

Advantages and Disadvantages

Advantages of music are that it

1. Can be low in cost. You can always sing without any equipment.
2. Often can be used to help discuss affective issues.
3. Is excellent for setting a mood.
4. Can allow for individual expression.

Disadvantages are that it

1. Often requires equipment, such as a piano, which may be difficult to obtain and move.
2. Is sometimes difficult to find correct music.
3. Poses difficulty in appealing to a variety of tastes.

Examples

Some examples of the use of music follow:

1. Sing songs with health messages.
2. Develop songs to reinforce health messages.
3. Start a group chant: "No matter what you say about me, I'm still a worthwhile person." While the group is chanting, walk around the room making negative statements about each person. Have the group continue chanting, ignoring the negative statements.
4. Use chants to reinforce various messages.
5. Play a funeral march to lead into a discussion about funeral customs and the purposes of a funeral.
6. Ask participants to make up health lyrics to popular songs.
7. Ask participants to bring in a sample of music that expresses something personal or special to them.
8. Ask participants how relationships are depicted in popular songs. Bring in examples to discuss.

Method/Intervention 20: Newsletters

We are all familiar with newsletters but often do not realize that they can be an important component of an educational intervention. They can provide vital information to target groups, such as location; set a climate for an upcoming workshop or class; serve to reinforce concepts presented in a workshop, or act as a reminder for action. The newsletter is often a very cost-effective way to deliver and reinforce information, encourage compliance, and increase the likelihood of attendance. The availability of personal computers makes this method accessible to most groups today. Figure 5-7 shows an example of a newsletter.

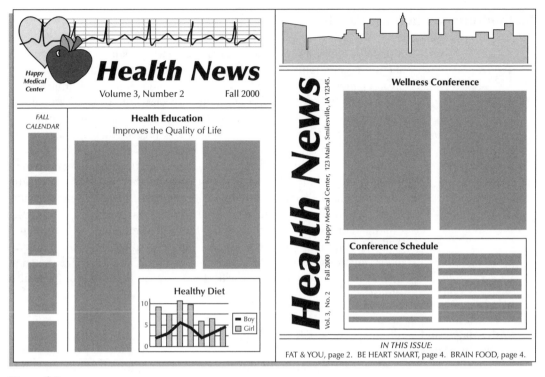

Figure 5-7
Example of Newsletter

Advantages and Disadvantages

Advantages of newsletters are that they

1. Have the potential for providing a considerable amount of information at relatively low cost.
2. Can target specific needs.
3. Can reinforce information presented in a program.
4. Can serve as a reminder to take action (boster).

Disadvantages are that they

1. Have high mailing costs and production costs.
2. Require some equipment—for example, they generally require access to a personal computer.
3. Can be very time-consuming to construct.
4. Require at least a minimal level of expertise.

Method/Intervention 21: Panels

A **panel** is a useful way for an audience either to explore differing opinions about the same topic or to examine varying issues within the same subject area. A panel can be used in both the school and community settings, made up of members of the local community (or class) or "experts" brought in from outside agencies. In the school setting a panel is an innovative way to motivate students to research an area and present their findings to the class in the context of a panel. The school health educator should always ensure that the school administration has full knowledge of any panels that include outside speakers. Using a panel in the community is a little more complicated, and great consideration must be given to certain factors when matching panel members with the community setting. For example, will the community members view the panel members as legitimate? Will the community give credence to "outside opinions"? Can the community members relate to the panelists in any way? These are all basic questions that must be considered with great care by the **community health educator.**

Advantages and Disadvantages

Advantages of panels are that they

1. Allow the audience to hear a diversity of opinions about the same subject.
2. Have the potential for critical debate among panelists, allowing the audience to learn about the issues in greater depth.
3. Allow the audience to hear more than one speaker, decreasing the likelihood of boredom.

Disadvantages are that they

1. Are often difficult to compile with just the right "mix." For example, one of the panelists might dominate the proceedings, or the members might be so antagonistic toward one another that nothing meaningful gets accomplished.
2. Require a moderator, as panelists have the potential of getting off track, either individually or collectively. Rules, such as allowed time to speak, opportunities for questions, and so on, should be considered before beginning.
3. Have the potential to lack closure. A good moderator can prevent this problem. In the classroom setting a moderator might ask the students to write a paragraph about what they have heard or their feelings about a topic in light of the panel discussion. In the community setting a moderator might briefly summarize the discussion or allow a few minutes for each panelist to review his or her position.

Example: Teenage Pregnancy A panel to help expectant teenage mothers and fathers anticipate problems they may encounter might include the following individuals:

- A teenage mother and father who have already been through the process and can describe their experiences.
- A representative of a local agency who can explain the available program resources, both financial and otherwise.
- A member of the local school system who can give information related to finishing school.

This list is not exhaustive, yet even a panel limited to these few people would be much more useful than a lecture from a single "expert" who has probably never experienced this particular problem. A link to local resources alone would make this panel a worthwhile and valuable health education strategy.

Method/Intervention 22: Peer Education

The **peer education** approach of presenting health education information has become very popular over the past few years. This approach, which consists of individuals or groups presenting workshops for their peers, can be a very effective and productive means by which to disseminate information. This method is commonly used on college campuses and in school and community settings. Peer education is a particularly useful method to use when funding for professional personnel is limited or when it is particularly important for the audience to be able to relate to the presenters. (See the example at the conclusion of this section.)

Advantages and Disadvantages Advantages of peer education are that it

1. Provides a modeling experience. Individuals often learn through modeling. Because peer educators are extremely similar to their audiences, the opportunity for modeling to occur is enhanced.
2. Has a greater effect than a solitary health educator. The peers have many more points of entry into a population than a professional and can thus reach more people.
3. Has the potential for providing continuing, informal education. Peers will become known in the community as sources of information and referral and will therefore have the opportunity to educate even when they are not offering a structured presentation.
4. Can influence people that professionals cannot. Peers can be "gatekeepers" to a population that would otherwise be unreached. The peers' values and interests are similar to those of their potential clients, and this can provide an effective entrée.

5. Affords an incredible opportunity for the personal growth and development of the peers themselves. We should not ignore this benefit by focusing exclusively on the recipients of the programming efforts (Goodhart, 1989).

Disadvantages of peer education are that it

1. Might sometimes lack credibility in the eyes of the audience because peer educators are not perceived as "experts."
2. Could provide inaccurate information or poor performance, resulting in the loss of program credibility, unless the peer educators are well trained and their programming is closely monitored.
3. Could be dangerously inadequate for programs requiring a high degree of sophisticated and technical information. Peer educators should not be asked to do more than they are capable of doing.

Example: Alcohol Abuse, Sexuality, and Stress Management Programs

Assume you have just been appointed community health educator at a college with an enrollment of 15,000. You are the only health educator on staff, and your supervisors would like you to begin implementing programming around the issues of alcohol abuse, sexuality, and stress management as soon as possible. After educating your supervisors as to what is humanly possible, you set about planning your strategy, which includes peer education.

Peer education can be an incredibly valuable programming strategy, particularly when staffing levels are low. Although finding interested, enthusiastic students to help is not usually a problem, training them to high standards of performance can be demanding. High standards, however, are crucial in

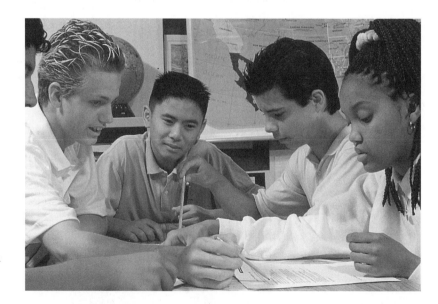

Peer education is a method that can solve low staff problems for administrators and can help students get extra credit for their efforts.

order to avoid fellow professionals questioning the wisdom of using "mere students" in a paraprofessional role. Once the programs are up and running, an additional suggestion would be to formalize the program by investigating the possibility of obtaining course credit for the students. Independent studies or internships through sympathetic academic departments is one possibility, but the health educator must ensure that the programs are sufficiently well developed to survive academic scrutiny and sometimes cynicism!

Method/Intervention 23: Personal Improvement Projects

Personal improvement projects can serve as incentives to make positive personal changes in a targeted health behavior. The objective is to provide clients with an opportunity to learn proper techniques for changing health behaviors such as those involved in nutrition and enable them to incorporate these new skills into a **healthy lifestyle.**

Components of a personal improvement project are to

1. Establish a contract with realistic objectives.
2. Chart these realistic objectives.
3. Chart actual progress.
4. Maintain some type of diary to explain progress.

Advantages and Disadvantages

Advantages of personal improvement projects are that they

1. Are low in cost.
2. Have the potential for actually influencing directly health behavior.
3. Can target specific needs, including behavioral objectives.
4. Can reinforce information presented in a program.
5. Require active application of principles.
6. Personalize health practices for every participant.

Disadvantages are that they

1. Require considerable individual attention.
2. Can be difficult to achieve.
3. Require considerable paperwork.
4. Some participants may not be sufficiently motivated. If this is a course, you may wish to provide an alternate assignment.

Examples

Examples of personal improvement projects follow:

1. Weight reduction—see Figure 5-8 for a sample project.
2. Regular exercise.

It is not the intention of this project merely to provide incentive for another crash-diet program. The objective is to provide you with an opportunity to gain a good knowledge of proper diet and nutrition practices and to enable you to incorporate them into your chosen lifestyle.

In order to ensure this, it is part of this assignment that you read proper background material and determine a course of action that fits your needs (this should include consultation with your physician if possible and for certain if any major weight reduction is contemplated). In your paper you should explain your selection of a diet plan, your goal, any problems you encountered, and include a graph of your progress as shown here. Weight data must be made on the same scales and measured at the same time of day to be "officially accurate." Before undertaking this project you must have a conference with your instructor.

Progress toward the objective should be charted. A personal computer can make charting progress easy.

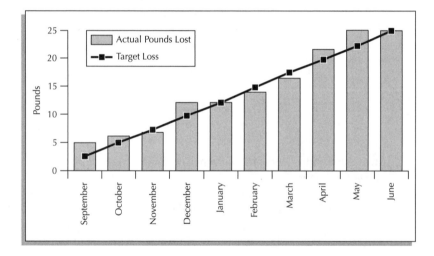

Figure 5-8
Personal Improvement
Project for Weight Loss

3. Increasing fruit and vegetable consumption.
4. Regular mental health breaks.
5. Smoking cessation.
6. Consistent seat belt use.

Method/Intervention 24: Problem Solving

The **problem-solution technique** requires scenarios that need a solution. These can be written or oral. Given the circumstances described, participants are asked to determine the best answer. Often there is no one, guaranteed acceptable answer. The purpose is to stimulate discussion and to expose participants to multiple points of view.

Advantages and Disadvantages

Advantages of using a problem-solution technique is that it

1. Can serve to create a questioning atmosphere.
2. Can demonstrate that often there is no one certain correct answer.
3. Sets the ground rules for participant interaction.
4. Develops questioning strategies.

Disadvantages are that it

1. Can be time-consuming.
2. Can make participants uncomfortable as they realize that there may be no clearly correct answer.

Examples

Two examples of problem solving follow:

1. A scenario such as that shown in Figure 5-9 can apply problem solving to a health problem such as cardiovascular disease.
2. A scenario such as that shown in Figure 5-10 can apply problem solving to a social and community problem such as gang violence.

Harvey Schwartz, a fat middle-aged diabetic, was seated in front of the TV smoking and feasting on a meal of french fries, shrimp, strawberry shortcake, and beer when his wife Hilda came in screaming about his lazy habits. He jumped to his feet and began shouting in return, then collapsed on the floor holding his chest. His funeral was the following Monday. He was buried alongside his father and brother, who died of heart attacks and strokes.

Which of the following do you feel contributed to Harvey's demise? Check the statements you agree with.

_____ *1. His understanding wife, Hilda Schwartz.*
_____ *2. His obese body.*
_____ *3. His culinary habits.*
_____ *4. His choice of beverage.*
_____ *5. His fine physical conditioning.*
_____ *6. His use of tobacco products.*
_____ *7. His genetic background.*
_____ *8. His youthful appearance.*
_____ *9. His foul-functioning pancreas.*
_____ *10. His job as a taxi driver in Brooklyn, New York.*

Figure 5-9
"The Demise of Harvey Schwartz," a Problem-Solution Scenario

> *Lamon Thomas and Bruce Chen, wearing their gang colors, are attending a high school dance together when Lamon gets into a verbal argument with another student. The other student is offended when Lamon asks the other student's girlfriend to dance. All participants have been drinking. Bruce comes over to aid his friend when a gun appears. In the struggle Bruce is shot twice and later dies.*
>
> *Which of the following do you feel contributed to Bruce's death? Check the statements you agree with.*
>
> _____ 1. *Lamon's asking the young women to dance.*
> _____ 2. *Bruce's getting involved with something that was not his business.*
> _____ 3. *The way the young men were dressed.*
> _____ 4. *Bruce's choice of beverage.*
> _____ 5. *Lack of metal detectors at the entrance.*
> _____ 6. *The availability of handguns.*
> _____ 7. *Poor supervision.*
> _____ 8. *Lack of parental control.*
> _____ 9. *Lack of stated policies.*
> _____ 10. *No police protection.*

Figure 5-10
"The Wrong Place at the Wrong Time," a Problem-Solution Scenario

It is important to note these problem solutions are designed so there is no clear answer to most questions posed. An important component of the activity is this planned disagreement that generally gives rise to a fairly heated discussion and disagreement. It is possible to make assumptions and then make an argument for agreeing or disagreeing with statements. The whole point of the activity is the discussion that follows. This element will drive some participants crazy. Many participants insist on getting the "right answer" and are distraught when told there are could be many correct answers depending on assumptions.

Method/Intervention 25: Puppets

Puppets can be a very powerful tool in health education, particularly with the young. They can be purchased or made at low cost. An easy-to-make puppet is the finger puppet, which consists of a small paper drawing that is cut out of paper and attached to a finger. The drawings, or paper dolls, can also be attached to long sticks. Making puppets can be used as an icebreaker or team builder. Alternatively, a doll can be used as a puppet, or one can simply draw on the hand.

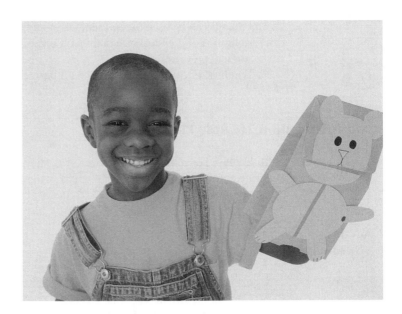

Puppets are inexpensive to create and a fun learning tool for children.

Advantages and Disadvantages

Advantages of puppets are that they

1. Are entertaining.
2. Can address difficult topics and the affective domain.
3. Allow participants to act out feelings without reprisals.
4. Can promote creative thinking skills.

Disadvantages are that they

1. Will not be effective if people refuse to participate.
2. Can bring out unintended emotions or outcomes.
3. Require the facilitator to be well prepared because of the uncertainty of outcome.
4. Can be threatening to some individuals.

Examples

Examples of ways to use puppets follow:

1. Puppets are effective in working with children to express feelings. Young children will often talk to a friendly puppet when they would not talk to an adult. This technique is used extensively with victims of child sexual abuse to elicit responses, a fact that indicates how powerful a tool puppets can be. Be certain you choose your questions carefully.
2. Puppets can be used to bring some entertainment to an adult group. Have a debate with your puppet. Tape a conversation, then play the tape as you provide the answers.

3. Puppets can be used to represent an organ or other body part in a demonstration of the effects of healthy and unhealthy practices or to explain a surgical procedure.
4. Purchase a readymade program with puppets and scripts.

Method/Intervention 26: Role Plays

Role plays are acting out assigned roles. There is no script as in a play, but participants are not free to act in any way they wish. They are assigned parameters with limited flexibility.

Advantages and Disadvantages

Advantages of role plays are that they

1. Require no equipment.
2. Can address difficult topics and the affective domain.
3. Can allow participants to act out feelings without reprisals.
4. Are interesting and entertaining.

Disadvantages are that they

1. Will fail if people refuse to participate.
2. Can bring out unintended emotions or outcomes.
3. Require that the facilitator be well prepared because of the uncertainty of outcome.
4. Can sometimes be difficult to control.
5. May not be taken seriously by participants.

Rules

Certain rules should be established for role plays:

1. Actors are acting out *assigned* roles. It must be understood that they are not playing themselves.
2. No put downs of actors should be allowed.
3. Do not stereotype casting.
4. Establish parameters for roles.
5. It should be understood that in real life it is rare that there is one clear-cut correct answer or role.

Debriefing

Debriefing is particularly important after role playing. Be sure to analyze the roles for realism and most common responses. Ask participants what are appropriate and realistic ways to handle the problems posed. Explore alternatives, asking for the likely consequences of each alternative. Finally, promote discussion on how we can achieve positive outcomes.

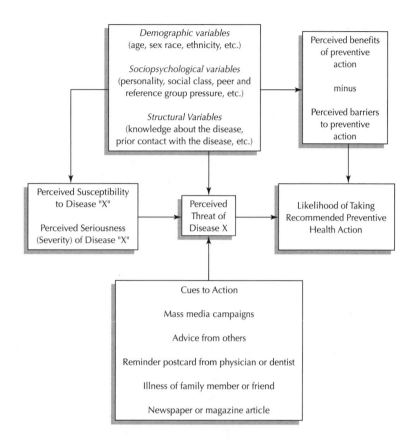

Figure 3-1
Health Belief Model.
From M. Becker, Ed.
(1974). *The Health Be-
lief Model and Personal
Health Behavior*
(p. 7). Thoroughfare,
NJ: Slack. Reprinted
with permission.

gree of seriousness of a given health problem. *Perceived benefits* are the beliefs a person has regarding the availability and effectiveness of a variety of
possible actions in reducing the threat of illness. *Perceived barriers* are those
costs or negative aspects associated with engaging in a specific health behavior. In addition, *cues to action* are viewed as necessary triggers of behavior.
Defined as instigating events that stimulate the initiation of behavior, these
cues may be internal, such as perceptions of pain, or external, such as feedback from a health care provider (Rosenstock, 1974). Cues to action and
perception of risk (susceptibility) are two elements that should always be
considered in method selection.

According to the model, in order for a person to take action to avoid illness, the positive forces need to outweigh the negative forces. Thus, the
health behavior is likely to occur, if an individual believes that

1. He or she is personally susceptible to the disease or illness.
2. The occurrence of the health problem is severe enough to negatively impact his or her life.

3. Taking specific actions would have beneficial effects.
4. The barriers to such action do not overwhelm the benefits. (Rosenstock, 1974)

In addition to those beliefs, the individual must be exposed to the cues for action just explained.

The health belief model has been applied to a variety of populations and a diversity of health issues, including alcoholism (Bardsley and Beckman, 1988), compliance with a diabetes regimen (Becker and Janz, 1985), breast self-examination (Champion, 1985), contraceptive behavior (Herold, 1983; Hester and Macrina, 1985), skin cancer (Glanz et al., 1999), and medication compliance among psychiatric outpatients (Kelly, Mamon, and Scott, 1987). Although it is true that the majority of studies are retrospective in nature and the predictive value of the model is still in doubt (Kegeles and Lund, 1982), some studies have used the model to make predictions (Stein et al., 1992; Harrison, 1992) with limited results.

Case Study: Bill

Bill is teaching a unit on AIDS to ninth-grade classes in a local high school. He is dismayed to find that his students are bored and restless, despite this being a topic related to sex. After class, Bill questions several students about their attitudes and discovers that although the students consider AIDS to be a serious disease, they feel that because they are heterosexual and do not use drugs the problem has little relevance to their lives. Bill ponders the issue of how to increase the students' perceived susceptibility to HIV and finally develops a strategy. With permission from school administrators, Bill shows his students a film that dramatically depicts the story of a high school student who contracts HIV from heterosexual sex. In addition, a local speakers bureau provides a speaker for Bill's classes. The speaker is a young woman who has contracted HIV through heterosexual intercourse while in college. Both activities have a sobering effect on Bill's students, and, at least in the short term, they no longer view AIDS as "someone else's problem." (See Case Studies Revisited page 75.)

Precede-Proceed Model

The PRECEDE model (Figure 3-2) was developed by Green et al. (1975) with financial support from the National Institutes of Health. It is a planning model for health education based on principles, both theoretical and applied, from epidemiology, education, administration, and the social/ behavioral sciences. The acronym PRECEDE stands for predisposing, reinforcing, and enabling causes in educational diagnosis and evaluation (Green et al., 1980). The model has been revised in an effort to accommodate the evolving nature and broader perspective of health promotion. The addition of a new set of steps called PROCEED (policy, regulatory, and organizational constructions in educational and environmental development) has been superimposed on the original model (Green and Kreuter, 1991) (Figure 3-3).

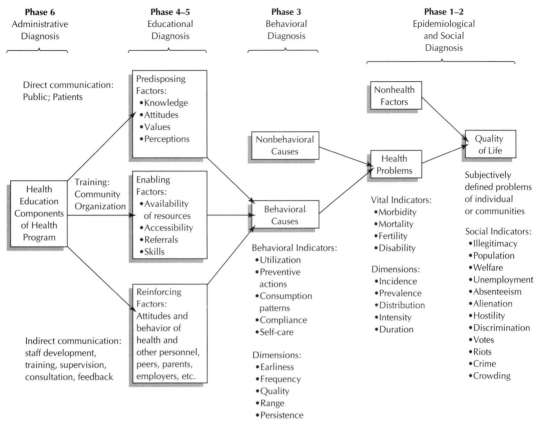

Figure 3-2
PRECEDE Framework. From L. W. Green, M. W. Kreuter, S. G. Deeds, & K. B. Partridge. (1980). *Health Promotion Planning: A Diagnostic Approach* (pp. 14–15). Palo Alto, CA: Mayfield Publishing Co. Reprinted by permission.

The PRECEDE model was designed to be acceptable to health educators with various philosophical and theoretical orientations and to be readily applicable across a variety of settings. It is intended to give structure and organization to health education program planning and evaluation. Application of this approach occurs in several phases and involves the diagnoses of variables in five domains: social, epidemiological, behavioral, educational, and administrative (Green et al., 1980). It is unique in that it begins with active engagement of the target population in defining the desired final outcome and works backward, asking what are the factors that must precede that result.

Phase 1 of the model is *social diagnosis*. An analysis of the social problems that exist in a community is a necessary prerequisite in assessing the quality of life of the target population. The purpose of this phase is to obtain maximum feasible participation in ascertaining the relationship between a

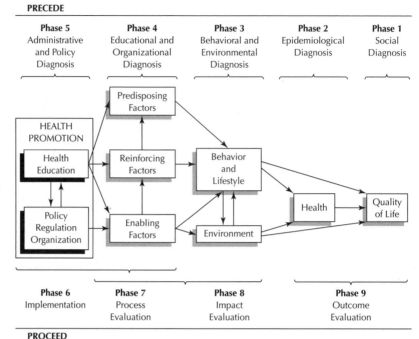

Figure 3-3
PRECEDE-PROCEED
Model. From L. W.
Green & M. W.
Kreuter. (1991). *Health
Promotion Planning: an
Educational and Envi-
ronmental Approach*
(2nd ed.). (p. 24, Figure
1.4). Mountain View,
CA: Mayfield. Re-
printed by permission.

given health problem and the social problems of the population. Phase 2,
epidemiological diagnosis, is an evaluation of the health problems associated
with the community's quality of life. Morbidity, mortality, fertility, and disability are the primary indicators of the health of a population (Green et al.,
1980).

Behavioral diagnosis, the third phase, attempts to identify the health-
related behaviors that have impact on the health problems isolated in the
epidemiological diagnosis. It is important at this stage to also acknowledge
the nonbehavioral factors, such as age, gender, and environment, that
may contribute to the health problem of interest. Behavioral factors are
then rated on a scale of importance and changeability. In the PRECEDE-
PROCEED model (Green and Kreuter, 1990, 1991), equal weight is given
to an environmental diagnosis as to a behavioral diagnosis at this stage in the
diagnostic process. Factors rated high in importance and changeability are
usually selected as the targets for intervention (Green et al., 1980).

In the fourth phase, *educational diagnosis*, the theories described previously are used to identify factors influencing the health behaviors stated in
the behavioral diagnosis. These are differentiated by three categories of influence: predisposing, enabling, and reinforcing factors. *Predisposing factors*
provide the motivation or rationale for the behavior, for example, knowledge, attitudes, values, and beliefs. *Enabling factors* include personal skills
and assets and community resources. Predisposing and enabling factors are

antecedent to the health behavior and allow for the behavior to occur. *Reinforcing factors* supply the reward, incentive, or punishment of a behavior that contribute to its maintenance or extinction. Similar procedures are applied to an organizational diagnosis of factors influencing the environment in the combined PRECEDE-PROCEED model. Each group of factors is analyzed in terms of importance and changeability, and priorities are established for the intervention. Based on the nature of the targets for intervention, educational methodologies are selected (Green et al., 1980).

The final phase of the process (phase five), *administrative diagnosis*, assesses budgetary implications, identifies and allocates resources, defines the nature of any cooperative agreements, and sets a realistic timetable for the intervention. Neglect of this important step can doom an otherwise viable intervention to failure. The PROCEED modifications (Green and Kreuter, 1991), at this point in the model, include an assessment of policies, regulations, and organizational factors that impact on the resourcing and implementation of health promotion programs and the development of strategies to effectively manage these influences. In addition, the revised PRECEDE-PROCEED model includes a discussion of implementation issues as well as process, outcome, and impact evaluation.

The PRECEDE-PROCEED Model now has had 25 years of use and refinement. Green has a web site (http://www.ihpr.ubc.ca/precede.html) that discusses the model and includes a list of references to the model. This list contains over 750 references of use in programs and in texts. It is certainly the most widely used planning model in the world and one of the few extensively used models developed by health educators.

The PRECEDE model has been used in a variety of settings with a number of different populations, including planning an adolescent school-based sexuality program (Rubinson and Baillie, 1981); analysis of school health education programs (Green and Iverson, 1982); and educational interventions for hypertension control (Green, Levine and Deeds, 1975, 1979; Levine, et al., 1979).

Transtheoretical Model or Stages of Change Model

The transtheoretical model (also known as the stages of change model) is predicated on the theory that behavior change is not an "either/or" phenomenon but instead exists on a continuum and is more of a process than an event, occurring in distinct stages. This model suggests that individuals move from *precontemplation* (the stage at which a person is either (1) unaware of any risk from specific behaviors or (2) aware of risk but unwilling to consider change in the forseeable future), to *contemplation* (the stage where the individual is considering a behavior change but is not yet actively involved in changing), to *preparation* (the stage during which the individual is making definite plans to change), to *action* (the stage in which the person actually initiates the behavior change by modifying some type of behavior or action), to *maintenance* (taking measures intended to sustain the changed behavior and decrease the likelihood of relapse) (Prochaska et al., 1994). Individuals may go through these stages several times before actually successfully maintaining or sustaining the behavior change. This model was initially used in the area of psychotherapy (Prochaska, 1979), but has since been successfully adapted for use in many other areas such as dietary patterns among African American women (Haire-Joshu et al., 1999), work site health promotion and dietary change (Glanz et al., 1998), smoking (DiClemente et al., 1991), sexuality and condom use (Grimley et al., 1995, Prochaska et al., 1994), weight control (Prochaska et al., 1992), and mammography (Rakowski et al., 1992).

Limitations and Future Directions

Among health education professionals and in the health education literature, there is much confusion over the terms *theory, model,* and *paradigm* (Parcel, 1984). Many of the "theories" described in professional journals are not theories at all, but rather constructs or models. In addition, those theories that do satisfy the criteria described by Strauss and Corbin (1990) are not specific to health concerns. Theories currently in vogue often fall short in their ability to accurately predict or explain much of the variance in health behavior. In addition, these theoretical frameworks fail to address the complexity of human health behavior, typically lack a description of the relationships among the variables in the theory, and do not account for interaction effects or synergism among the constructs. Poorly operationalized variables and constructs and a lack of valid measures are also limitations of existing theories. Someone planning an intervention must sort out as much as possible the constructs to be employed before selecting the methods.

It has been suggested that the essence of the health education discipline is to understand and identify methods of managing the influence of multiple variables on health behavior, whether this behavior be health destructive or health generating (Toohey and Shireffs, 1980). We can contribute to the scientific basis of health education by utilizing and testing theories and models as appropriate. These theories and models can be important tools in method selection as they potentially can lead us to more effective health education interventions.

Programs would be much stronger if they utilized what we know of models and theories in making selections of methods/strategies for interventions. To advance our knowledge, we must more thoroughly test these models and theories. Seldom in research do we test a single method in isolation. It is true that there have been evaluation projects that have tested the impact of a pamphlet or TV media spot, but for the most part it is evident to most researchers that success requires not only adequate contact time but also multiple methods.

Almost any single method can be applied according to any model or theory, but it is most unlikely that any one method can truly test a model. It is only when methods are packaged together in units or curriculum programs that we have the possibility of influencing the attitudes and behaviors of our target populations. According to Donnermeyer and Davis, untangling the connections between a specific curriculum or activity and health behaviors will be very challenging. "In addition, attempting to isolate effects may miss a more important research pursuit: measuring the cumulative influence of these experiences" (Donnermeyer and Davis, 1998; p. 157).

There are many other issues to consider in method selection. One important consideration is the educational domain.

Educational Domains

An important consideration is the characteristics of the objectives we are seeking to achieve. Most health education programs work in more than one "domain" as defined in the classic, *Taxonomy of Educational Objectives*. The three major domains are cognitive, affective, and psychomotor. *Cognitive* refers to the recall and synthesis of information. *Affective* refers to the change of an attitude. *Psychomotor* refers to the performance of a physical skill. Sometimes skills are also included as a domain. Examples include refusal skills or the ability to analyze the unscientific nature of appeals used in health advertising.

There is disagreement as to the relationship of these domains and health behavior. Knowledge, attitudes, physical performance, and skills all have important relationships, but they act in different ways at different times and with different people. Knowledge can change behavior at times and at other times seems to have no relationship. Most people, if they know their partner is HIV positive, will take extra precautions or avoid sexual contact altogether. However, although most of us know the relationship of diet to heart disease and cancer, we will still elect to eat high-fat, low-fiber foods on occasion. Several highly respected health educators, for example, are overweight. What motivates one person may not motivate another. A model or theory may never explain the behavior of some individuals. Therefore, it is probably wise to use a variety of methods addressing as many domains as practical. (See Chapter 2 on the subject of writing objectives.)

Characteristics of Learner and Community

We must always consider the characteristics of the individuals and groups we are working with, namely the following:

Age
Gender
Reading ability
Language skills/proficiency in English

Biases and beliefs held
Readiness to learn
Cultural and ethnic background
Motivation to learn

Successful application of the previously mentioned theories and models depends on how these characteristics are addressed. For example, if this is a court-ordered alcohol education program, you may have good attendance in terms of the number of bodies, but it is usually a great challenge to get the minds in those bodies interested and attentive. Most community workshops mix ability groups, making it a further challenge to maintain interest levels.

Group Size   The size of the group will play an important role in method selection. Large groups, say over 100, make individual interaction difficult. Methods must be selected keeping in mind the size of the group. Lecture is a way to share a considerable amount of cognitive information in a short time but usually is not effective for reaching affective or psychomotor objectives. Small groups offer flexibility in many ways but also put more pressure on the individual to participate.

Contact Time   The time you have to spend with a group will play a major role in the selection of appropriate methods. Certain methods simply cannot be used in a short period of time. Many activities require a certain amount of trust to be successful. Developing trust often involves icebreaking activities, which usually require time in order to create openness among the participants. Short workshops do not lend themselves to these activities.

Case Study: James   James is conducting a two-hour workshop on alcohol abuse with 20 individuals who have been referred to this mandatory workshop for drinking and driving offenders. James has not worked with this type of group before and decides to use an icebreaker exercise designed to reveal personal details of the participants. The group members immediately become hostile and barrage poor James with comments like, "I don't want to be here anyway," "This information is no one's business but mine," "Just get on with the facts and let's all get out of here!" James cuts short the icebreaker and concludes the workshop as quickly as possible with a less than successful lecture on the dangers of alcohol abuse and driving. (See Case Studies Revisited page 75.)

Budget   Quality health education need not be expensive, but it does require an appropriate budget. To compete successfully with unhealthy media messages and long-held unhealthy habits, we need and deserve a chance through a reasonable budget. Do you have enough money to use the best methods for the health educational program? If you have limited resources, can you still achieve your objectives, or would you be better off limiting the number of programs but improving the quality of the programs offered?

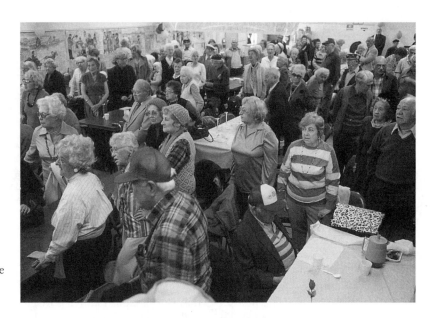

Be sure that the size of your group is appropriate for the type of program you are conducting.

Quality health educators should receive quality salaries for their time and that requires an appropriate budget. Photocopies, videotapes, computer software, and other tools of the health educator all cost money.

Resources/Site/ Environment

You must consider all the resources you have at your disposal. Do you have good facilities to break out into small groups? If you have access to a microcomputer lab, it opens up totally new possibilities. Will you have a quiet space for presentations? What about parking or transportation? If you have access to well-appointed teaching facilities, it opens up the use of many methods. This is especially true of those methods that include technology. Do the participants have Internet access? Of course, many quality health education programs have been offered without any facilities by reaching into homes or utilizing community settings. You work with what is available, and often the local setting is much better for achieving your objectives.

Characteristics of the Educational Provider

If you are the primary provider, what are your strengths as a health educator? What methods are you uncomfortable using? Although you should be willing to take some chances if you are to be successful, it is important you not set yourself up for disaster by selecting a method that will make you so uncomfortable that you cannot do a credible job. If certain methods seem central to achieving your objectives, it may be vital to employ them. Therefore, you may need to practice the method so you can be effective in using it, or perhaps you should bring in an outsider to conduct the method. Using such guests can often increase your comfort with a method while providing a needed activity for your target population. Again, the important principle is to use the correct method given your objectives.

SALLY FORTH   HOWARD & MACINTOSH

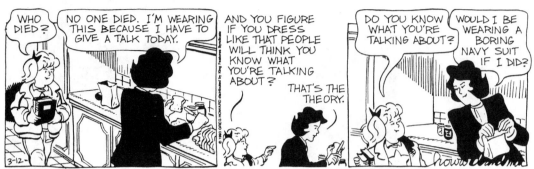

Reprinted with special permission of North America Syndicate. © 1993.

Cultural Appropriateness

It is most important that you consider the cultural characteristics of the group you are targeting. Many programs have failed because of this issue. The best protection is to establish an advisory group from the group being targeted. This small group can review your methods and give you some idea of what response to expect from the participants. Another, less formal way to get some idea is to sit down with a few participants prior to the event and ask them if they think the method would work and be appropriate. (See also Chapters 8 and 9.)

Using a Variety of Methods

Why use a variety of methods? Following are some reasons.

1. It makes it more likely you will achieve your objectives.
2. It may prevent disruptive behavior.
3. It may maintain participant interest.
4. It is more fun for the presenter and learner.
5. Not all learners respond positively to the same methods.

Remember, in health education we are often working with hard-to-reach groups, and anyone gets tired of the same presentation method. Always do what you can to make your presentation interesting, and you will have a better chance of achieving your objectives. By keeping people interested you will also minimize disruptive behavior, such as demonstrated lack of attention or even outright hostility. During community workshops some participants may actually walk out. The first time you have a large number of people walking out on your presentation, you will be very upset, but the problem may simply be a lack of variety or poor method selection. Variety is more fun for you too. You will lose interest yourself if you do things the same way each time. Try new methods, and you will find your task much more enjoyable.

Some Comments on Method Choice

At the elementary and secondary levels, straight lecture or textbook methods are *considered nonfunctional* (Fodor and Dalis, 1974, p. 53).

Each instructor must develop his or her own technique of facilitating. Learning is greatly increased if students are motivated and interested in what they are doing. One of the major criticisms of health education programs is that they are dull. Developing a caring, humanistic approach toward students should help health teachers make their classes more exciting and challenging for the students. The learning process can and should be made enjoyable and interesting (NEA-AMA, 1966).

Any teaching technique or procedure must actively involve the learner if it is to be effective. Active participation can be either direct or vicarious. In direct participation, the student is physically involved in the activity; in vicarious, he or she is a viewer of an activity that is going on in another place or another time. Either way, the goal is for the individual to be affected positively and provided perceptions and experiences contributing to the attainment of desirable long-range cognitive, affective, and action goals (Kime, Schlaadt, and Tritsch, 1977, p. 96).

Different learning opportunities should not be used for the sake of variety alone. True, a variety of learning is of value in that variety tends to break the monotony for the teacher as well as for the student but there are other important reasons for using different learning opportunities: (1) to meet a variety of objectives, (2) to meet a variety of student needs and interests, and (3) to stimulate a variety of senses (Oberteuffer, et al., 1972, pp. 138-139).

One of the most important generalizations that emerges from systematic comparisons of programs and experiments with positive results and those with

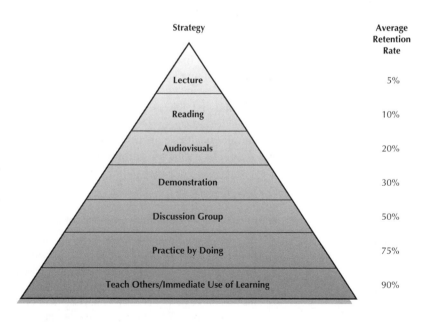

Figure 3-4
Learning Retention According to Strategy. From M. Cohen. (1991). *A comprehensive approach to effective staff development: Essential components.* Presented at Education Development Center, meeting for Comprehensive School Health Education Training Centers. Cambridge, MA. Adapted with permission.

Strategy	Average Retention Rate
Lecture	5%
Reading	10%
Audiovisuals	20%
Demonstration	30%
Discussion Group	50%
Practice by Doing	75%
Teach Others/Immediate Use of Learning	90%

negative findings (no effect) is that the greater the variety in educational methods used, the more likely the program or experiment will show positive results. This generalization applies both with individuals and with populations. At the individual level, variety in education methods apparently helps to surround the learner with communications appealing to different senses and modes of learning that are mutually supportive (Green, 1976, p. iv)

Cohen (1991) believes that learning is related to the method selected as shown by the pyramid in Figure 3-4. The more active and involved the learner becomes, the more likely he or she will learn. Hence, the least effective strategy is simple lecture, with no learner activity, and the most effective involves the learner in teaching others and thus immediately applying what has been learned to the fullest extent.

Packaging the Total Intervention Strategy

How your methods fit together to form your intervention package is important in achieving your objectives. Are the methods complementary and reinforcing? Do the methods break up the time together so that you can more easily hold the attention of your intended audience? Have you appealed to different styles of learning? Have you applied as many educational principles as possible, such as reinforcement, repetition, and practice?

Common Mistakes in Method Selection

Beware of the following common mistakes in method selection.

1. Selecting a method that you personally like but that is not the best method for achieving your stated objectives.
2. Underestimating the time required to conduct a method properly.
3. Overestimating the time required to conduct a method properly.
4. Selecting an inappropriate method for the characteristics of the group.
5. Not reinforcing key points.

Principles of Engagement

The Centers for Disease Control and Prevention have developed a set of principles of engagement to promote quality community involvement in community health projects. These principles, presented in Table 3-1, can and should be applied to community health programs.

Table 3-1
Principles of Community Engagement

Before Starting a Community Engagement Effort . . .

1. Be clear about the purposes or goals of the engagement effort, and the populations and/or communities you want to engage.

2. Become knowledgeable about the community in terms of its economic conditions, political structures, norms and values, demographic trends, history, and experience with engagement efforts. Learn about the community's perceptions of those initiating the engagement activities.

For Engagement to Occur, It Is Necessary to . . .

3. Go into the community, establish relationships, build trust, work with the formal and informal leadership, and seek commitment from community organizations and leaders to create processes for mobilizing the community.

4. Remember and accept that community self-determination is the responsibility and right of all people who comprise a community. No external entity should assume it can bestow to a community the power to act in its own self-interest.

For Engagement to Succeed . . .

5. Partnering with the community is necessary to create change and improve health.

6. All aspects of community engagement must recognize and respect community diversity. Awareness of the various cultures of a community and other factors of diversity must be paramount in designing and implementing community engagement approaches.

7. Community engagement can only be sustained by identifying and mobilizing community assets, and by developing capacities and resources for community health decisions and action.

8. An engaging organization or individual change agent must be prepared to release control of actions or interventions to the community, and be flexible enough to meet the changing needs of the community.

9. Community collaboration requires long-term commitment by the engaging organization and its partners.

Source: U.S. Department of Health and Human Services (1997). Principles of Community Engagement. CDC/ATSDR Committee on Community Engagement. Atlanta, GA: U.S. Public Health Service.

 For more information and tools related to this chapter visit www.jbpub.com/healtheducation.

EXERCISES

1. Select one of the theories/models or elements of a theory/model described in this chapter and apply it (them) to a specific health intervention. For example, consider HIV education for a community youth group. You could apply the health belief model as a whole, elements of the health belief model, or maybe you want to focus on self-efficacy of condom use. State the health issue on which you will focus, select the theory/model/element, and then briefly outline an intervention, describing the methods that will operationalize the theory.

2. One of the educational principles related to motivating the learner states: *Fear and punishment have uncertain effects upon learning. They may facilitate or hinder learning.* You are conducting a workshop for middle-aged women on preventing cervical cancer. Briefly describe how this educational principle could have an impact on your workshop.

3. One of the educational principles related to the needs and abilities of the learner states: *The lower the educational level, the greater is reliance on oral or picture media.* You are conducting a workshop for 10-year-old children on safety in the home. Briefly describe how this educational principle could have an impact on your presentation, and give concrete examples of how you would incorporate this principle.

4. You are planning to conduct a series of community workshops on weight control. List four *characteristics of the learner* that should be considered in planning, and briefly describe why each is important.

5. Interview a health educator regarding what models and theories he or she uses in the practice of health education.

CASE STUDIES REVISITED

Case Study Revisited: John

John has much to learn about workshop conduct and method selection. John sent out 100 invitations . . . how many people should he expect to attend? If health educators get a 50 percent attendance rate from invitations, they are usually thrilled! Is it likely that low-income individuals will be willing or even able to travel to an upscale hotel outside their community? John's attendance might have improved had he conducted the workshop at a site in the target community. Because of a personal interest in a strategy, John may have selected an inappropriate method for this population. Did he consult local community leaders about his presentation and discuss the most effective approaches he could utilize? Probably not. When health educators work with groups that they are unfamiliar with, it is essential that research or consultation of some type be performed in order to optimize effective strategy selection. (See page 47 and Chapters 8 and 9.)

Case Study Revisited: Marcel

Marcel deserves a good deal of credit for being intuitive about the concerns of the group. It takes courage to realize that the presentation is not going as planned and then making the conscious decision to stop and reorganize the material. It is probably unrealistic to expect Marcel to whip out a health locus of control instrument that he conveniently had in his back pocket! However, the important point being made is that health theory plays an important role in determining the most effective ways of delivering health messages and information. When preparing presentations, such theories should be considered and elements of relevant models utilized to increase the effectiveness of the intervention. If nothing else, this approach forces the presenter to consider the very specific intent of the presentation and facilitates the development of behavioral objectives. (See page 51.)

Case Study Revisited: Nancy

Like Marcel in the previous case study, Nancy should receive credit for recognizing a problem and then confronting the issue with the intent to make a program more effective. In some instances the easiest way to deal with a problem is to ignore it . . . ultimately ignoring the fact that an intervention might have become totally ineffective. Nancy identified a problem and devised a strategy to alleviate her difficulties. Health educators working in the area of addictions should be aware that there exists in the field of prevention and treatment a belief by some that only individuals who have experienced addiction themselves can fully relate to the problem. Although this philosophy is not necessarily held by the majority, this issue needs to be considered by health educators when planning interventions of this nature. Nancy's experience is not an unusual one. (See page 53.)

Case Study Revisited: Don

Don did a good job of taking into account the important elements of self-efficacy and behavioral intent when considering the impact of his workshop. It would have been much easier to simply go through the mechanics of teaching CPR and at the conclusion of the workshop make the assumption that most individuals were sufficiently trained. Utilizing a simulation helped participants gauge their individual skill levels and the pretest/posttest questionnaires allowed Don to evaluate an often-ignored element of CPR training: are people likely to use their training in a real-life situation? (See page 53.)

Case Study Revisited: Jessica

Jessica's approach is one that is based on health education theory and is an approach that has become commonplace in drug education today. The emphasis, particularly in schools, is to spend less time on didactic, factual learning and more time on developing practical skills to avoid becoming involved in drug abuse. Elements of health education models such as self-efficacy, locus of control, and behavioral intent are all utilized in an attempt to equip the individual to combat risky health behavior. Jessica's method selection allows participants to experience and develop their own skills on a personal level rather than simply hearing facts about drugs in an impersonal, abstract manner. (See page 57.)

Case Study Revisited: Bill

Bill is another good health educator who is aware enough to realize when his approach might need an adjustment to make a program more effective. In theoretical terms his students were demonstrating extremely low perceived susceptibility to HIV/AIDS. This lack of concern is endemic among adolescents, and Bill was perceptive enough to know that he needed to change his plans. Bill's strategy was to show a dramatic film about AIDS and bring in a speaker who was HIV positive. Both methods had two key elements in common . . . the major character in the film and the guest speaker were very close in age to Bill's students and both had contracted HIV through heterosexual sex—something Bill's students had failed to take seriously before exposure to these strategies. Bill successfully applied his knowledge of health education theory to enhance his program delivery. (See page 62.)

Case Study Revisited: James

James obviously had not made a good match between his strategy selection and learner characteristics. In addition, using a revealing icebreaker exercise in a short, once-only workshop where trust could never be established was an error and not a good use of limited contact time. This example points to the necessity of thoroughly examining all the elements of learner characteristics and presentation conditions (group size, contact time) before proceeding with an intervention. Too many health educators have had to learn the hard way . . . through painful experience. (See page 68.)

SUMMARY

Selecting the appropriate educational intervention is vital to achieving your objectives.

1. The selection of a method should always take into account the objectives to be achieved.

2. Some other important considerations are
Educational principles
Theory and model application
Educational domain
Characteristics of the.learner

Group size
Contact time
Budget
Resources/site/environment
Characteristics of the educational provider
Cultural appropriateness
Using a variety of methods
Packaging the total intervention strategy

3. Principles of community engagement can greatly enhance the likelihood of success.

REFERENCES

Ajzen, I., & Fishbein, M. (1973). Attitudinal and normative variables as predictors of specific behaviors. *Journal of Personality and Social Psychology, 27,* 41–57.

Ajzen, I., & Fishbein, M. (1980). *Understanding Attitudes and Predicting Social Behavior.* Englewood Cliffs, NJ: Prentice-Hall.

American Association for Health Education, National Commission for Health Education Credentialing, I., & Education, S. f. P. H. (1999). *A Competency-Based Framework for Graduate-Level Health Educators.* Allentown, PA: The National Commission for Health Education Credentialing, Inc., American Association for Health Education, and the Society for Public Health Education.

Bandura, A. (1977). Self-efficacy: Toward a unifying theory of behavioral change. *Psychological Review, 84,* 191.

Bandura, A. (1977). *Social Learning Theory.* Englewood Cliffs, NJ: Prentice-Hall.

Bandura, A. (1986). The explanatory and predictive scope of self-efficacy theory. *Journal of Social and Clinical Psychology, 4,* 359–373.

Bardsley, P., & Beckman, L. (1988). The health belief model and entry into alcoholism treatment. *International Journal of the Addictions, 23,* 19–28.

Becker, M. (Ed.). (1974). *The Health Belief Model and Personal Health Behavior.* Thoroughfare, NJ: Slack.

Becker, M., & Janz, N. (1985). The health belief model applied to understanding diabetes regimen compliance. *Diabetes Educator, 11,* 41–47.

Casey, T.A., Kingery, P.M., Bowden, R.G., & Corbett, B.S. (1993). An investigation of the factor structure of the Multidimensional Health Locus of Control scales in a Health Promotion Program. *Educational and Psychological Measurement, 53,* 491–498.

Champion, V. (1985). Use of the health belief model in determining frequency of breast self-examination. *Research in Nursing and Health, 8,* 373–379.

Clark, N.M., & Dodge, J.A. (1999). Exploring self-efficacy as a predictor of disease management. *Health Education & Behavior, 26* (1), 72–89.

Cornish, E. (1980). Toward a philosophy of futurism. *Health Education, 11,* 10–12.

Creswell, W.H. (1984). Health education issues. In L. Rubinson & W. F. Alles (Eds.), *Health Education: Foundations for the Future.* St. Louis: Times Mirror/Mosby.

Cummings, K.M., Becker, M.H., & Maile, M.C. (1980). Bringing the models together: An empirical approach to combining variables used to explain health outcomes. *Journal of Behavioral Medicine, 3,* 123–145.

Dalkey, N., & Helmer, O. (1963). An experimental application of the Delphi method to the use of experts. *Management Science, 9,* 458.

Dennison, D. (1977). Activated health education. *Health Education, 8,* 24–25.

Dennison, D. (1984). Activated health education: The development and refinement of an intervention model. *Health Values, 8,* 18–24.

Dennison, D., Frauenheim, K.A., & Isu, L. (1983). The DINE microcomputer program: An innovative curricular approach. *Health Education, 14.*

Dennison, D., Prevet, T., & Affleck, M. (1980). *Alcohol and Behavior: An Activated Health Education Approach.* St. Louis: C.V. Mosby.

DiBlasio, F.A. (1986). Drinking adolescents on the roads. *Journal of Youth and Adolescence, 15,* 173–189.

DiClemente, C., Prochaska, J.O., Fairhurst, C., Velicer, W., Velasques, M., & Rossi, J. (1991). The process of smoking cessation: An analysis of precontemplation, contemplation, and preparation stages of change. *Journal of Consulting Clinical Psychology, 59,* 295–304.

Donnermeyer, J.F., & Davis, R.R. (1998). Cumulative effects of prevention education on substance use among 11th grade students in Ohio. *Journal of School Health, 68*(No. 4), 151–157.

Eiser, J.R. (1985). Smoking: The social learning of addiction. *Journal of Social and Clinical Psychology, 3,* 357–446.

Fishbein, M. (Ed.). (1967). *Readings in Attitude Theory and Measurement.* New York: Wiley.

Fodor, J., & Dalis, G. (1974). *Health Instruction.* Philadelphia: Lea and Febiger.

Frazer, G.H., Kukulka, G.G., & Richardson, C.E. (1988). An assessment of professional opinion concerning critical research issues in health education. In J. H. Humphrey (Ed.), *Advances in Health Education: Current Research* (Vol. 1). New York: AMS Press.

Gilbert, G.G. (1981). *Teaching First Aid and Emergency Care.* Dubuque, IA: Kendall/Hunt.

Glanz, K., Lew, R.A., Song, V., & Cook, W.A. (1999). Factors associated with skin cancer prevention; Practices in multi-ethnic population. *Health Education, 26*(3), 344–359.

Glanz, K., Patterson R.E., Kristal, A.R., Feng, Z., Linnan, L., Heimendinger, J., & Hebert, J.R. (1998). Impact of work site health promotion on stage of dietary change: The working well trial. *Health Education and Behavior, 25*(4), 448–463.

Green, L. (1976). *Determining the Impact and Effectiveness of Health Education as it Relates to Federal Policy.* Washington, D.C.: Office of the Deputy Assistant Secretary for Planning and Evaluation/Health, HEW.

Green, L.W., & Iverson, D. (1982). School health education. *Annual Review of Public Health, 3,* 321–328.

Green, L.W., & Kreuter, M.W. (1990). Health promotion as a public health strategy for the 1990s, *Annual Review of Public Health* (Vol. 11). Palo Alto, CA: Annual Reviews, Inc.

Green, L.W., & Kreuter, M.W. (1991). *Health Promotion Planning: An Educational and Environmental Approach.* Mountain View, CA: Mayfield.

Green, L.W., Kreuter, M.W., Deeds, S.G., & Partridge, K.B. (1980). *Health Education Planning: A Diagnostic Approach.* Palo Alto, CA: Mayfield.

Green, L.W., Levine, D.M., & Deeds, S.G. (1975). Clinical trials of health education for hypertensive outpatients: Design and baseline data. *Preventive Medicine, 4,* 417–425.

Green, L.W., Levine, D.M., Wolle, J., & Deeds, S.G. (1979). Development of randomized patient education experiments with urban poor hypertensives. *Patient Education and Counseling, 1,* 106–111.

Grimley, D, Prochaska, J.O., Velicer, W.F., & Prochaska G. (1995). Contraception and condom use adaption and maintenance. A stage paradigm approach. *Health Education Quarterly, 22*(1), 20–35.

Haire-Joshu, D., Auslander, W.F., Houston, C.A., & Williams, J.H. (1999). Staging of Dietary Patterns Among African American Women. *Health Education & Behavior, 26*(1), 90–102.

Harrison, J.A., Mullen, P.D., & Green, L.W. (1992). A meta-analysis of studies of the Health Belief Model with adults. *Health Education Research* Mar 7(1):107–16.

Herold, E. (1983). The health belief model: Can it help us understand contraceptive use among adolescents? *Journal of School Health, 53,* 19–21.

Hester, N., & Macrina, D. (1985). The health belief model and the contraceptive behavior of college women: Implications for health education. *Journal of American College Health, 33,* 245–252.

Jessor, R., & Jessor, S. (1977). *Problem Behavior and Psychosocial Development: A Longitudinal Study of Youth.* New York: Academic.

Jillson, I.A. (1985). The national drug abuse policy delphi: Progress report and findings to date. In L. A. Turoff (Ed.), *Delphi Method: Techniques and Applications*. Reading, MA: Addison-Wesley.

Kelly, G., Mamon, J., & Scott, J. (1987). Utility of the health belief model in examining medication compliance among psychiatric outpatients. *Social Science Medicine, 25*, 1205–1211.

Kerlinger, F.N. (1973). *Foundations of Behavioral Research*. New York: Holt, Rinehart, and Winston.

Kime, R., Schlaadt, R., & Tritsch, L. (1977). *Health Instruction: An Action Approach*. Englewood Cliffs, NJ: Prentice-Hall.

King, K., Price, J.H., Tellojahann, S.K., & Wahl, J. (1999). High school teachers' perceived self-efficacy in identifying students at risk for suicide. *Journal of School Health, 69*(5), 202–207.

Kirscht, J. (1974). The health belief model and illness behavior. In M. Becker (Ed.), *The Health Belief Model and Personal Health Behavior*. Thoroughfare, NJ: Slack.

Kuhn, J. (1970). *The Structure of Scientific Revolutions*. Chicago: University of Chicago Press.

Levenson, H. (1974). Activism and powerful others: Distinction within the concept of internal-external control. *Journal of Personality Assessment, 38*, 377–383.

Levine, D.M., Green, L.W., Deeds, S.G., Smith, C., Chwalow, A.J., & Finlay, J. (1979). Health education for hypertensive patients. *Journal of the American Medical Association, 241*, 1700–1703.

Levine, D.M., Morisky, D.E., Bone, L.R., Lewis, C., Ward, K.B., & Green, L.W. (1982). Data-based planning for educational interventions through hypertension control programs for urban and rural populations in Maryland. *Public Health Reports, 97*, 107–112.

Maiman, L., & Becker, M. (1974). The health belief model: Origins and correlates in psychological theory. In M. Becker (Ed.), *The Health Belief Model and Personal Health Behavior*. Thoroughfare, NJ: Slack.

McGuire, W. (1981). Behavioral medicine, public health and communication theories. *Health Education, 12*, 8–13.

Mullen, P., & Iverson, D. (1982). Qualitative methods for evaluative research in health education programs. *Health Education, 13*, 11–18.

Oberteuffer, D., et al. (1972). *School Health Education*. New York: Harper and Row.

Parcel, G., & Meyer, M.P. (1978). Development of an instrument to measure children's health locus of control. *Health Education Monographs, 6*, 149–159.

Parcel, G., Nader, P.R., & Rogers, P.J. (1980). Health locus of control and health values: Implications for school health education. *Health Values, 4*, 32–37.

Parcel, G.S. (1984). Theoretical models for application in school health education research. *Special combined issue of Journal of School Health 54, 39–49 and Health Education 15*, 39–49.

Prochaska, J.O. (1979). *Systems of Psychotherapy: A Transtheoretical Analysis*. Homewood, IL: Dorsey Press.

Prochaska, J.O., Norcross, J., Fowler, J., Follick, M., & Abrams, D. (1992). Attendance and outcome in a worksite weight control program: Processes and stages of change as process and predictor variables. *Addictive Behavior, 17*, 35–45.

Prochaska, J.O., Redding, C.A., Harlow, L.L., Rossi, J.S., & Velicer, W.F. (1994). The transtheoretical model of change and HIV prevention: A review. *Health Education Quarterly, 24*(4), 471–486.

Rakowski W., Dube, C., Marcus B., Prochaska, J., Velicer W., & Abrams, D. (1992). Assessing elements of women's decisions about mammography. *Health Psychology, 11*, 111–118.

Rosenstock, I. (1974). Historical origins of the health belief model. In M. Becker (Ed.), *The Health Belief Model and Personal Health Behavior*. Thoroughfare, NJ: Slack.

Rosenstock, I.M., Stretcher, V.J., & Becker, M. (1988). Social Learning Theory and the Health Belief Model. *Health Education Quarterly, 15*, 175–183.

Rotter, J.B. (1954). *Social Learning and Clinical Psychology*. Englewood Cliffs, NJ: Prentice-Hall.

Rubinson, L., & Alles, W.F. (1984). *Health Education: Foundations for the Future*. Prospect Heights, IL: Waveland.

Rubinson, L., & Baillie, L. (1981). Planning school-based sexuality programs utilizing the PRECEDE model. *Journal of School Health, 51*, 282–287.

Scaffa, M. (1992). *The Development of a Comprehensive Theory in Health Education: A Feasibility Study*. Unpublished doctoral dissertation, University of Maryland.

Shireffs, J.A. (1984). The nature and meaning of health education. In L. Rubinson & W.F. Alles (Eds.), *Health Education: Foundations for the Future*. St. Louis: Times Mirror/Mosby.

Stainbrook, G., & Green, L.W. (1982). Behavior and behaviorism in health education. *Health Education, 13,* 14–19.

Strauss, A., & Corbin, J. (1990). *Basics of Qualitative Research: Grounded Theory Procedures and Techniques.* London: Sage.

Suggested School Health Policies (5th ed.) (1966). NEA-AMA Committee.

Tarabokia, J.R. (1985). *Forecasts by Selected Professional Health Educators and Their Implications for Health Education: A Delphi Application.* Unpublished doctoral dissertation, Brigham Young University.

Toohey, J.V., & Shireffs, J.H. (1980). Future trends in health education. *Health Education, 11,* 15–17.

Travis, R. (1976). The delphi technique: A tool for community health educators. *Health Education, 7,* 11–13.

U.S. Department of Health and Human Services (1997). Principles of Community Engagement.

CDC/ATSDR Committee on Community Engagement. Atlanta, GA: U.S. Public Health Service.

Wallston, K.A., & Wallston, B.S. (1978). Preface to health locus of control. *Health Education Monographs, 6,* 101–105.

Wallston, K.A., Wallston, B.S., & DeVillis, R. (1978). Development of the multidimensional health locus of control scales. *Health Education Monographs, 6,* 160–170.

Wallston, K.A., Wallston, B.S., Kaplan, G.D., & Maides, S.A. (1976). Development and validation of the health locus of control scale. *Journal of Consulting and Clinical Psychology, 44,* 580–585.

Wodarski, J. (1987). Evaluating a social learning approach to teaching adolescents about alcohol and driving: A multiple variable evaluation. *Journal of Social Science Research, 10,* 121–144.

Wolfgang, J., & Dennison, D. (1981). The effects of a heart health education workshop. *Journal of School Health, 51,* 356–359.

Presentation and Unit Plan Development

Entry-Level and Graduate-Level Health Educator Competencies Addressed In This Chapter

Responsibility III:	Implementing Health Education Programs
Competency A:	Exhibit competence in carrying out planned educational programs.
Competency B:	Infer enabling objectives as needed to implement instructional program in specified settings.
Competency C:	Select methods and media best suited to implement program plans for specific learners.
Responsibility IV:	Evaluating Effectiveness of Health Education Programs
Competency A:	Develop plans to assess achievement of program objectives.
Competency B:	Carry out evaluation plans.
Competency C:	Interpret results of program evaluation.
Competency D:	Infer implications from findings for future program planning.
Responsibility V:	Coordinating Provision of Health Education Services
Competency D:	Organize inservice training programs for teachers, volunteers, and other interested personnel.

Note: the competencies listed above, which are addressed in this chapter, are considered to be both entry-level and graduate-level competencies by the National Commission for Health Education Credentialing, Inc. They are taken from *A Framework for the Development of Competency Based Curricula for Entry Level Health Educators* by the

Method Selection in Health Education

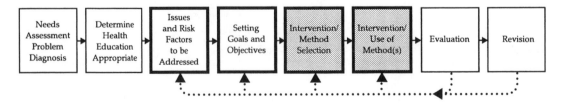

Heavy-bordered boxes indicate subjects addressed in this text; shaded boxes indicate subjects(s) of current chapter.

National Task Force for the Preparation and Practice of Health Education, 1985; and *A Competency-based Framework for Graduate Level Health Educators* by the National Task Force for the Preparation and Practice of Health Education, 1999.

This chapter will discuss the components of lesson/presentation plans and unit plans in curriculum development.

OBJECTIVES   After studying the chapter the reader should be able to

- Develop an appropriate lesson/presentation plan for a given setting.
- Construct a unit of instruction for a given setting and population.
- Describe the strengths and weaknesses of using lesson/presentation plans and unit plans for instructional organization.

KEY ISSUES   Preparing a presentation/lesson plan

Preparing a unit plan

Strengths and weaknesses of lesson/presentation plans and unit plans

Lesson/Presentation Plans

Curriculum development involves much more than the design of lesson/presentation plans and unit plans. However, the development of these types of plans is the foundation of a comprehensive curriculum. Comprehensive curriculum development is outside the parameters of this text, and there are many outstanding books dedicated to the topic. This text focuses on just the plans, the starting point of curriculum development.

Preparing properly for a presentation requires careful organization. You must take into account all the issues used to select or write your objectives and carefully review what objectives are appropriate for your workshop, presentation, or class. **Lesson/presentation plans** should be written in a format that any health educator could use, given some preparation time, and present the materials well. If properly constructed, the presentation should capture the essence of what the author intended no matter who is the user. Figure 4-1 shows a recommended format.

There are many suggested formats for lesson/presentation plans. Check with your agency or school to see if there is a required or recommended format. All suggested formats include the basic components of background information, introduction, objectives, developmental section (body or core), conclusion/culmination and evaluation. It is also recommended that you try to anticipate problems by preparing an alternative plan (often referred to as **Plan B**).

LESSON/PRESENTATION PLAN FORMAT

Name: _____

Grade Level/Comm. Setting: _____

Date: _____ Topic/Unit: _____

Lesson Title: _____

Age of Target Population: _____ Demographics: _____

Objectives (Consider cognitive, affective, and psychomotor):
_____
_____
_____

Introduction (a statement of what you will be doing and why):
_____
_____
_____

Developmental Section (this section may be several pages):

Content Outline	Method/Strategy	Estimated Time Needed	Materials Needed
	Name Game	20 minutes	None
I. XXXX 　A. XXX 　B. XXX 　C. XXXXX			
II. XXXXXXXXXXX 　A. XXXX 　B. XXXXX 　C. XX 　　1. XXXXXXXXXXXXXXXXX 　　　XXXXXXXXXXXXXXXX 　　2. XXXXXXXXXX 　　3. XXXXXXXXXXXXXXXX	Lecture/ Discussion	15 minutes	Overhead Projector
III. XXXXXXXXXXX 　A. XXXXX 　B. XXXX 　　1. XXXXXXXXXXXXXXX 　　2. XXXXXX 　　3. XXXXXXXXXXXXX 　　4. XXXXXXX 　　5. XXX	Guided Imagery—see attachment	30 minutes	Tape Recorder Tape of Sounds Script—see attachment
XX. XXXXXX 　A. XXXXXXXXXX 　B. XXXXX 　　1. XXXXXXXXX 　　2. XXXXX	Game Bingo— see attached for rules	20 minutes	Bingo Cards Pencils Questions Prizes

Culmination (Summary of the key points this lesson and what will happen next):
_____
_____

Anticipated problems and possible solutions (plan B):
_____
_____
_____

Evaluation (How will you determine if you have been successful):
_____
_____
_____

Figure 4-1 Sample Lesson/presentation Plans.

Case Study: Shane

Shane is ill and asks a colleague at his agency to take over for the day. On his agenda is a presentation to students at Hillsboro Public High School regarding HIV infections. Mary, the colleague asked to fill in, is well versed in HIV and AIDS issues, having formerly worked for the State Public Health Epidemiology Division. Mary can find only brief notes so she grabs some slides on Kaposi's sarcoma and other diseases associated with AIDS and heads to the high school. She provides a very graphic presentation on sexual behaviors, including anal intercourse, and, of course, a very visual show on the effects of the diseases. Shane is surprised some days later when he is reprimanded for the presentation and told he is no longer welcomed at the high school. (See Case Studies Revisited page 102.)

Background

The initial section, which may be thought of as the background for the plan, includes basic information that will assist in determining strategy selection: the setting for the presentation (community or school), the presentation topic, the approximate number of participants, and as much demographic information about the participants as can be obtained (age, ethnicity, socioeconomic status, etc.)

Introduction

The introduction is where you capture the interest of the target audience. Give a welcome, and provide reasons for covering the information. Include some local statistics, if appropriate, and logical statements regarding the issues addressed that will get the group enthusiastic about the topic.

Objectives

The objectives are the specific objectives you hope to achieve with this lesson/presentation. They must be stated in specific terms (see Chapter 2). You may have only one objective, or you may have several. However, contact time must be taken into account, since you cannot achieve some objec-

Your presentation will go smoothly and will hold your audience's interest if you have thoroughly researched the demographics of your participants.

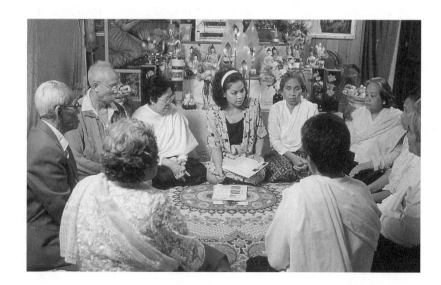

tives in a short time frame. You must be realistic in what you set out to achieve. You might be able to achieve several cognitive objectives in a short time or one or two psychomotor objectives but generally not both. It is important to review educational principles and remember some important issues such as the need to repeat key points and the need to use multiple approaches to accommodate differences in learning styles.

Developmental Section The developmental section is the core of the lesson plan and includes all strategies and the appropriate information to carry them out. Sufficient information must be supplied in outline or text format so *any health educator, given some preparation time, could conduct the lesson or presentation.* Time estimates and needed materials should be included. This section is often multiple pages. All the information needed for any health educator to conduct the lesson should be included. Content materials or directions might be attached, especially if photocopying materials is easier than rewriting the information.

Conclusion The conclusion/culmination is the ending of the lesson/presentation and should include a summary of the key issues covered (reinforcement) and directions for the next meeting. If this is a one-time workshop or the final workshop of a series, it should include a thorough review of key points and an opportunity for feedback and questions. This would also be the time to administer an evaluation questionnaire.

Anticipated Problems Obviously, we cannot anticipate every problem that might occur when making a presentation, but we can anticipate some common ones and plan to deal with them. It is important that we learn to do this as well as possible. Good planning will increase our self-confidence, allowing us to focus on the lesson. We should consider the possibility of audiovisual failures or a group's unwillingness to participate, for example, and develop an alternate plan for such events.

Some common problems often encountered in lesson/presentation preparation include the following:

1. Not enough material (people often speak faster when nervous, or anticipated group discussion does not materialize).
2. Methods inappropriate for group (group unwilling to participate).
3. Little variety in methods employed (group acts bored and restless).
4. No evaluation or feedback system built in (no way to determine value or make improvements).

Evaluation The evaluation is an integral part of any lesson plan. If our objectives are well stated and achievable, evaluation should be straightforward. Short time frames influence evaluation in that we must often use the majority of time for the intervention. However, it is always important that we conduct as much evaluation as possible. Contact time will have a major impact on evaluation time. If this is a one-time, one-hour presentation, a simple anonymous evaluation form or even a few oral questions may be all that is necessary. If this is the final presentation in a series, then a much more elaborate assessment tied to your objectives is in order. The type of evaluation techniques employed will be a function of the objectives, available time, type of group, and resources. Consider outcome and process evaluation techniques. As a general rule, 15 percent of time should be spent on evaluation.

Fundamental Principles

Presenting successfully requires the same skills as teaching successfully; it is simply the setting that is different. Why do we assume that the community health educator who has to plan five one-hour workshops on drug prevention will not have to follow the same sound principles of planning and methods delivery as the teacher who has to prepare a five-lesson unit also on drug prevention? Yes, the rules and constraints in the school classroom might influence the teacher's planning, but the fundamental principles remain the same in the school and community settings.

To be an effective health educator, particularly at the entry level, good presentation skills are essential. In order to optimize presentation skills, thoughtful planning must occur at both the individual lesson/presentation level and at the series or unit level. Anyone who has sat through a stunningly boring presentation in the classroom or in the community should consider how much time the presenter spent on thoughtful planning and method selection . . . probably very little! This important phase of health educator preparation involves all people in this field, regardless of the setting.

Case Study: Michael

Michael, a young, enthusiastic health educator, had recently been hired by the local health department. His first assignment was to plan and implement a series of five one-hour workshops on general health issues for a senior citizens' community group. In college Michael had taken a methods and materials course, but he had put little effort into studying the construction of lesson/presentation planning or unit development. He had argued that only school health majors needed that knowledge, and the last thing that Michael wanted was to be a teacher! Michael asked all the right initial questions related to group size, demographic background, location, time, available equipment and so on. He then jotted down a few notes for the first meeting, grabbed an available videotape, arranged for the use of a VCR, and was on his way to the first workshop. Michael's first presentation left a lot to be desired. He lectured far too long, boring many of the participants, and was unable to show the videotape on the VCR that the group had gone to great pains to borrow. When asked what the ensuing workshops would cover, Michael was unable to answer, mumbling something about covering whatever the group wanted. The following week only one of the group's members showed up, and eventually the series of workshops was canceled.

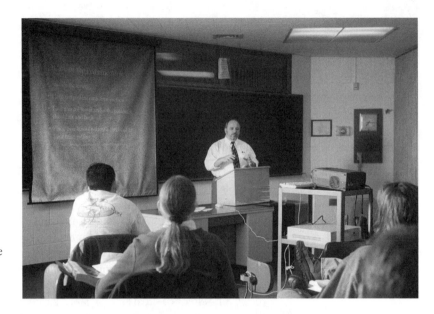

A thoughtful and prepared presentation style is the key to maintaining your audience's attention.

Not surprisingly, Michael was asked to meet with his supervisor! (See Case Studies Revisited page 102.)

Unit Plans

There are many ways to organize for instruction. Whenever you have more than a few hours of contact time with a target population group, you should consider organizing for instruction in a unified manner. We will use the term **unit plan** to describe an orderly self-contained collection of activities educationally designed to meet a set of objectives. Other terms are *curriculum plans, modules, and strands.* All such systems seek to organize materials so that they are more than the sum of their parts and have a high likelihood of achieving the stated objectives. They are meant to be more than a collection of lesson plans. As coordinated activities that build on one another, it is hoped they will be able to influence even challenging issues such as attitudes or behaviors.

Depending on the time and other resources available, the unit plan can be a powerful tool if implemented as constructed. But there must be a significant amount of contact time allowed—usually more than five hours—and a fairly consistent participating group. A lesson/presentation plan might be more appropriate than a unit plan if you are working with a group of people for only a short period of time. Whether you are planning a major three-day community workshop or 20 hours of classroom contact time in a school setting, you need to provide for have a significant amount of contact time for your intervention so that you can build one component onto another.

Reinventing the Wheel

Unit plan construction is a challenging endeavor. Although good units already exist for a wide variety of health topics, the challenge is finding one that meets your particular objectives. Federal, local, and state governments have supported the development of many curriculum projects that include multiple units. Many of the voluntary agencies have curriculum materials designed to meet their health objectives, which are sometimes available free or at low cost. Others are more extensive and are sold by vendors, sometimes at considerable cost. If you are working on a curriculum development project, it is most helpful to review what is available, as without such a review you are committing the sin of reinventing the wheel. Try contacting local health educators for people who can help you. Professional organizations can also put you in touch with good contacts. Even if you decide your project or population group is distinctive enough that it requires a new unit, it is most helpful to review how others have approached the issues and objectives.

Sources include professional organizations as well as vendors. Working with university health educators is a good way to locate materials and Internet sites. Any national professional health meeting is replete with vendors showing their curriculum projects and related materials. Many vendors will sell copies of their curriculum guides or complete packages which include all needed materials, such as videotapes, and some will develop custom units for you. Costs often are high, but you may acquire materials that are far better than you could develop on your own. If you wish to use part of the materials, you will need to negotiate permission from the vendor and generally a fee will be required.

Noteworthy Use of Your Tax Dollars

The federal government has supported the development of many curriculum projects over the years. These often cost taxpayers millions of dollars. Because of budget cuts and changing priorities, many of the projects have ended up in closets and are rarely used. Today most government agencies encourage vendors to take these projects and use them. The vendors turn them into a marketable products and copyright the materials, sometimes making good profits. In one way this seems like a ripoff of public funds, but without such practice these good materials might well end up gathering dust. If you can find a government copy, you can use the materials without violating any copyright law.

Unit Construction Guidelines

The components of a unit plan are as follows:

1. Overview
2. Statement of purpose
3. Long-range goals, general objectives, or key concepts
4. Behavioral objectives

5. Outline of content
6. Methods/strategies/learning opportunities
7. List of materials
8. Evaluation activities
9. List of available resources and materials
10. Block plan

*The greatest medications
are those swallowed by
the mind.*
—Mohan Singh

Each will be discussed in detail.

Overview

Begin with an overview, a paragraph or two describing the setting of where the unit will be offered. Include the ages of participants or grade level, number of meetings and duration, economic situation, and cultural environment. Identify the actual location(s) by name where the health education program will be conducted. Pertinent demographics should be included. (See Chapter 2 for information on needs assessment.)

Statement of Purpose

The *statement of purpose* is a description of why this content is part of the curriculum for this target population. Footnote any statistics or generalizations used to support the need for this unit. Write this section as if you were trying to convince an outsider of the need for this unit. Use statistics whenever possible to support the need for this specific target population.

Long-Range Goals, General Objectives, or Key Concepts

The very broad outcome intentions for the unit may be expressed as *long-range goals, general objectives, or key concepts.* These are optimal behaviors you hope to achieve and need not be easily measurable. (See Chapter 2.)

Behavioral Objectives

The *behavioral objectives* are stated in behavioral terms—that is, in cognitive, affective, and psychomotor terms—according to recognized authority or as covered by the instructor. Often your agency, hospital, or school will have a specific format. These are the specific objectives to be achieved and should include an indication of how they will be measured. (See Chapter 2.)

Outline of Content

An *outline* of the content to be presented should include all items. This detailed outline can be supplemented by an appendix with more detail or photocopies of the overheads to be used. The content in the outline should be presented in a logical order, though not necessarily in the order of presentation to be followed in the unit plan.

Methods/Strategies/ Learning Opportunities

Methods, strategies, and learning opportunities are the component of greatest importance. Selection of the best methods to reach one's objectives is essentially what this book is all about. Selection should take place after reviewing all practical options. Each method should be selected based on the objectives to be achieved, and each should be named and described in detail in such a way that it could be utilized by any health educator. All directions and rules should be included. Since these directions may be lengthy, the details might be on attached photocopies. Proper citations and permissions should be obtained. It is helpful to list after each method which specific objective(s) it is likely to achieve. This will help insure that all objectives are addressed and that methods are selected for the correct reasons.

List of Materials

Included should be a complete *list of materials* needed by the health educator (e.g., overhead projector) and those needed by each participant (e.g., paper). In many settings you cannot count on the participants arriving with anything, so it is necessary to provide all that is needed. Many an activity has been ruined by three participants sharing a pencil.

Evaluation Activities

Evaluation activities are based on your stated objectives. For example, in a community setting you might use anonymous self-assessments. In a school setting you might include five quizzes, of ten multiple-choice questions each, and one final, an essay variety worth 40 percent, and so on. Include activities to measure *knowledge*, *attitudes*, and *behavior*. Use a variety of assessment techniques appropriate for the target population. Be certain to include *teacher/facilitator evaluation* activities for the assessment of the instructor.

List of Available Resources and Materials

A *list of resources and materials* should include only those materials (books, articles, films) known to be of good quality and availability. Include complete titles, costs, and the Internet site or phone number at which prices and orders can be obtained.

Block Plan

The term **block plan** comes from the days when teachers would divide the day into "blocks" of time. This item is a breakdown of your suggested sequence, specifying the amount of time to be spent on each activity. Since learning opportunities are explained in detail elsewhere, they need only be listed here. Give consideration to the proper sequence for your material.

Unit Plan Samples

Unit plans can be and often are, hundreds of pages. The following samples are only representative of the type of information to be included and are incomplete for even a short unit plan. It is suggested that the reader review complete unit plans developed by professionals as well.

Sample Overview (Well-Baby Program)

The unit plan for a Well-Baby Program is targeting pregnant women who have applied for the "HELP NOW" program of King Sam County of Anystate. The program will accept the first 50 women who sign up. Based on county statistics, it is estimated that the group will range in age from 13 to 40, with the majority of participants being under 20 years of age. Most will be English speaking, with approximately two thirds reading at above a fifth grade level. Approximately half are expected to be African American and the

Let the health educator be as a coconut floating upon tropic seas and letting down roots on a foreign strand, that others may harvest their own nuts.
—Mohan Singh

other half white. Group size will be approximately 25, and participants will self-select their group according to their schedule. Only a small number of participants are employed, and the site is in the community, so transportation is not expected to be a problem. Day care, however, is an issue, since 50 percent of the participants have one or more children and less than 25 percent have a spouse or partner living with them.

This overview section will generally be less than one page and lays out the estimated demographics of the group.

Sample Statement of Purpose (Drug Prevention Program)

The unit for a Drug Prevention Program was developed because of an identified need in the community. The program is modeled on one that has proved to be successful in other communities similar to "Anytown," USA, which has shown rather dramatic increases in drug use by school-age children. According to the Anytown Department of Health annual survey, the number of students using marijuana was as follows:

	1990	1995	2000
4th Grade	2%	6%	9%
6th Grade	3%	8%	9%
8th Grade	11%	13%	16%
11th Grade	14%	14%	18%
12th Grade	13%	16%	27%

Cocaine use has shown a similar trend as follows:

	1990	1995	2000
4th Grade	1%	2%	3%
6th Grade	1%	3%	3%
8th Grade	2%	5%	8%
11th Grade	1%	7%	10%
12th Grade	2%	8%	14%

Alcohol use has remained a serious problem:

	1990	1995	2000
4th Grade	11%	12%	13%
6th Grade	11%	13%	13%
8th Grade	22%	25%	38%
11th Grade	21%	27%	40%
12th Grade	32%	48%	64%

State studies indicate a strong relationship between the use of these drugs and the increase in violence, unwanted pregnancies, AIDS, and low school performance. Studies show that 90 percent of cases of unprotected intercourse occurred during the use of drugs, including alcohol, by both males and females. Last year three seniors scheduled to graduate died in an alcohol-related auto accident three weeks before commencement. This unit is needed in our schools and should be implemented as part of our comprehensive school health education program.

All statistics in the statement of purpose should be referenced and be as recent as available.

Local statistics should be used when appropriate. The U.S. Health Goals for the Year 2010 are often helpful, as are local newspaper reports.

Sample Goals (Child Abuse Prevention) Goals for a Child Abuse Prevention Program are as follows:

1. Participants will acquire a set of workable and practical stress management techniques.
2. Participants will develop good parenting skills.
3. Participants will develop efficacy in the presented parenting skills.

Three or four general goals are usually adequate to express the general nature of a program unless it is a very long unit. Many units are 10 hours or less in total contact time. Schools often have longer units that might average 20 contact hours each.

Sample Objectives (Stress Management) Objectives for a Stress Management Program are as follows:

Cognitive 1. Participants will be able to identify personal sources of stress according to the guidelines presented in the program.
2. Participants will be able to define stress, eustress, and stress management according to the handouts provided.

Affective 1. Participants will show a willingness to learn more about stress management by voluntarily signing up for future programs.
2. Participants will show an increase in self-efficacy according to their self-ratings of utilization of presented stress management techniques.

Psychomotor 1. Participants will be able to demonstrate Jacobson progressive relaxation as shown in class.
2. Participants will be able to demonstrate the Jones breathing techniques as presented in class meeting 4.

The number of objectives will depend largely on the contact time and resources available. The number is really not important. The important consideration is that they be appropriate, achievable, and clearly stated. Most units of 20 hours or more have 15 or 20 objectives.

Sample Outline (Nutrition)

The outline for a Nutrition Program is as follows:

I. Dietary Guidelines for Americans
   A. Recommendations to help people maintain good health and/or improve it.
   B. A good diet is based on variety and moderation.
   C. Moderation means not eating large amounts of foods high in fat (saturated fatty acids and cholesterol).
   D. A risk factor is a condition that may increase the chance that something (usually negative) might be experienced by someone.
   E. For some people, certain types of diets are risk factors for chronic health conditions, such as heart disease, cancer, and high blood pressure.
   F. The Seven Dietary Guidelines
      (1) Eat a variety of foods.
         (a) No one food can supply all the essential nutrients needed for maintaining good health.
         (b) Should include foods from a variety of food groups.
         (c) Creates a balanced diet.
      (2) Maintain desirable weight.
         (a) Desirable weight will vary according to many factors such as age, health, gender, and so on.
         (b) Avoid sudden, potentially dangerous, aggressive dieting.
         (c) Calorie intake and expenditure must be balanced to maintain weight.
      (3) Avoid too much fat, saturated fat and cholesterol.
         (a) A small amount of fat is needed in your diet.
         (b) Risk of heart attack is increased by diets high in fat.
         (c) How foods are prepared will influence the fat content of food.
      (4) Eat foods with adequate starch and fiber.
         (a) Starch is a complex carbohydrate.
         (b) Carbohydrate-rich foods provide many essential nutrients and fiber.
         (c) Dietary fiber is plant material which humans cannot digest.
         (d) Grain products and starchy vegetables are good sources of starch.
         (e) Whole grain products, fruits, vegetables, nuts, and dry beans contain fiber.
         (f) How the food is prepared will affect the fiber content.
      (5) Avoid too much sugar.
         (a) Sugars are carbohydrates; some present in food naturally, some added.
         (b) Added sugars provide calories/energy, but almost no nutrients.
         (c) High-sugar diets can increase the risk of developing tooth decay.

(d) High-sugar foods often take the place of more nutritious foods in your diet.

(e) Through careful food selection and preparation, you can control sugar levels.

(6) Avoid too much sodium.

(a) Sodium is an essential nutrient.

(b) Helps the body maintain normal blood volume and pressure, helps muscle function.

(c) High sodium increases risk of hypertension, heart attacks, strokes, and so on.

(d) Sodium is added to many foods as a flavor enhancer.

(e) Food labels can help to identify high-sodium foods.

(f) Through careful food selection and preparation, you can control sodium levels.

(7) For teens: avoid alcoholic beverages.

For adults: if you drink alcohol, do so in moderation.

(a) People who drink alcohol and drive increase their risk for unintended injuries.

(b) Heavy alcohol use can contribute to liver disease and some forms of cancer.

(c) Alcohol can add calories to your diet, but almost no nutrients.

(d) There are many nonalcoholic beverage alternatives.

II. Reading a Nutrition Label

A. Found on food package/container. . . .

The outline should include the details of all items to be covered. It can be supplemented by an appendix with more detail, including photocopies of the overheads to be used. The content to be covered should be presented in a logical order though not necessarily in the order of presentation to be followed in the unit plan. If the contact time is, say, 20 hours, this section could be 30 or 40 pages.

Sample Methods (Nutrition)   The methods for a Nutrition Program are as follows:

1. *Lecture 1*

   Will cover outline parts I and II.

   Overheads will be used for reinforcement.

   Objectives addressed

   Cognitive objectives 1, 2, 7, and 8

2. *Lecture 2*

   Guest speaker, who is a registered dietitian, will cover outline parts III and V, including food labeling.

   Objectives addressed

   Cognitive objectives 2, 3, and 4

   Affective objectives 1

3. *Nutrition relay*
   See Appendix D for rules and questions.
   Objectives addressed
   Cognitive objectives 1, 2, 3, 4, 6, 8, 9, 10, 11, and 12
4. *Demonstration and cooking*
   See Appendix E for recipes and lists of ingredients.

Facilitator will demonstrate proper cooking of vegetables followed by an opportunity for all to enjoy a meal that they have prepared. Prior notification is required, and special material is needed.

It is most important that activities be selected with achieving objectives in mind. This is the most crucial component of a unit, assuming the objectives are appropriate and well stated. The number of methods is dictated by the contact time and the objectives to be achieved. A variety of learning styles should be addressed, as well as the characteristics of the target population.

Sample Materials (Any Unit)   Materials for an unspecified unit plan follow:

Facilitator
1. Extra pencils and paper
2. Blackboard
3. VCR and monitor (VHS format)
4. Chalk

Participant
1. Paper and pencil

Sample Evaluation (HIV/AIDS Workshop)   Evaluation for an HIV/AIDS Workshop is as follows:

Outcome Evaluation
1. Pretest and posttest on content of workshop.
2. Post-workshop survey of behaviors.
3. Postconference short survey of health behaviors in six months.

Process Evaluation
1. Post-workshop evaluation of facilitator performance and rating of workshop components.

The quantity and to some extent the quality of evaluation strategies will depend on the contact time for the workshop and for evaluation. Evaluation strategies should be tied to the objectives.

Sample Resources (First Aid)   Resources for a First Aid Program are as follows:

1. Doe, John. 1999. *First Aid.* J&J Publishers, Anytown. $29.95
2. American First Aid Society Film Series (five short videotapes)
   National Headquarters, Anytown U.S.A.
   Cost $1,250 set or $15 rental each

CLOSE TO HOME JOHN McPHERSON

Every high school student's worst enemy:
the essay question.

*Your unit objectives
must be reasonable in
order to be effective.*

3. First Aid Chart
   American First Aid Society Film Series
   National Headquarters, Anytown U.S.A.
   800-222-2222
   $49.95

List only those materials you know to be useful and important to the success of the unit.

**Sample Block Plan
(Any Topic)**

*The health educator who
plays roulette must first
invent the wheel.*
—Mohan Singh

The following table shows a block plan for an unspecified unit plan.

The block plan is how the total intervention fits together. Use of educational principles should be evident, including pacing, variety, and reinforcement. There is no need to review method or content in this section, as it has already been developed in the outline and method sections.

Day 1	Day 2	Day 3	Day 4	Day 5
Introduction Statement of Purpose Lecture 20 minutes	Introduction Review of last meeting What we will do today 10 minutes	Introduction Review of last meeting What we will do today 10 minutes	Introduction Review of last meeting What we will do today 10 minutes	Introduction Review of last meeting What we will do today 10 minutes
Get-acquainted activity Get it off my back 20 minutes	Skit Communications 10 minutes	Lecture Discussion on communication strategies 25 minutes	Role play Communications Stop and discuss as needed 45 minutes	Videotape on communication strategies 20 minutes
Lecture Discussion on the need for communications 25 minutes	Debriefing Overview of communication strategies 45 minutes	Problem-solving activity 15 minutes	Debrief review methodology 10 minutes	Debriefing of videotape 10 minutes
		Debriefing 10 minutes		Role play Communications 20 minutes
Summary review next meeting 10 minutes	Summary review next meeting 10 minutes	Summary review next meeting Self-assessment 15 minutes	Summary review next meeting 10 minutes	Summary review next meeting Evaluation 15 minutes

 For more information and tools related to this chapter visit
www.jbpub.com/healtheducation.

EXERCISES

Exercise 1: You Be the Judge! Take a look at the following lesson/presentation plans and critique them. Consider the appropriateness and feasibility of the objectives, the variety of the teaching methods, and the general "completeness" of the lesson/presentation plan. (Please note that in the interests of time and space the "content" section of the plans are highly abbreviated. A greater depth of information would ordinarily be required.)

Lesson/Presentation Plan 1 **Group:** 25 seventh-grade students, mixed ability
Unit: Addictive behaviors (four sessions)
Topic: Cigarette smoking (first session)
Time: 50 minutes

Objectives

1. Students will understand that smoking is an unhealthy habit.
2. Students will understand the harmful effects of smoking.
3. Students will decide to stop or not begin cigarette smoking.

Introduction

Students will write down all the reasons why people their age begin smoking cigarettes.

Development

Content	Method	Time	Materials
1. Reasons why people begin smoking	Q & A	10 minutes	None
2. Physical effects of smoking	Lecture	20 minutes	Overhead
3. Smoking and addiction	Lecture	15 minutes	Slides

Note: Would include attachments with content details.

Conclusion

Verify that students have understood the basic concepts of the lesson by asking them questions about the material covered in class. Students will respond orally.

Lesson/Presentation Plan 2

Group: 35 older adults (aged 60 to 65) in community group setting
Topic: Nutrition (one session only)
Time: 1 hour

Objectives

1. Participants will be able list the four major food groups.
2. Participants will be able to describe the contents of a well-balanced meal.
3. Participants will appreciate the relationship between nutrition and health and make a commitment to improve their diets.

Introduction

Facilitator will uncover four dishes (or photographs) at the front of the room to reveal four meals. Each dish will be described, and participants will be asked to rank-order each dish according to its nutritional value.

Development

Content	Method	Time	Materials
1. Describe the four major food groups	Lecture	15 minutes	None
2. Discuss suggested daily caloric intake	Q & A	15 minutes	Pamphlets
3. Suggested healthy-food preparation	Videotape	25 minutes	TV and VCR
4. Question time	Respond to questions	5 minutes	None

Note: Would include attachments with content details.

Conclusion

Distribute pamphlets related to nutrition and healthy-food preparation.

Critique of Lesson Plan 1

Objectives

The first problem with this lesson plan is that the objectives are poorly stated. The first two objectives are more like goals in that they are written in a very general and nonmeasurable sense. The verb *understand* is not appropriate for use in objective writing unless it is followed by another verb that reflects the degree or specificity of "understanding," such as *list* or *describe*. The problem with the third objective, "Students will decide to stop or not begin cigarette smoking," is that it is unrealistically optimistic. Again, as a goal for a lesson, this type of statement would not be out of place. However, to suggest that a 50-minute lesson could have such a dramatic, immediate impact on health behavior is to set up the health educator and the program for failure. When individuals begin smoking or fail to stop smoking, the behavioral objectives have not been met, and critics of the program might justifiably question the validity of continued support for such an ineffectual program. This objective could be made appropriate by qualifying it as follows: "Students will *be able to cite reasons* for stopping or not beginning cigarette smoking."

Development

The lesson has a promising beginning by quickly involving the students in the learning process. They write down reasons why people their age begin smoking cigarettes and then, through question and answer, the responses are verbalized. Unfortunately for the teacher and the students, that is the end of student involvement! For the majority of the lesson (35 minutes) the teacher intends to lecture to this class of seventh graders . . . good luck! In addition, the use of audiovisual equipment such as the overhead and slide projectors, which require semidarkness and are not traditionally known for scintillating lessons, could exacerbate the problems. When developing a lesson/presentation plan, the instructor needs to pay particular attention to the target population. In this case, seventh-grade students require teaching methods far more diverse than simply lecture. Break up a 35-minute block by using methods that are more interactive and interesting and yet still permit the dissemination of important information (see Chapter 5).

Conclusion

The teacher has allowed for some type of summary, or wrap-up, in the form of verbal responses to questions. This conclusion may allow the teacher to get a sense of how effective the lesson has been, and it is a method often used, yet it could be criticized as being somewhat haphazard. A better conclusion would be to allow a little more time and finish with a very brief pencil and paper test. Alternatively, teams could be organized and some type of game format utilized to review the information (see Chapter 5).

Critique of Lesson Plan 2

Objectives

The first two objectives are quite good in that they are measurable, fairly precise, and seemingly achievable. They could be even better if a qualifier of standard was added: "list four major food groups *according to . . .*" and "describe the contents of a well-balanced meal *according to . . .*" This way the parameters and criteria of the objectives are specifically stated. There are a few problems with objective 3. First, the verb *appreciate* is too vague; it should be followed by a verb that quantifies the objective. For example:

> Participants will appreciate the relationship between nutrition and health by listing five positive effects that a sound diet can have on health, according to the workshop.

Also, the third objective is actually two objectives within one. This is not an uncommon problem with individuals who are inexperienced in objectives design. We have already discussed the difficulty with using ambivalent terms like *appreciate*, but now the facilitator has added another objective related to committing to an improvement in diet. Such a commitment is not a bad objective if a qualifier is added:

> Participants will make a commitment to improve their diets *by voluntarily joining a relevant support group.*

However, this objective cannot simply be tacked on to the end of another; it must be given its own importance. It is quite possible that participants will be able to list five positive effects of a good diet and yet will refuse to join a support group. In this case, has the instructor succeeded or failed to achieve the objective? Keep objectives simple, and beware of linking two objectives together by use of the word *and.*

Introduction

The intended introduction is an excellent attention getter and is a practical and effective way for the facilitator to both gain the audience's attention and lead into the subject matter of the workshop. Unfortunately, the presentation plan shows no evidence of any follow-up of this introduction in the development section. Warm-up exercises in the classroom and introductions in the community presentation are usually effective when they are innovative and capture the attention of the participants, but they have to be connected to be the development section of the lesson/presentation, so that their relevance and connection to the main topic become obvious. In this specific instance, the facilitator planned an extremely innovative introduction by bringing actual meals to the workshop to enable a practical comparison. After being rank-ordered, the meals could have been incorporated into the discussion of the major food groups and the preparation of nutritious meals. This inclusion would have added a real-life feel to the workshop, and the presentation would have tied together more effectively.

Development

The biggest weakness of this presentation plan is the passivity of the learning process. The participants are simply not actively involved in the workshop, and concerns about boredom and distraction must be considered. If the facilitator is an outstanding speaker who can hold the attention of audiences, then these concerns might be minimized. The question-and-answer period is the only part of the plan that calls for group participation, and even this method affords only a low level of participation.

The facilitator intends to show a 25-minute videotape. In contrast to the school setting, where the discipline issue could be problematic, with this population fatigue might be a concern. Will the videotape be riveting enough to even keep the audience awake, especially after several minutes of lecturing preceding the videotape? Health education films are often dull and boring and should be used only if they impart important information, are relevant to the audience, and are at least minimally interesting. A more fundamental question might be, is a 25-minute videotape too long to use in a one-hour workshop? Many experienced presenters might feel that unless the videotape is of exceptional importance, it is in fact too long to be used in such a brief workshop. A more effective approach might be to view only parts of the videotape, so that at least some of the value of the tape could be utilized.

Allowing five minutes to answer questions is almost certainly not enough, particularly in the light of so much information being disseminated without any substantial discussion. The videotape would undoubtedly raise issues and concerns, and allowing only five minutes for responding to questions is simply poor planning.

Conclusion

There is no conclusion! The facilitator has allowed no time for it, nor for any type of evaluation. In an attempt to perhaps reinforce the material covered in the workshop, the facilitator plans to distribute pamphlets. Distributing pamphlets is common practice and can be an effective means to achieve several goals. This process, however, should not replace the summary or conclusion of a presentation and obviously plays no part in evaluation. In addition to some type of evaluation (however informal), dealing with what the audience has learned and how the facilitator has performed, the facilitator should also be concerned about the effectiveness of the videotape and whether or not using nearly half the workshop time showing the videotape is worthwhile. Obtaining participant feedback on the videotape is one way to achieve this end.

Both of these presentation plans have some obvious problems. They are good examples of how crucial thoughtful planning is to the success of any presentation. Think about the type of class or workshop you would like to be involved in as a participant; conversely, remember some of the characteristics of the most boring and ineffective classes or presentations you have sat through. Do not perpetuate poor presentation methods! Thorough planning and method consideration can minimize your chances of boring someone else to death!

Exercise 2: Now You Try!

Using your newfound knowledge of lesson/presentation planning, consider the following scenarios and develop an appropriate lesson/presentation plan for each. Remember to include achievable objectives and a variety of methods.

1. You are teaching the first of a four-session unit on cigarette smoking to a class of 25 seventh graders of mixed ability. The class period is 50 minutes long.
2. You are conducting a single, once-only workshop on hypertension for a group of 20 older adults (age 50 to 65). The group is racially diverse and includes both men and women. The workshop lasts for one hour and fifteen minutes.
3. You are teaching the final session of a three-session unit on sexuality and communication, including the subject of date rape, to a group of 20 tenth-grade high school students. The class period is 50 minutes long.
4. You are completing a two-session workshop on bicycle and traffic safety for a group of 18 ten-year-old children from a local youth group. Each session is one hour long, and all the children have brought their own bicycles with them.

CASE STUDIES REVISITED

Case Study Revisited: Shane
Shane and Mary have made numerous errors in planning. Shane has failed to construct an appropriate lesson plan with clear objectives, methods, and content. Mary has made several inappropriate decisions regarding content and format. Shane failed to make the school standards clear to his substitute for the day. The regular teacher at the high school should also assume some of the blame since she failed to share the school standards with the substitute. Generally, the regular teacher is held accountable for the presentation of any guest speaker, and that means she must communicate the standards of the school and school district to any speaker. (See page 82.)

Case Study Revisited: Michael
Michael's attitude that school and community health educators need to develop different sets of skills is all too common among many health education students. Regardless of what we call the "entity," the planning and delivery is virtually the same for both school and community health educators. When Michael stands up in front of a community group for an hour-long presentation and then declares that he does not teach, one has to wonder what he has been doing! (See page 85.)

SUMMARY

1. Lesson/presentation plans are vital to insure coverage of important objectives in a purposeful manner.

2. Lesson/presentation plans and unit plans are important to insure fidelity to the intention of the program developers.

3. A backup plan should be developed for components of a lesson plan that require the cooperation of the target group.

4. Evaluation is important for the improvement of any lesson or unit plan.

5. Unit plans are very useful for programs with more than five hours of contact time and are much more than a collection of lesson plans.

6. It is important to avoid the sin of reinventing the wheel. There are many good resources for purchase or to be shared via the Internet.

REFERENCES

Ames, E.E., Trucano, L.A., Wan, J.C., & Harris, M.H. (1992). *Designing School Health Curricula; Planning for Good Health*. Dubuque, IA: W.C. Brown.

Arends, R.I. (1991). *Learning to Teach*. New York: McGraw-Hill.

Bates, I.J., & Wider, A.E. (1984). *Introduction to Health Education*. Palo Alto, CA: Mayfield.

Bedworth, A.E., & Bedworth, D.A. (1992). *The Profession and Practice of Health Education*. Dubuque, IA: W.C. Brown.

Bender, S.J., Neutens, J.J., Skonie-Hardin, S., & Sorochan, W.D. (1997). *Teaching Health Science: Elementary and Middle School* (4th ed.). Boston: Jones and Bartlett Publishers.

Breckon, D.J., Harvey, J.R., & Lancaster, R.B. (1994). *Community Health Education: Settings, Roles and Skills for the 21st Century* (3rd ed.). Gaithersburg, MD: Aspen Publication.

Carroll, L. (1946). *Alice in Wonderland and Through the Looking Glass*. New York: Grosset and Dunlap.

Galli, N. (1978). *Foundations and Principles of Health Education*. New York: Wiley.

Goodlad, J.I. (1984). *A Place Called School: Prospects for the Future*. New York: McGraw-Hill.

Greenberg, J.S. (1988). *Health Education: Learner-Centered Instructional Strategies*. Dubuque, IA: W.C. Brown.

Greene, W.H., & Simons-Morton, B.G. (1984). *Introduction to Health Education*. New York: Macmillan.

Hellison, D. (1978). *Beyond Balls and Bats: Alienated (and Other) Youth in the Gym*. Washington, DC: AAHPER Publications.

Hoff, R. (1988). *I Can See You Naked*. New York: Andrews and McMeel.

Joyce, B., & Weil, M. (1986). *Models of Teaching*. Englewood Cliffs, NJ: Prentice-Hall.

Lazes, P.M., Kaplan, L.H., & Gordon, K.A. (1987). *The Handbook of Health Education*. Rockville, MD: Aspen.

Mayshark, C., & Foster, R. (1966). *Methods in Health Education*. St. Louis: C.V. Mosby.

McKenzie, J.F., Pinger, R.R., & Kotecki, J.E. (1999). *An Introduction to Community Health* (3rd ed.). Boston: Jones and Bartlett Publishers.

Meeks, L., Heit, P., & Page, R. (1996). *Comprehensive School Health Education* (2nd ed.). Backlick, OH: Meeks Heit Publishing Company.

Read, D.A. (1997). *Health Education: A Cognitive-Behavioral Approach*. Boston: Jones and Bartlett Publishers.

Rubinson, L., & Alles, W.F. (1984). *Health Education: Foundations for the Future*. Prospect Heights, IL: Waveland.

Scott, G.D., & Carlo, M.W. (1979). *On Becoming a Health Educator*. Dubuque, IA: W.C. Brown.

U.S. Department of Health and Human Services. (1980). *Promoting Health Prevention Disease Objectives for the Nation*. Washington, DC: U.S. Public Health Service.

U.S. Department of Health, E., and Welfare. (1979). *Healthy People: The Surgeon General's Report on Health Promotion and Disease* (Vol. Publication 79-55071). Washington, DC: U.S. Public Health Service.

Wilgoose, C.E. (1972). *Health Teaching in Secondary Schools*. Philadelphia: W.B. Saunders.

Methods of Instruction/Intervention

Entry Level and Graduate Level Health Educator Competencies Addressed In This Chapter

Responsibility III: Implementing Health Education Programs
  Competency A: Exhibit competence in carrying out planned educational programs.
  Competency C: Select methods and media best suited to implement program plans for specific learners.
  Competency D: Monitor educational programs, adjusting objectives and activities as necessary.

Method Selection in Health Education

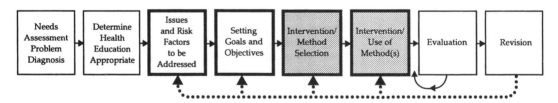

Needs Assessment Problem Diagnosis → Determine Health Education Appropriate → Issues and Risk Factors to be Addressed → Setting Goals and Objectives → Intervention/ Method Selection → Intervention/ Use of Method(s) → Evaluation → Revision

Heavy-bordered boxes indicate subjects addressed in this text; shaded boxes indicate subjects(s) of current chapter.

Note: The competencies listed above, which are addressed in this chapter, are considered to be both entry-level and graduate-level competencies by the National Commission for Health Education Credentialing, Inc. They are taken from *A Framework for the Development of Competency Based Curricula for Entry Level Health Educators* by the National Task Force for the Preparation and Practice of Health Education, 1985; and American Association for Health Education, National Commission for Health Education Credentialing, I., & Education, S. F. P. H. (1999). *A Competency-Based Framework for Graduate-Level Health Educators.* Allentown, PA: The National Commission for Health Education Credentialing, Inc., American Assoc. for Health Education, and the Society for Public Health Education.

OBJECTIVES   After studying the chapter the reader should be able to

- Describe the major advantages and disadvantages of using each method
- Describe how to use each method
- Provide a rationale for using each method
- Match methods with objectives

KEY ISSUES   Method description   Advantages
                 When to use   Disadvantages
                 How to use   Examples

Using Methods as a Framework

An arsenal of methods is available to us in health education. It is important we consider the objectives first and then focus on the methods to meet those objectives within the context of the resources we have at our disposal. This chapter will focus on the many methods available to the health educator, some of which are as follows:

1. Getting-acquainted activities
2. Audiotapes
3. Audiovisual materials
4. Brainstorming
5. Case Studies
6. Computer-assisted instruction
7. Cooperative learning and group work
8. Debates
9. Displays and bulletin boards
10. Educational games
11. Experiments and demonstrations
12. Field trips
13. Guest speakers
14. Guided imagery
15. Humor
16. Lecture
17. Mass media
18. Models
19. Music
20. Newsletters
21. Panels
22. Peer education
23. Personal improvement projects
24. Problem solving
25. Puppets
26. Role plays
27. Self-appraisals
28. Service learning
29. Simulations
30. Theater
31. Value clarification
32. Word games and puzzles

Each method should be considered a "framework." Every possible method should be considered for each objective to be achieved. An important step in making the decision is to use the preceding list of activities/methods and consider how each one might conceivably be employed to meet your objectives. This will force you to consider the many options available for achieving your objectives and make it less likely you will pick a method for inappropriate reasons.

Case Study: Pam   Pam has been asked to develop a health education program for the local community. During her years in college the only teaching method she experienced was lecture. She therefore develops and emulates an intellectual lecture presentation on the evils of drugs for the five parents of adolescents who are believed to have drug problems. When the parents seem uninterested in her approach, she is disappointed. One of the parents suggests she just sit down and talk with them. Another parent, who is a physician, says they are all aware of the evils of drugs but need help in relating to their children. (See Case Studies Revisited page 172.)

Of all the beasts in the jungle, we most often resemble the crashing boar.
—Mohan Singh

This chapter will present a variety of methods and one or more examples of the application of the method. The reader should remember that the methods presented can be converted to other subject matter with relative ease. To reiterate, each method is a framework that can and should be adapted to meet your needs. Always think of how each method might be applied to meet your objectives. Health educators often "crash" into a method without thinking through what is the best method to achieve the desired outcome. Table 5-1 presents a matrix helpful in method selection. We will examine each of the methods listed there in detail. Note the varied roles of the **facilitator.**

Method/Intervention 1: Getting-Acquainted (Icebreaker) Activities

Getting-acquainted activities, also called *icebreakers*, can be used to set the tone for a workshop or class. These activities should be easy to follow and fun. They range from having participants introduce themselves to more complex activities designed to show what will be covered or why the lesson is being presented. They should be selected very carefully, with the objectives and **target population** characteristics in mind. It is often said that the first fifteen minutes of any presentation sends a message of what is to follow. Send a positive message that this will be a good presentation! Start on time, and be enthusiastic. Always be polite and interested in the people present. Try to address people by name. Encourage all to participate, and participate as much as possible yourself. Your active participation sets the tone for the group.

Advantages and Disadvantages   Advantages of getting-acquainted activities are that they

1. Can serve to create an atmosphere of mutual trust and respect.
2. Can help the facilitator learn the names and interests of participants.

Table 5-1 Methods Selection Matrix

Method	Cognitive Objectives	Affective Objectives	Psychomotor Objectives	Time Required Minutes	Ages/Years	Size/Suggested Max	Budget	Community Setting	School Setting	Comments
1 Getting-acquainted activities	X	P	P	15+	All	None	Low	X	X	
2 Audiotapes	X	P	P	15+	All	None	Low	X	X	Equipment required
3 Audiovisual materials	X	P	P	15+	All	None	Mod	X	X	Equipment required
4 Brainstorming	X			20+	All	20	Low	X	X	
5 Case studies	X	X		30+	All	20	Low	X	X	
6 Computer-assisted instruction	X	P		30+	10+	Ratio	High		X	Equipment required
7 Cooperative learning	P	P	P	30+	All	20	Low	X	X	
8 Debates	P	P		30+	All	30	Low	X	X	
9 Displays/bulletin boards	X			30+	All	None	Low	X	X	Special materials required
10 Educational games	X			20+	All	30	Low	X	X	
11 Experiments and demonstrations	X		X	30+	All	Ratio	Mod+		X	Equipment required
12 Field trips		P		60+	All	Ratio	Mod	X	X	
13 Guest speakers	X	P		30+	All	None	Low+	X	X	
14 Guided imagery		X	P	30+	All	None	Mod	X	X	Equipment required
15 Humor	X	X		2+	All	None	Low	X	X	
16 Lecture	X			5+	All	None	Low	X	X	
17 Mass media	X			5+	All	None			X	Access required
18 Models	X		P	5+	All	None	Low+	X	X	Equipment required
19 Music	P	X		5+	All	None	Low	X	X	Equipment required
20 Newsletters	X			120+	All readers	None	Mod	X	X	Equipment and duplication required

continued

Table 5-1 *continued*

Method	Cognitive Objectives	Affective Objectives	Psychomotor Objectives	Time Required Minutes	Ages/Years	Size/Suggested Max	Budget	Community Setting	School Setting	Comments
21 Panels	P	X		30+	All	None	Low	X	X	
22 Peer education	P	X		120+	All	Ratio	Mod	X	X	Special training needed
23 Personal improvement projects		X	P	600+	10+	None	Low+	X	X	Requires adequate time
24 Problem solving	P	P		30+	All	25	Low	X	X	
25 Puppets	X	X		30+	All	25	Low+	X	X	Equipment required
26 Role plays		X	P	30+	10+	25	Low	X	X	
27 Self-appraisals		X		15+	10+	None	Low	X	X	Handout or computer required
28 Service learning	X	X	P	120+	All	None	Mod	X	X	Consider insurance
29 Simulations	X	X	X	30+	10+	25	Mod+	X	X	Special materials required
30 Theater	X	X		30+	All	None	Mod	X	X	Scripts required
31 Value clarification		X		30+	14+	30	Low	X	X	
32 Word games and puzzles	X			10+	10+ readers	None	Low	X	X	Handout required

X = Yes common use.
P = Possible.
Blank = uncommon.

Sample debriefing questions (that should be outlined by facilitator before role play follow:

1. Was the situation realistic?
2. What would be the likely outcome of the actions of the big brother/sister?
3. What are other options?
4. What are the issues here? (drug use, dating older man, some unknown, sexuality, no supervision, etc.)
5. What are realistic objectives?
6. How can we reach these objectives?

Example 1: Drug Prevention/ Education

Following are several possible role plays for the subject of drug prevention/education.

1. Two parents discuss the marijuana joint one parent has found in their son's room. They must decide what action to take.
2. You (age 21 and a college student) walk into your home unexpectedly and find your younger sister (age 15) home alone with an older (age 19) boy. The couple is in the kitchen drinking beer and there are some red capsules on the table that are obviously illegal drugs. They both act nervously when you walk in and try to hide the drugs. Your mother (single-parent family) is working and will not be home for several hours.
3. Parents are teaching their child about drug abuse. You are sitting in the kitchen at home.
4. You find someone in the next dorm room smoking marijuana.
5. Intoxicated date wants to drive you home.
6. You are at a party where two friends urge you to try pot or LSD or some other illicit drug.
7. Your friend gives you his locker combination so you can retrieve the book you loaned him last night. While getting the book you notice several bags of drugs in his locker. This guy has been a pretty good friend and has never offered you or sold you drugs. What do you do?

Example 2: Violence Prevention

Following are two possible role plays on the subject of preventing violence.

1. A friend who lives in a very tough part of town has brought a handgun to school for protection. You spot it when you are having lunch together, and he explains he needs it for protection. He says he does not need it at school but has nowhere else to hide it. You often bring your mom's car to school. He suggests leaving it in the trunk of your car during the day.
2. A good friend of your son is arrested for assault and carrying a concealed weapon (knife).

Example 3: Sexuality Education

Following are three possible role plays on the subject of sexuality education.

1. Parent finds diaphragm belonging to 16-year-old daughter.
2. Parent discovers condoms in purse of 14-year-old daughter.
3. Parent discovers condoms on dresser of 14-year-old son.

Example 4: Ecology Social Responsibility

Following are two possible role plays on the subject of ecology social responsibility.

1. Your son or brother pours oil into the street drain after changing your oil.
2. Your friend dumps trash out of the car window.

Method/Intervention 27: Self-Appraisals

Self-appraisal is a technique to encourage personal assessment as an important step in personal behavior change. It involves some form of personal assessment, which can range from a checklist of a few items to a diary and computer analysis kept for a long time. The key element is to encourage self-

SELF-ASSESSMENT OF PRESENTATION (REVIEW OF VIDEO TAPED PRESENTATION)

Name: _____

Date video reviewed: _____

Overall impression of presentation:
_____
_____
_____
_____

Some things I did well:
_____
_____
_____
_____
_____
_____

Some things I should work on:
_____
_____
_____
_____
_____
_____

Figure 5-11
Example of Self-Appraisal Form for Video Presentation

inspection as a first step in behavior change. Self-appraisal is sometimes coupled with personal improvement projects. Figures 5-11 and 5-12 present forms for self-appraisal.

Self-appraisal can be used effectively as an evaluation tool for **community health education** program. We can label an anonymous assessment a self-appraisal and make it acceptable. If we call it a test, participants may walk out.

Advantages and Disadvantages

Advantages of self-appraisals are that they

1. Allow individual assessment.
2. Are an important first step in personal behavior change.

NEEDS ASSESSMENT   SELF-ASSESSMENT

Name: _____ Year in School: _____

Local Phone: _____

Specialization? School or Community, Worksite or other: _____

If Grad Student degree program and major interests: _____

Are you currently employed? Yes No
If yes what approximately how many hours do you work a week? _____

TEACHING/PRESENTATION EXPERIENCE (PAST FIVE YEARS)
1. Teaching or working with children _____ (Contact hours with you as the primary instructor)

2. Teaching or working with adults _____

LESSON/PRESENTATION PLANNING
1. How many lesson/presentation plans have you personally written? _____

2. Have you been trained in writing behavioral objectives? _____ If yes – what system was used? _____

EQUIPMENT USE
Have you successfully used (feel comfortable in using) the following?
_____ 1. Overhead Projector
_____ 2. E-mail
_____ 3. Film Projector
_____ 4. Video Disk Player
_____ 5. Computer Projection System
_____ 6. Video Tape Camera & Recorder
_____ 7. CD ROM & Computer
_____ 8. Slide Projector
_____ 9. Personal Computer-model _____
                 Preferred Word Processing Software _____
_____ 10. Internet – finding health information.

Figure 5-12
Example of Self-Appraisal Form for Needs Assessment

3. Provide excellent focus to start a workshop or class.
4. Interesting and entertaining.

Disadvantages are that they

1. Require development of instruments.
2. Can be misinterpreted.
3. May require medical testing.
4. Can be expensive if using a commercial vendor.

Examples   Examples of ways to use self-appraisals follow:

1. Use to test health education knowledge.
2. Use to appraise health risks.
3. Use to evaluate food intake—24-hour recall.
4. Use as post-workshop assessment.
5. Use as a stress audit.

Method/Intervention 28: Service Learning

Service learning is the notion that one learns through doing and can acquire good personal values through service to others. This method also provides real service to the community. Some school districts require such service of all students and have even gone so far as to make it a graduation requirement. East Carolina University, through its Department of Health Education and Promotion, has operated a large service learning program for many years. The program is promoted through many courses on campus. An amazing 9,000 of the total 18,000 students on campus in a recent year provided service to local groups and agencies through the program. All participants are covered by insurance, and only agencies with negotiated contracts ensuring supervision and an appropriate experience are included.

Service learning is not a new notion, of course, but it has been gaining popularity at many institutions of learning. Not that long ago educational institutions were encouraged to be value-neutral, but often today they are actively encouraged to teach basic values such as treating others with respect and responsibly giving back to the community.

Advantages and Disadvantages   Advantages of service learning are that it

1. Generally requires little equipment.
2. Is able to address affective objectives.
3. Provides real service to the community.

Disadvantages are that it

1. Is often unpredictable in outcome.
2. Can place participants at risk and often requires insurance.
3. Requires close supervision and time-consuming cooperation with community agencies.

Examples
1. Require a given number of service hours in a health related agency before being eligible to graduate from high school.
2. Require a given number of service hours in a specific agency as part of a health education course.

Method/Intervention 29: Simulations

Simulations are activities that take on the appearance of some real-life phenomenon. They allow participants to observe and even participate in an event without the risk of injury that would occur in the real event and in a very controlled manner. An example would be an injury simulation kit, providing realistic-looking blood and ways to make people look wounded. Participants can treat injuries as they would in real-life situations.

According to Cruickshank (1972), a simulation is "the end product, the model resulting from the process of simulating. The simulation is contrived experience used to expose someone to a certain prescribed set of circumstances based on a model. It is usually to teach a role, function, or operation. By using simulation, it is possible to attain the essence of something without its reality."

Rationale The common application of simulations to emergency care such as first aid is useful for the following reasons:

1. They provide examples of real-life emergency care situations.
2. They provide an opportunity for the practical application of skills covered in the classroom.
3. They provide practice in the analysis and evaluation of emergency situations without the risk of injury resulting from judgment errors.
4. They provide an alternative teaching strategy for the instructor.
5. They provide an evaluation technique for instructors.
6. They provide students with practice in performing skills under stress and thus increase self-confidence.

Advantages and Disadvantages Advantages of simulations are that they

1. Provide an element of realism.
2. Can address some difficult-to-teach issues such as comfort levels of performance.

3. Provide variety.
4. Can provide opportunities for repetition of important skills.

Disadvantages

1. Generally are time-consuming.
2. Can be expensive.
3. Are often difficult to use with large groups.

Examples   Some examples of simulations follow:

1. First-aid instruction—see Figures 5-13 through 5-17.
2. Fire alarm and building evacuation.

> 1. *You must treat this* **like a real-life situation**. *Nothing will be assumed—you must do all that you would in a real-life situation. To receive credit for any procedure, it must actually be completed. The only exceptions to this are procedures that cannot be done in the classroom such as making a phone call, and they must be explained.*
> 2. *You may use only material* **provided** *in the testing area.*
> 3. *You may not use any notes or cards.*
> 4. *For assistance you may use only those people provided, and you* **must give them explicit directions** *for any aid they administer. No undirected assistance or information is to be given by other students or victims.*
> 5. **Time will be an important factor in life-threatening situations**. *A reasonable time will be allowed for less severe injuries, but do not waste time. (After using a situation several times, an instructor will have an idea of how long it should take to complete and may wish to set a time limit.)*
> 6. *In situations where you want to take a pulse, you must actually take a reading. (Victims will also be taking their own pulse so that assessment can be properly made.)*
> 7. *Bleeding tags will be marked mild, moderate, or severe. Mild bleeding will require direct pressure and elevation for credit. Moderate bleeding will require the same plus proper use of pressure points where appropriate. Severe bleeding will require the use of all three aforementioned techniques plus proper use of a tourniquet. This is done only as a grading convention and is not meant to imply that proper first aid would be guided only by estimates of blood flow.*

Figure 5-13
First Aid Instructions for Participants. From Gilbert, G.G. (1981). *Teaching First Aid and Emergency Care.* Dubuque, IA: Kendall/Hunt.

(Text continues on page 165)

SAMPLE SIMULATION SITUATION 1

Information Supplied to First-Aider.
Situation:
    You are home with your younger sister (age 11) when you hear her crying. You find her on the front porch.
Where:
    Your home.
Miscellaneous Information:
    No one else is home.

Position of Victim:
    Seated.
Special Instructions for Victim:
    Cry, but answer questions. You fell and scraped your knee. You have no other injuries.
Supplied Materials:
    Home materials box.
Tags:
    1. Moderate bleeding (1)–knee.

Figure 5-14
Sample Simulation
Situation 1

SAMPLE SIMULATION EVALUATION 1

Scraped Knee

Name of First-Aider   Grader

	Yes Well Done	Yes Adequate	No
1. Was the victim properly examined and questioned for all possible injuries?	4, 3	2, 1	0
2. Was the victim given verbal encouragement?	2	1	0
3. Was moderate bleeding controlled and bandaged properly?	7, 6, 5, 4	3, 2, 1	0
a. Direct pressure (2) b. Elevation (2) c. Proper bandage (3)			
4. Was proper shock treatment given?	2	1	0
Comments:			

Add _____
Deductions _____
Total _____
Possible _____15_____

The evaluator circles the appropriate point value and adds the points up for grading. These can be used to determine pass or failure or a letter grade. Multiple situations must be developed prior to class (see Gilbert, 1981) so all participants have different situations.

Figure 5-15
Sample Simulation
Evaluation 1

SAMPLE SIMULATION SITUATION 2

Information Supplied to First-Aider.
Situation:
    You are the first to arrive at the scene of a single-car automobile accident.
Where:
    Freeway (interstate).
Miscellaneous Information:
    Several other people stop, but no one has first-aid training. There appears to be no danger of fire.

Position of Victim:
    Victim is face down on front seat (use two chairs).
Special Instructions for Victim:
    You are unconscious and will remain so.
Supplied Materials:
    1. Coats.
    2. Bandaging materials.
    3. Water.
    4. Splints.
Tags:
    1. Moderate bleeding (1)–forehead.
    2. Moderate bleeding (1)–nose (nose bleed).

Figure 5-16
Sample Simulation
Situation 2

SAMPLE SIMULATION EVALUATION 2

Bleeding

Name of First-Aider	Grader		
	Yes Well Done	Yes Adequate	No
1. Was the victim examined carefully for all injuries?	4, 3	2, 1	0
2. Was moderate bleeding of the forehead controlled properly? a. Direct pressure (4) b. Bandaged properly (3)	7, 6, 5, 4	3, 2, 1	0
3. Was victim removed from the car? (If removed–give credit if good explanation for removal given and proper technique applied.)	0	0	4
4. Was note made of possible head injury (medical personnel notified and movement minimized?)	5, 4, 3	2, 1	0
5. Was proper aid sent for?	2	1	0
6. Was the victim treated for shock?	3, 2	1	0
Comments:			

Add _____
Deductions _____
Total _____
Possible _____25_____

Figure 5-17
Sample Simulation
Evaluation 2

3. Application of CPR.
4. Simulation games in which community member roles are simulated.

Method/Intervention 30: Theater

Theater has been commonly used in many health education programs. It differs from role plays in that it employs a script that dictates all dialogue and action. These plays can be purchased or developed, and often professional actors or para-professional student actors are enlisted to make the presentation. Generally a follow-up discussion guide with questions for the audience is included.

Theater can be very powerful. Several plays have been developed in the AIDS/HIV prevention area (Denman 1996), and some university student health centers are using student actors to provide plays on date rape. Because there is an established script, presentations can be reviewed very carefully for content. It is therefore easy to determine if the play fits the objectives being sought and if it fits any model or theory being employed in reaching the target population.

Advantages and Disadvantages

Advantages of theater are that it

1. Generally requires little equipment.
2. Is able to address difficult topics in a controlled manner.
3. Can address the affective domain.
4. Allows good control over content.

Disadvantages are that it

1. Requires the use of actors, who may be difficult to find or afford.
2. May require a stage and related equipment.
3. May be ineffective if poor acting detracts from the message.

Examples

Examples of theater use follow:

1. Purchase health-specific scripts.
2. Develop scripts as a classroom project.
3. Use scripts constructed by a community group.

Sample Script

"The Babysitter's Dilemma"
Scene
Jane has been babysitting the Johnson children, who are now asleep. Jane is dressed like a typical teenager. Mr. and Mrs. Johnson return home from the party they were attending. Scene takes place in living room and adjoining

kitchen. Stage should include living room with couch and chair plus adjoining kitchen with counter table and chairs. Jane is sitting reading when Mrs. Johnson walks in the front door.

Mrs. Johnson: Hi, dearie. Sorry we are late, but the party was so much fun we lost track of the time.

Jane: The kids went to bed about 9:30, as you asked, Mrs. Johnson, but I don't think they fell asleep until much later.

Mrs. Johnson: Don't worry, dearie, they can sleep in tomorrow since it is Saturday. In fact, it *is* Saturday—what time is it?

Jane: It is almost 3 AM.

Mr. Johnson comes through the front door looking a bit disheveled and appears to have been drinking.

Mr. Johnson Had a little trouble getting the car into the garage. Oh, Christ, I forgot the babysitter. Come on, cutie, I'll take you home. Where are my keys?

Mrs. Johnson: Maybe you left them in the car, dear. [*Mrs. Johnson takes off her coat and shoes.*]

Mr. Johnson: Oh yeah, that is probably where they are. Honey, you go to bed and I'll be right back. Come on, cutie—how old did you say you were?

Mr. Johnson looks her up and down with interest, in an inappropriate manner.

Jane: Maybe I should call my parents?

Mr. Johnson: Nonsense. It is too late, and I am not tired. I am feeling good.

Jane: My parents have a rule that if I work past 1 AM, that they pick me up.

Mr. Johnson: That is a silly rule. You will just wake them up for no reason.

Mrs. Johnson: We don't want to upset her parents. Let her call home if she wants.

Mr. Johnson: This is ridiculous! What do we have to drink? Do we have any bourbon?

Jane moves to the kitchen and calls her parents.

Jane: Mom, the Johnsons just got home from the party, and I need you to pick me up. Thanks, Mom. I'll be ready as soon as you can make it.

Mr. Johnson [using a stern, directive voice]: Why don't you call them back and tell them I can drive you home? I am not going to give you a tip unless I drive you home. It isn't right for your parents to come.

Mrs. Johnson has moved to the kitchen and is cleaning up.

Jane: My Mom and Dad have strict rules, and I must follow them since I am only 15. Mrs. Johnson, let me help you clean up.

Jane moves to kitchen and begins cleaning. Mr. Johnson acts huffy, fixes himself a drink, and sits, watching the ladies clean up. A few minutes later Jane hears a car and moves to the window.

Jane: It is my Dad, and I have to go. [*She heads for the front door.*]
Mr. Johnson [*standing up and getting out his wallet*]: Here you go, Jane. There is a nice tip. I hope there are no misunderstandings. We may need you next week.
Jane: Thank you, Mr. Johnson. [*She hurries out the door.*]

Follow-up discussion.

1. Did Jane do anything that contributed to the problem?
2. What other options did Jane have? What might be the consequences of these behaviors?
3. What if Jane did not have parents at home? What could she have done?
4. Should Jane return to babysit again?

Method/Intervention 31: Value Clarification

Value clarification is a method designed to help people understand how they have reached decisions. It has the potential of teaching *rational decision-making skills.* This method had great popularity in the 1960s and 1970s. It fell into disfavor under charges that it taught no values and allowed free choice even when the correct choice was clear to "any rational person." The method was often misused, and this contributed to its being banned in some settings. It is a useful tool if used properly. Many of the principles can be applied well under the title developing decision-making skills.

Advantages and Disadvantages

Advantages of value clarification are that it

1. Is low in cost.
2. Can deal with feelings and emotions.
3. Allows for individual and group expression.

Disadvantages are that it

1. Can be controversial.
2. Requires that the instructor be prepared to deal with emotional responses.
3. Is unpredictable in outcome.

Rules

Rules for value clarification should be established as follows:

1. No put downs are to be allowed.
2. The rights of others to different opinions are to be respected.

According to Raths, Harmin, and Simon (1966, p. 30), true values are those which do the following:

Choosing	1.	Freely
	2.	From alternatives
	3.	After consideration of the consequences of each alternative

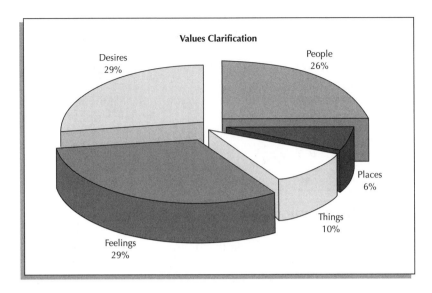

Figure 5-18
Pie Chart for Value
Clarification Exercise

Prizing	4.	Cherishing, being happy with choice
	5.	Willing to affirm the choice publicly
Acting	6.	Doing something with the choice
	7.	Repeatedly, in some pattern of life

Example: Health Education Decision   Use value clarification to help participants make a health education decision by asking them to do the following:

1. List five major factors that influenced you to go into health education. These can be people, places, things, feelings, or desires.
2. Draw a large circle.
3. Divide the circle into pie slices for each of your "influencers," and make the proportion of each slice appropriate to the amount of influence (see Figure 5-18).

Now lead a group discussion by asking participants these questions:

1. Are these rational and positive ways to make a decision?
2. How would the pie chart look if you went about this decision the most rational way?
3. Are you proud of your decision?

Method/Intervention 32: Word Games and Puzzles

Word games are entertaining and are very useful in increasing vocabulary. They are commonly used with elementary school children, with people studying English as a second language, or with any area that introduces a considerable number of new vocabulary words. These activities include crossword puzzles, anagrams, and other word games.

Advantages and Disadvantages

Advantages of word games are that they

1. Are low in cost.
2. Are fun.
3. Serve as good productive filler for individuals who finish work fast or need additional stimulation.
4. Are excellent for improving vocabulary.

Disadvantages are that they

1. Generally address only the cognitive domain.
2. Require time to develop.
3. Require equipment to reproduce.

Examples

Two examples of word games follow:

1. Crossword puzzle for health education methods and interventions—see Figure 5-19.
2. Anagram for drug classifications—see Figure 5-20.

Promising Methods by Topic

As we have stated many times, we encourage you to consider all methods that might meet your objectives. Following is a list of methods by topic which have either had some success, or the authors recommend the exploration of this method for the listed content area.

Drug Education

Debates
Experiments and demonstrations
Mass media
Panels
Peer education
Role plays
Value clarification

Human Sexuality

Debates
Guest speakers
Panels
Peer education
Puppets

ACROSS

3 a classification of national background can be from any ethnic group.

5 a precise statement of intended outcome and must be stated in measurable terms.

8 An orderly self-contained collection of activities educationally designed to meet a set of objectives.

9 Belief or expectation by an individual that they can carry out the desired behavior.

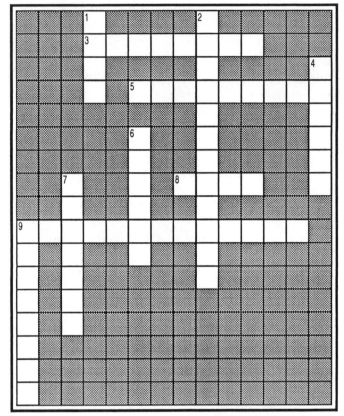

Created using Crossword Creator, Centron Software Technolgies, Inc., Version 1.12, 1992.

DOWN

1 Certified Health Education Specialist

2 The overall strategy to achieve stated objectives.

4 One component of intervention - can be used interchangeably with strategy.

6 Author of text.

7 Author of text.

9 One component of the intervention. Can be used interchangeably with method.

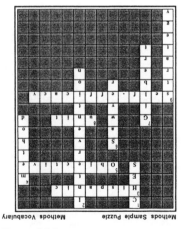

Methods Vocabulary   Methods Sample Puzzle

Figure 5-19
Crossword Puzzle on Health Education Methods/Interventions

Change the following names into drug classifications.

Name	Drug Classification
Minee Haptma	*Amphetamine*
Bet Arbitura	*Barbiturate*
Lum Stanti	*Stimulant*
Ant Pedress	*Depressant*

See the methods selection matrix in Chapter 3.

Figure 5-20
Anagram on Drug
Classifications

Role plays
Value clarification

**Environmental
Health**

Debates
Experiments and demonstrations
Field trips
Guest speakers
Panels

**Consumer
Health/Nutrition**

Computer-assisted instruction
Guest speakers
Mass media
Personal improvement projects
Self-appraisals

First Aid

Computer-assisted instruction
Guest speakers
Simulation

*For more information and tools related to this chapter visit
www.jbpub.com/healtheducation.*

EXERCISES

Take a look at the following situations. Construct *one* behavioral objective for each situation, and then select *one* appropriate method to fulfill the objective. Give a brief justification as to why you selected a particular method, and explain how the method would facilitate achieving the objective.

1. You are teaching the first class in a five-part unit on nutrition for approximately 25 seventh-grade students.

2. You are conducting a one-hour, once-only workshop for a community group of women (approximately 20 women aged 35 to 45) on the subject of menopause.

3. You are facilitating the first in a series of eight workshops on smoking cessation for a community group of 10 adults.

4. You are teaching the final class in a five-part unit on HIV/AIDS for a group of 25 tenth-grade students.

5. You are facilitating the second of six one-hour workshops for approximately 10 college students on the subject of body image/weight management.

6. You are teaching the first in a three-part unit on environmental health for an eighth-grade class of approximately 20 students.

CASE STUDIES REVISITED

Case Study Revisited: Pam
Pam needs help in her method selection. She needs to review her objectives and select more appropriate methods. She has selected an inappropriate method for the target population and has failed to take advantage of an excellent opportunity for small-group techniques.

There is an arsenal of methods available to us in health education. It is important we consider the objectives first and then focus on the methods to meet those objectives within the context of the resources we have at our disposal. (See page 106.)

Case Study Revisited: Pat
The fundamental question that should be asked is whether or not a debate on such a volatile subject as abortion should even be considered. High school students are notoriously opinionated and quite often totally unreceptive to opposing views, making an abortion debate a disaster waiting to happen. Pat was also incredibly naïve in thinking that a debate would change anyone's position on such a difficult and personal topic as abortion. One debate technique sometimes used is to have individuals research and present arguments that are diametrically opposed to their own viewpoint. This ensures that participants consider the "other side" in relation to their own opinions. However, abortion is such a personal and polarized issue that discretion, in the form of simply not debating such a topic, may indeed have been the better part of valor in this instance. (See page 121.)

Case Study Revisited: Meshah
Meshah could have done a couple of things to make the field trip more effective. Time could have been built into the day's events to allow for questions, although if someone on-site is coordinating the visit, that might prove difficult to control. Another strategy might be to provide the students with a list of questions that they need to have answered by the end of the visit. This could even be made into a type of informational scavenger hunt to encourage active participation. Clearly, Meshah could have used the bus ride home as a time to process the day's events and clarify any points of confusion, although in fairness to Meshah, a bus full of tired or boisterous students might not be the optimal

place to process information! A football discussion might indeed be a sound plan, saving the post-visit processing or scavenger hunt analysis until the next class period. There is no one right way to implement strategies, but the likelihood of success with any single method relies heavily on the planning and thought that precedes the activity. (See page 136.)

SUMMARY

This chapter has reviewed over 30 categories of methods that can be employed by a health educator. Each has advantages and disadvantages that should be taken into account when making a selection for inclusion in any health education program.

REFERENCES

American Association for Health Education, National Commission for Health Education Credentialing, I., & Education, S. F. P. H. (1999). *A Competency-Based Framework for Graduate-Level Health Educators*. Allentown, PA: The National Commission for Health Education Credentialing, Inc., American Association for Health Education, and the Society for Public Health Education.

Ames, E.E., Trucano, L.A., Wan, J.C., & Harris, M.H. (1992). *Designing School Health Curricula: Planning for Good Health*. Dubuque, IA: W.C. Brown.

Arends, R.I. (1991). *Learning To Teach*. New York: McGraw-Hill.

Bates, I.J., & Wider, A.E. (1984). *Introduction to Health Education*. Palo Alto, CA: Mayfield.

Bedworth, A.E., & Bedworth, D.A. (1992). *The Profession and Practice of Health Education*. Dubuque, IA: W.C. Brown.

Carlyon, W., & "Carlyon, P. (1987). "Humor As a Health Education Tool," in Peter M. Lazes, Laura Hollander Kaplan, and Karen Gordon. (1987). *The Handbook of Health Education, p. 115*. Rockville, MD: Aspen.

Carroll, L. (1946). *Alice in Wonderland and Through the Looking Glass*. New York: Grosset and Dunlap.

Cruickshank, D. (1972). *Simulation and Gaming*. Unpublished mimeographed handout.

Davis, W., Feller, K., & Thaut, M. (1992). *Introduction to Music Therapy*. Dubuque, IA: W.C. Brown.

Denman, S., Davis, P., Pearson, J., & Madeley, R. (1996). HIV theatre in health education: An evaluation of *Someone Like You. Health Education Journal, 55*, 156–164.

Doyle, E.I., Beatty, C.F., & Shaw, M.W. (1999). Using cooperative learning groups to develop health-related cultural awareness. *Journal of School Health, 69*(No.2), 73–74.

Feldman, R.H., & Humphrey, J.H. (1989). *Advances in Health Education: Current Research* (Vol. 2). New York: AMS Press.

Galli, N. (1978). *Foundations and Principles of Health Education*. New York: Wiley.

Gilbert, G.G. (1981). *Teaching First Aid and Emergency Care*. Dubuque, IA: Kendall/Hunt.

Gilbert, G.G., & Ziady, M. (1986). *Experiments and Demonstrations in Smoking Education*. Washington, D.C.: U.S. Department of Health and Human Services, Office on Smoking and Health.

Gold, R.E. (1991). *Microcomputer Applications in Health Education*. Dubuque, IA: W.C. Brown.

Goodhart, F. (1993). Generating enthusiasm among peer educators. *Journal of American College Health, 41*(No. 6), 295.

Goodlad, J.I. (1984). *A Place Called School: Prospects for the Future*. New York: McGraw-Hill.

Goodwin, S.C. (1998). Bringing urban legends into the classroom. *Journal of School Health, 68*(No. 3), 114–115.

Greenberg, J.S. (1988). *Health Education: Learner-Centered Instructional Strategies*. Dubuque, IA: W.C. Brown.

Greene, W.H., & Simons-Morton, B.G. (1984). *Introduction to Health Education*. New York: Macmillan.

Gronlund, N. (1991). *How to Write Instructional Objectives* (4th ed.). New York: Macmillan.

Hellison, D. (1978). *Beyond Balls and Bats: Alienated (and Other) Youth in the Gym*. Washington, D.C.: AAHPER Publications.

Hoff, R. (1988). *I Can See You Naked*. New York: Andrews and McMeel.

Joyce, B., & Weil, M. (1986). *Models of Teaching*. Englewood Cliffs, NJ: Prentice-Hall.

Krathwohl, D.R., Bloom, B.S., & Masia, B.B. (1964). *Taxonomy of Educational Objectives: The Classification of Educational Goals. Handbook II: Affective Domain*. New York: David McKay.

Kreuter, M.W., Lezin, N.A., & Green, L.W. (1998). *Community Health Promotion Ideas That Work A Field-Book for Practitioners*. Sudbury, MA: Jones and Bartlett Publishers.

Lazes, P.M., Kaplan, L.H., & Gordon, K.A. (1987). *The Handbook of Health Education*. Rockville, MD: Aspen.

Loya, R. (1984). *Health Education Teaching Ideas: Secondary*. Reston, VA: American Alliance for HPERD.

Mayshark, C., & Foster, R. (1966). *Methods in Health Education*. St. Louis: C.V. Mosby.

Pfeiffer, J.W., & Jones, J.E. (1970). *A Handbook of Structured Experiences for Human Relations Training* (Vol. 2). Iowa City, IA: University Associates Press.

Pfeiffer, J.W., & Jones, J.E. (1971). *A Handbook of Structured Experiences for Human Relations Training* (Vol. 3). Iowa City, IA: University Associates Press.

Popham, W.J., & Baker, E.L. (1970). *Establishing Instructional Goals*. Englewood Cliffs, NJ: Prentice-Hall.

Raths, L., Harmin, H., & Simon, S.B. (1966). *Values and Teaching*. Columbus, OH: Charles E. Merrill.

Read, D.A., Simon, S.B., & Goodman, J.B. (1977). *Health Education: The Search for Values*. Englewood Cliffs, NJ: Prentice-Hall.

Rubinson, L., & Alles, W.F. (1984). *Health Education: Foundations for the Future*. Prospect Heights, IL: Waveland.

Scheer, J.K. (1992). *HIV Prevention Education for Teachers of Elementary and Middle School Grades*. Reston, VA: AAHE/AAHPERD.

Scott, G.D., & Carlo, M.W. (1979). *On Becoming a Health Educator*. Dubuque, IA: W.C. Brown.

Sculley, J., & Byrne, J. (1987). *Odyssey*. New York: Harper and Row.

Suess, D., Geisel, T.S., & Geisel, A. (1973). *The Lorax*. New York: Random House.

Synovitz, L.B. (1999). Using puppetry in a coordinated school health program. *Journal of School Health*, 69(No. 4), 145–147.

Taffee, S.J. (1986). *Computers in Education* (2nd ed.). Guilford, CT: Dushkin Publishing Group.

U.S. Department of Health and Human Services. (1980). *Promoting Health Preventing Disease Objectives for the Nation*. Washington, D.C.: U.S. Public Health Service.

U.S. Department of Health, Education, and Welfare. (1979). *Healthy People: The Surgeon General's Report on Health Promotion and Disease* (Publication 79-55071). Washington, D.C.: U.S. Public Health Service.

Wilgoose, C.E. (1972). *Health Teaching in Secondary Schools*. Philadelphia: W.B. Saunders.

Zannis, M.A. (1992). *Health Educators' Use of Microcomputer Technology in Graduate Programs*. Unpublished doctoral dissertation, University of Maryland, College Park, MD.

Personal Computers and the Internet

Entry-Level and Graduate-Level Health Educator Competencies Addressed in This Chapter

Responsibility III: Implementing Health Education Programs
  Competency A: Exhibit competence in carrying out planned educational programs.
  Competency C: Select methods and media best suited to implement program plans for specific learners.

Responsibility VI: Acting as a Resource Person in Health Education
  Competency A: Utilize computerized health information retrieval systems effectively.
  Competency D: Select effective resource materials for dissemination.

Responsibility VII: Communicating Health and Health Education Needs, Concerns, and Resources
  Competency C: Select a variety of communication methods and techniques in providing health information.

Note: The competencies listed above, which are addressed in this chapter, are considered to be both entry-level and graduate-level competencies by the National Commission for Health Education Credentialing, Inc. They are taken from *A Framework for the Development of Competency Based Curricula for Entry Level Health Educators* by the National Task Force for the Preparation and Practice of Health Education, 1985; and *A Competency-Based Framework for Graduate Level Health Educators,* by the National Task Force for the Preparation and Practice of Health Education, 1999.

Method Selection in Health Education

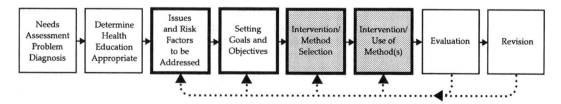

Heavy-bordered boxes indicate subjects addressed in this text; shaded boxes indicate subjects(s) of current chapter.

| OBJECTIVES | After studying this chapter the reader will be able to |

- Describe the development and importance of technology in health education.
- Summarize the steps necessary to go "online" via a personal computer.
- List the uses of a personal computer in the health education profession.
- Describe the components and process of evaluating Web sites.
- Correctly cite a source of information retrieved from a Web site.
- Describe the process involved in decoding an electronic address, or URL.
- Describe the components and process of properly using chat rooms.
- Describe the uses of distance education in health education.
- Locate the email addresses of health educators using HEDIR.

KEY ISSUES

Internet access	PCs and health education
Internet search	Distance learning
Evaluating web sites	Chat rooms
Citing Web sources	Bulletin boards

Perhaps one of the most explosive technological advances of the twentieth century has been the development of almost limitless access to information through the use of personal computers and the Internet. Less than a decade ago, searching for information about any subject usually involved a trip to a local library and a walk through the dusty stacks of books, hoping that the volume in question had not already been borrowed by another inquisitive patron. Although libraries today still fulfill an important role as providers of the printed word, even these institutions have altered their focus to include Internet access. According to a 1997 national survey of U.S. libraries, at least 60 percent of libraries provide online services to the public (Bertot, McClure, and Fletcher, 1997). Today vast numbers of individuals all over the world seeking information of all types turn as a matter of course to their personal computers and literally search the world for answers to their questions. The explosion of personal computer usage in the United States is an indicator of habits changed forever. In the mid 1980s only about 8 percent of Americans had a personal computer in their home, but by 1997 that number had increased to nearly 42 percent. In addition to home computer ownership, computer experts estimate that as many as 41.5 million American adults are regular users of the Internet and World Wide Web. Perhaps most important for health educators is the statistic that nearly 50 percent of those individuals accessing the Web are seeking information related to health issues (Eng et al., 1998).

Although many people today are now extremely facile using the Internet, it should not be assumed that all individuals share such high levels of enthusiasm, understanding, or expertise in accessing and utilizing the information superhighway. To that end, the next section of this chapter is in-

<table>
<tr><td colspan="2" align="center">**SOME VERY BASIC DEFINITIONS**</td></tr>
<tr><td>Access Provider</td><td>This is the service company that provides you access to the Internet. This service is invariably for a fee.</td></tr>
<tr><td>Browser</td><td>This is software that allows you to examine Internet resources. Examples include Netscape, Internet Explorer and America On-Line.</td></tr>
<tr><td>E-Mail</td><td>Electronic mail. Messages sent to another person using a computer. Currently no cost (above the access provider fee).</td></tr>
<tr><td>Home Page</td><td>This is the first page of an Internet site. It usually provides information on what is available at the site.</td></tr>
<tr><td>Search Engine</td><td>This is the software designed to conduct searches on the Internet. They are usually directories of resources on the Internet compiled by the company. Each uses different logic and it is important to examine how each works. Examples are Yahoo, Lycos, Webcrawler and Alta Vista.</td></tr>
<tr><td>Uniform Resource Locators (URLs)</td><td>These are the Internet addresses found on the location bars at the top or bottom of your browser.</td></tr>
<tr><td>World Wide Web</td><td>This is a collection of hypertext servers that allow text, graphics, and sound to be mixed together. It is often used as a term to describe the entire Internet, although strictly speaking, this is not accurate.</td></tr>
</table>

Figure 6-1
Some Very Basic
Definitions

tended to be useful to the uninitiated. It provides a brief description of the Internet, definitions of Internet-related terms, (see Figure 6-1), and a simple guide of how to get online. If you consider yourself to be a computer expert and a seasoned veteran of the electronic superhighway, *skip this section.*

Case Study: Robyn Robyn has been asked to facilitate a prenatal workshop for a community group of expectant mothers. Robyn has been extremely busy lately, feeling overwhelmed with the numerous projects with which she has been involved. As the evening of the workshop date arrives, she has not yet pulled together materials for her presentation. Racing against time, Robyn decides to perform a rapid Internet search for relevant resources. Her search results in a myriad of sites, of which she selects a few that look the most promising and interesting. Hastily making photocopies of the information, Robyn heads to her workshop. The session begins well, with introductions, an explanation of the purpose of the workshop and the dissemination of the first Internet-generated handout—a discussion about diet during pregnancy. Robyn's growing confidence is abruptly punctured as an astonished and increasingly irate participant loudly notes that the author of the handout was a doctor who had lost his license to practice medicine for promoting his own diet plan that was judged to be unsafe and, in two instances, potentially fatal. Robyn, obviously shocked, stammers an apology and quickly moves on to another handout, fervently hoping that lightning won't strike twice! What steps could Robyn have taken to avoid this problem? (See Case Studies Revisited page 201.)

Getting Started

To begin using the Internet you must have access to a computer, phone, and modem or other direct connection, as well as an access provider, browser, and a little knowledge. The computer doesn't necessarily have to be new or expensive, but generally it will need to have at least 32 megabytes ("megs") of RAM (a type of memory called *random access memory*) to function effectively. The brand of the computer does not matter. Today personal computers utilize one of two major types of operating systems. IBM, Dell, Compaq, and Gateway generally use a Windows format, which utilizes the Microsoft operating system. Macintosh, manufactured by Apple, uses its own operating system. Most Internet screens look pretty much the same on either operating system.

Generally, the modem needs to have a speed of at least 28.8 kilobytes (K) (most computers today come with a 56 K modem). To gain entry to the Internet, you will also need an access provider and a browser. Examples of providers include America Online, Microsoft Internet Explorer, Compuserve, your school system, a local cable television company, a university, or some other local provider. These providers will supply access using a browser such as Netscape Navigator or Internet Explorer. There is generally a charge for access ranging anywhere from $18 a month for unlimited access (fee dependent on how many months or years you sign up for) to $30 per month plus $2.95 an hour after the first five hours. Most of the examples cited are "dial up" providers that necessitate the use of a telephone line. Many cable television companies now offer an Internet connection in addition to television service. The user rents a modem and connects to the Internet through a cable, resulting in a much faster connection (no dial up) and quicker downloading but also a larger monthly fee, around $40 plus installation costs. The more expensive providers will obviously offer more services for the dollar, and as a consumer you'll have to decide whether or not you need all the "bells and whistles" or can operate effectively with a more basic service.

These provider access packages usually include an email (electronic mail) account. Email is particularly useful in that a user can send messages just about anywhere in the world in a matter of moments—a great improvement over the regular mail system, known as "snail mail" by the technology crowd. In addition, at the time of this writing, there is usually no charge for sending email above and beyond the cost of the access itself. Installing the software to begin your Internet account is usually simple and is mostly just a matter of following on-screen instructions.

Now That You Are Online

Once you have made the connection to the Internet, you have access to a wealth of information from every corner of the world. This information can range from U.S. government sources, such as the Centers for Disease Control and Prevention, census databases, and the White House, to great libraries and museums from around the globe. In addition, you can use your email connection to correspond with business contacts, friends, and relatives.

Conducting a Search

Using your browser, you can access information by entering the electronic site address, if you know it. It is important to enter the address carefully, as computers are unforgiving. You must know the exact address, including the appropriate case for all the text. If you don't know the electronic address, you can perform a search with a *search engine*, a special program (Yahoo is one) that uses the words you give it *(keywords)* to locate documents containing those words. Your browser will connect you to a search engine, and then you will often be given a choice of other engines. Each engine uses a slightly different logic to conduct searches, but basically they have all set up a directory of sites by keywords found in site addresses or site abstracts. Most of these search engines update their directories regularly, but you will find that many sites have shut down, are off-line (turned off), or are overloaded with people seeking information. Because each search engine approaches its task a little differently, using more than one search engine might prove to be an effective strategy.

Selecting a Search Engine

Browsers will generally default to a specific search engine. Remember that the default may not be the best search engine for your needs. The browser company may be receiving payment to default to a certain search engine. Select the search engine *you wish to use*. Most browsers allow you to set your own default search engine. It is also good to set up your own directory of search engines.

There are now search engines that search multiple search engines, such as Metacrawler. Macintosh has a product called Sherlock that will allow you to develop your own search engine. You can search the Internet and set up your directory on any topic much as the search engine companies do. This customized search will often take several hours to complete.

Worksheet for Internet Search

What is the topic of your search? _____

What words or phrases describe your needs? Be specific as possible.

Review the tips for the search engine you have selected.

Figure 6-2
Worksheet for Internet Search

When you are connected to the search engine, you conduct a search as you would with any library database. Enter as specific a title or term as you can. For example, entering a very general term like *cancer* will locate thousands of sites and make the examination of these search results very time-consuming. Selecting the term *breast cancer* will narrow the response but will still elicit numerous sites. Some search engines ask you to use specific syntax like ". . ." to select only sites that have *all* the terms that you stipulated. Figure 6-2 offers a worksheet for preparing a search.

Once an interesting or relevant site has been accessed, you should keep a record of the site location so that you can quickly return to that site at any time. In Netscape and some other browsers, this feature is called *Bookmarks*. In Internet Explorer it is called a *Favorite*. The next time you want to use a particular site there will be no need to search again. You will simply go to "Bookmarks" or "Favorites," select the desired site, and with one click the site will be accessed . . . unless of course its been shut down, always a possibility in the ever changing world of the Internet!

Most use boolean logic (see Figure 6-3), which looks for common words (overlapping) found in titles or abstracts. Boolean operators are AND, OR, and AND NOT. If two or more words are submitted, most engines assume an AND search and will look for listings with all words included. If this does not occur, try using quotation marks before and after a phrase and/or + signs between words. You can also use minus ($-$) signs in many searches, denoting do not include this word.

For a title search, generally typing the title of the work followed by a colon and then a keyword (or t:word) results in retrieving only documents with that word(s) in that title.

Give it a try, and if you get too many sites ("hits"), narrow your search further. Most search engines will give you a relevance score, often 0–100 or stars. Use more than one search engine, and compare the number of sites and relevance scores you obtain. Try not to get sidetracked, as you will of-

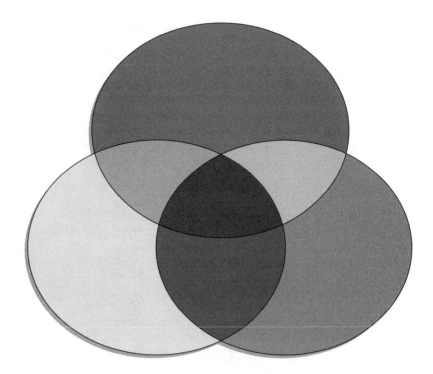

Figure 6-3
Much of the search process is based on the principle of Boolean Logic.

ten find other interesting information, and, if you're not careful, hours will pass without your having completed a thorough search. Use your time wisely!

Caveat Emptor

Although through the Internet we have the opportunity to access a wealth of current, accurate, state-of-the-art data, we can also be confronted with just the opposite . . . outdated, inaccurate, biased, controversial, and often unfounded information. Anyone who has access to the Internet can develop a Web site, and although many people assume information published on the Web to be accurate, the mere existence of a site means nothing with regard to legitimacy or objectivity. Many Web sites provide information that is vague as to its source or authorship. Some sites are blatantly biased; others appear to be legitimate but carry subtly prejudicial messages.

The Internet is a multibillion-dollar marketing tool, so users should be aware of the potential association between information and commercially marketed products. What makes the Internet unique with regard to legitimacy of information is that there is no screening device between the site developer and the user. Research or academic libraries, for example, have developed mechanisms whereby journals, books and other resources have already been evaluated for inclusion in the library as legitimate resources.

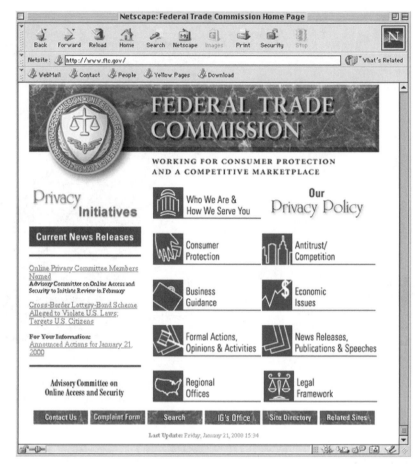

Figure 6-4
The Federal Trade
Commission Web Site.
The FTC provides con-
sumers with information
about bogus businesses
on the Internet.

When you search for information on any given topic in such a library, any
index or database that you access has been developed by a scholarly organization with an eye to maintaining strict standards of accuracy and legitimacy. No such screening device exists on the Internet; therefore, the user is
exposed to an incredible diversity of material, often ranging from the sub-
lime to the ridiculous. Clearly this is a case of *caveat emptor*, or buyer beware!

The Feds Strike Back!

The Federal Trade Commission (FTC), the government watchdog organization responsible for monitoring, among other things, false claims developed by manufacturers and distributors of health and medical products, has
created an innovative learning device. Instead of issuing boring, ineffective
warnings about being fooled by unscrupulous "snake oil salesmen," the

FTC has joined the game. A 1999 campaign has seen the FTC develop several bogus Web sites supposedly selling miracle cures and treatments like NordiCalite (weight loss), ArthritiCure (arthritis treatment), and Virility Plus (impotence) (see Figure 6-4). The screens describe the miraculous effects of the products and urge the consumer to purchase them immediately. When the consumer clicks on to the last screen to obtain the payment information, a screen explains that the Web site was developed by the FTC and is selling a nonexistent product, advising the site user that many hundreds of Web sites exist that either collect money without sending a product or sell products that have no medicinal or health value and are being supported by false or exaggerated claims. This is an extremely innovative way to use the Internet to educate consumers about the dangers of purchasing from an unknown Web site.

According to *The Washington Post* (1999) the FTC visited about 800 sites over a two-year period that contained questionable medical or health claims. The owners of these sites were sent an email warning that they were potentially violating federal law. When these same sites were rechecked some months later, approximately 62% were unchanged. Moreover, although the FTC charged 91 Internet sites with fraudulent advertising in a four-year period, the number of new sites proliferates on a daily basis. This would seem to suggest that creating more educated and sophisticated consumers might be a more productive and effective route than legal action. The FTC (1999) advises consumers to beware of marketing that includes the following techniques:

- Claiming the product will quickly cure a variety of ailments.
- Using words such as "scientific breakthrough," "secret ingredient," or "ancient remedy."
- Using impressive-sounding "medicalese."
- Claiming the government, scientists, or the medical profession have conspired to suppress the product.
- Including undocumented case histories or testimonials citing miraculous results.
- Advertising the product as available from only one source

Evaluating Internet Sites

This is an incredibly important concern given that millions of people are using the Web on a daily basis, and a high proportion of these users are seeking health-related information. Without some type of filtering device between the user and the site, how do we evaluate the legitimacy and accuracy of information obtained from the Internet, and what types of issues should users consider? A list of such criteria was developed by Betsy Richmond (1996) of the McIntyre Library at the University of Wisconsin-Eau Claire shown in Table 6-1.

Table 6-1 Ten Cs for Evaluating Internet Resources

1. *Content.* What is the intent of the content? Are the title and author identified? Is the document "juried?" Is the content "popular" or "scholarly," satiric, or serious? What is the date of the document or article? Is the "edition" current? Do you have the latest version? (Is this important?) How do you know?

2. *Credibility.* Is the author identifiable and reliable? Is the content credible? Authoritative? Should it be? What is the purpose of the information, that is, is it serious, satiric, humorous? Is the URL extension .edu, .com, .gov or .org? What does this tell you about the "publisher?"

3. *Critical Thinking.* How can you apply critical thinking skills, including previous knowledge and experience, to evaluate Internet resources? Can you identify the author, publisher, edition, etc. as you would with a "traditionally" published resource? What criteria do you use to evaluate Internet resources?

4. *Copyright.* Even if the copyright notice does not appear prominently, someone wrote, or is responsible for, the creation of a document, graphic, sound or image, and the material falls under the copyright conventions. "Fair use" applies to short, cited excerpts, usually as an example for commentary or research. Materials are in the "public domain" if this is explicitly stated. Internet users, as users of print media, must respect copyright.

5. *Citation.* Internet resources should be cited to identify sources used, both to give credit to the author and to provide the reader with avenues for further research. Standard style manuals (print and online) provide some examples of how to cite Internet documents, although standards have not yet been formally established.

6. *Continuity.* Will the Internet site be maintained and updated? Is it now and will it continue to be free? Can you rely on this source over time to provide up-to-date information? Some good .edu sites have moved to .com, with possible cost implications. Other sites offer partial free use, and charge fees for continued in-depth use.

7. *Censorship.* Is your discussion list "moderated?" What does this mean? Does your search engine or index look for all words, or are some words excluded? Is this censorship? Does your institution, based on its mission, parent organization, or space limitations, apply some restrictions to Internet use? Consider censorship and privacy issues when using the Internet.

8. *Connectivity.* If more than one user will need to access a site, consider each user's access and "functionality." How do users connect to the Internet, and what kind of connection does the assigned resource require? Does access to the resource require a graphical user interface? If it is a popular (busy) resource, will it be accessible in the time frame needed? Is it accessible by more than one Internet tool? Do users have access to the same Internet tools and applications? Are users familiar with the tools and applications? Is the site "viewable" by all Web browsers?

9. *Comparability.* Does the Internet resource have an identified comparable print or CD-ROM data set or source? Does the Internet site contain comparable and complete information? (For example, some newspapers have partial but not full text information on the Internet.) Do you need to compare data or statistics over time? Can you identify sources for comparable earlier or later data? Comparability of data may or may not be important, depending on your project.

10. *Context.* What is the context for your research? Can you find "anything" on your topic, that is, commentary, opinion, narrative, statistics and your quest will be satisfied? Are you looking for current or historical information? Definitions? Research studies or articles? How does Internet information fit in the overall information context of your subject? Before you start searching, define the research context and research needs and decide what sources might be best to successfully fill information needs without data overload.

Source: Richmond, B. (1996). *10 Cs for Evaluating Internet Resources,* McIntyre Library, University of Wisconsin-Eau Claire (richmoeb@uwec.edu). Used with permission.

NOTEWORTHY   **Internet Example: Just Who *is* Telling the Truth?**

Access the Internet and go to www.jbpub.com/healtheducation. Follow the links to read *Ten simple, compelling claims to frame arguments against drug legalization* and *A response to DEA statements.*

You will find two entirely opposite views, with point-by-point rebuttals of established government arguments related to the issue of drug legalization. Which statements are true? How can the viewpoints be so different? Surely, a government (.gov) Web site is more credible than a private organization (.org) site? Check out the statements, and you be the judge. How could you best utilize information of this type that is seemingly so contradictory?

Another way to approach a critical evaluation of Internet sites is to examine how scholars evaluate print media, then apply the same criteria to "electronic information." Elizabeth Kirk (1996) developed six basic categories of such criteria: authorship, publishing body, point of view or bias, referral to or knowledge of the literature, accuracy or verifiability of details, and currency. With Kirk's permission, we will now present these (adapted) criteria:

1. *Authorship* is perhaps the major criterion used in evaluating information. Is the author well-known in the field? Is the author a name that is recognized? If not, make sure that

- The author is mentioned in a positive fashion by another author or another person you trust as an authority.
- You found or linked to the author's Web/Internet document from another document you trust.
- The Web/Internet document you are reading gives biographical information, including the author's position, institutional affiliation and address.
- Biographical information is available by linking to another document; this enables you to judge whether the author's credentials allow him or her to speak with authority on a given topic.
- If none of the above, there exist an address and telephone number as well as an email address for the author so that further information can be requested on his or her work and professional background. An email address alone gives you no more information than you already have.

2. *The Publishing Body* should also be considered in evaluating a document. Ask the following questions to assess the role and authority of the "publisher," which in this case means server (computer) where the document is located.

- Is the name of any organization given on the document you are reading? Are there headers, footers, or a distinctive watermark that show the document to be part of an official academic or scholarly Web site? Can you contact the site Webmaster from this document?

NOTEWORTHY   ## Seal of Approval

Several organizations are trying to help with the evaluation of Internet sites. One notable example is the HONcode developed by the Health On the Net Foundation, which was established in 1996 after an international conference in Geneva on the medical use of the Internet. The code was developed to direct proper use of the Internet in sharing health information. A "seal" of approval was adopted for sites that comply with the standards. Although there are a significant number of adopters, even a brief look at Internet sources demonstrates only a small percentage of sites adhere to these rules.

- If not, can you link to a page where such information is listed? Can you tell that it is on the same server and in the same directory (by looking at the URL)?
- Is this organization suitable to address the topic at hand?
- Can you ascertain the relationship of the author and the publisher/server? Was the document that you are viewing prepared as part of the author's professional duties (and, by extension, within his or her expertise)? Or is the relationship of a casual or for-fee nature, telling you nothing about the author's credentials within an institution?
- Can you verify the identity of the server where the document resides? Internet programs such *dnslookup* and *whois* will be of help.

3. *Point of View or Bias* of the author and publisher must be kept in mind as information is rarely neutral. Because data are used in selective ways to form information, they generally represent a point of view. For this reason, when evaluating information on the Internet, it is important to examine who is providing the information. Steps for evaluating point of view are based on *authorship* or *affiliation* are as follows:

- First note the URL of the document. Does this document reside on the Web server of an organization that has a clear stake in the issue at hand?
- If you are looking at a corporate Web site, assume that the information on the corporation will present it in the most positive light.
- If you are looking at products produced and sold by that corporation, remember that you are looking at an advertisement.
- If you are reading about a political figure at the Web site of another political party, you are reading the opposition.
- Does this document reside on the Web server of an organization that has a political or philosophical agenda?
- If you are looking for scientific information on human genetics, would you trust a political organization to provide it?

4. *Referral to or Knowledge of the Literature* should be assessed. Note the context in which the author situates his or her work; it reveals what the author knows about his or her discipline. This allows you to evaluate the author's scholarship or knowledge of trends in the area under discussion. The following criteria serve as a filter for all formats of information:

- The document includes a bibliography.
- The author alludes to or displays knowledge of related sources, with proper attribution.
- The author displays knowledge of theories, schools of thought, or techniques usually considered appropriate in the treatment of his or her subject.
- If the author is using a new theory or technique as a basis for research, he or she discusses the value or limitations of this new approach.
- If the author's treatment of the subject is controversial, he or she knows and acknowledges this.

5. *Accuracy or Verifiability of Details* is an important part of the evaluation process, especially when you are reading the work of an unfamiliar author presented by an unfamiliar organization or presented in a nontraditional way. Criteria for evaluating accuracy include

- For a research document, the data that were gathered and an explanation of the research method(s) used to gather and interpret it are included.
- The methodology outlined in the document is appropriate to the topic and allows the study to be duplicated for purposes of verification.
- The documentation relies on other sources that are listed in a bibliography or includes links to the documents themselves.
- The document names individuals and/or sources that provided unpublished data used in the preparation of the study.
- The background information that was used can be verified for accuracy.

6. *Currency*, meaning the timeliness of the information, is extremely important, for some subjects. Consequently, the regularity with which the data are updated should be noted. Apply the following criteria to ascertain currency:

- The document includes the date(s) at which the information was gathered (e.g., US Census data).
- The document refers to clearly dated information (e.g., "Based on 1990 US Census data").
- Where there is a need to add data or update it on a constant basis, the document includes information on the regularity of updates.
- The document includes a publication date or a "last updated" date.
- The document includes a date of copyright.
- If no date is given in an electronic document, you can view the directory in which it resides and read the date of latest modification.

(Developed by Elizabeth E. Kirk, Electronic and Distance Education Librarian, Milton S. Eisenhower Library, The Johns Hopkins University. Used with permission.)

Understanding and Decoding URLs

One of the most important features to examine when searching for resources on the Internet is the **Uniform resource locator (URL),** which is, in effect, the electronic address of the Web site. URLs usually appear in a standard format, so, with a little information, analyzing their components is relatively straightforward. The following discussion of URLs is adapted with permission from material supplied by Elizabeth Kirk (1997).

Understanding the different elements of URLs will help you know what to expect before you click on a link. Also, you will be able to ascertain what kind of organization or institution the information is coming from. In some cases, you may be able to reconstruct someone's email address from a URL.

Here is how the URL is constructed:

Transfer protocol://servername.domain/directory/subdirectory/filename.filetype

Every URL must have at least the first two elements (the information directly before and after the //). Here are some examples:

http://milton.mse.jhu.edu:8001/research/education/url.html
ftp://milton.mse.jhu.edu/pub/research.txt
gopher://milton.mse.jhu.edu/databases/

Part One: Transfer Protocol

The first part of the URL indicates what type of information is being transferred and, usually, what port (or "door") to the server is being accessed. Here are the most common types:

- *Hypertext* (http): the standard format for the World Wide Web.
- Gopher format: text-only precursor of the Web; still good for text-based information.
- *File transfer protocol* (ftp): a computer file that is about to be sent to your computer!
- *Newsgroup* (news): something like a special-interest bulletin board.

Part Two: Servername.domain

When you perform a simple click of your mouse, your Web browser sends a message to a *server,* or computer where a Web site resides, asking it to send you information. The transfer protocol tells your computer and the server what formats of information need to be interpreted and with what particular features (e.g., "I am using Lynx, so please don't send me images"). The servername.domain is the address of the server itself: your message has to go somewhere. Most server addresses have three or sometime four parts:

- Actual name of the machine
- Domain (the institution/organization/enterprise/whatever where the machine is located).

- Domain type educational, commercial, network, organizational, governmental, military applicable only in (United States and United Kingdom).
- Country where the machine is located (not always applicable in the United States).

Most servers have a name of some kind. It is a fallacy that all Web servers are called "www." Many are, but that is simple matter of choice. The domain is key to understanding where the information is coming from. Is it an educational institution, or is it a commercial service such as Prodigy? This is an important consideration when you are trying to evaluate an electronic document. Don't forget, the Internet is vanity publishing on its largest scale. This doesn't mean that documents coming from someone's personal commercial account are not valuable: it means that you have to apply your critical thinking skills.

Part Three: Directories and Subdirectories

Once you have been admitted to a server to get to a document, or *page*, you need to know where you are going. Servers act just like your home computer: you keep your word processing program in a separate *directory* from your modem software. In fact, your computer probably keeps the processing program in a separate *subdirectory* in the word processing directory. The third part of the URL takes you directly to the directory and subdirectory where the pages you want are located.

When you see a directory or subdirectory that begins with a tilde (~) and looks like a person's name, or that follows a directory called "/users/" or "/people/" and looks like a person's name, it is probably a Web page on someone's personal Internet account. You can reconstruct the account name and address and send that person an email message. Here are some examples of how email addresses can be constructed from URLs:

URL	Email Address
http://server.state.edu/~jsmith/mypage.html	jsmith@server.state.edu
http://www.company.com/users/jsmith/metoo.html	jsmith@company.com
http://bigmachine.neighborhood.net:8001/people/jsmith/myturn.html	jsmith@bigmachine.neighborhod.net

These rules are not infallible, but they hold true most of the time. If the address is wrong, your message will be returned as "undeliverable," so you will know that the reconstructed address did not work.

Part Four: Filename.filetype

The last part of the URL specifies the individual document. If you go to the home page of any particular organization, there is a good chance that your URL does not include a file name. However, when you click on anything linking to that page, it will probably have one. Some standard file types are

- .html or .htm: *hypertext* (the standard for the Web)
- .gif, .jpg, .bmp: image types (formats of visual images)
- .zip, .tar: compressed files (proceed with caution: these are specially compressed files that will be downloaded onto your hard drive; you need to know if your computer can interpret them, and you need to have an "unzipping" utility).

(Developed by Elizabeth E. Kirk, Electronic and Distance Education Librarian, Milton S. Eisenhower Library, The Johns Hopkins University. Used with permission.)

Correctly Citing Web Sources

The Internet has become a major source of information and resources for many individuals who need to research specific topics. While the library has historically been the first research "port of call" for most people, the speed, efficiency, and global nature of the Internet has revolutionized the way research is conducted. When using the Internet you are obligated to reference materials cited just as you would for any other source (see Figure 6.5). It is unethical and usually a violation of copyright law to use the work of another

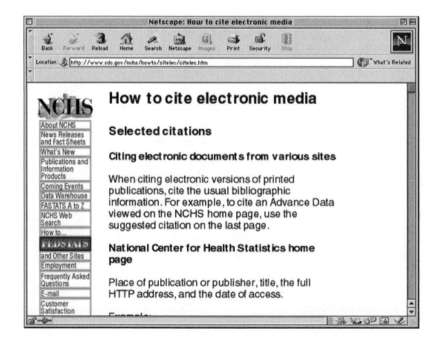

Figure 6-5
The need to cite electronic resources will become increasingly common.

without proper citation. Refer to newest version of the style manual you are using for your paper or publication. Professional researchers, scholars, and students are familiar with citing references from printed information such as journal articles, government publications, and books. However, citing information taken directly from Web sites is a relatively recent endeavor, and although it is similar in nature to traditional referencing, there are a few noticeable differences. You cite the Web site or other address used in addition to the usual information, and give the date the site was used. Some manuals recommend including the time as well. Refer to the newest version of the style manual you are using for your paper or publication.

One of the most commonly used style of references is that of the American Psychological Association (APA). The following examples are taken from the APA's Web page.

- **Journal article:** Jacobsen, J.W., Mulick, J.A., & Schwartz, A.A. (1995). A history of facilitated communication: Science, pseudoscience, and antiscience: Science working group on facilitated communication. *American Psychologist, 50,* 750–765. Retrieved January 25, 1996 from the World Wide Web: http//www.apa.org/monitor/peacea.html
- **Newspaper article:** Sleek, S. (1996, January). Psychologists build a culture of peace. *APA Monitor,* pp1, 33 [Newspaper, selected stories on line]. Retrieved January 25, 1996 from the World Wide Web: http//www.apa.org/monitor/peacea.html
- **Abstract:** Rosenthal, R. (1995). State of New Jersey v. Margaret Kelly Michaels: An overview [Abstract]. *Psychology, Public Policy, and Law, 1,* 247–271. Retrieved January 25, 1996 from the World Wide Web: http//www.apa.org/journals/ab1.html
- **Action alert posted by APA's Public Policy Office:** American Psychological Association. (1995, September 15). *APA public policy action alert: Legislation would affect grant recipients* [Announcement posted on the World Wide Web]. Washington D.C.: Author. Retrieved January 25, 1996 from the World Wide Web: http//www.apa.org/ppo/istook.html

World Wide Web pages:
Dewey, R. (1996). APA publication manual crib sheet. [On-line]. Available.[http://www.psych-web.com/resource/apacrib.htm.accessed 5/9/98.
_____ Doe, Pat T. (1996) Sentient microfilaments Home Page. [On-line].
Available:http://something.princeton.edu/pub/harnad/psyc.95.3.26/consciousness/11.html.

- **Gopher:** _____ Doe, Pat T. (1996) Sentient microfilaments: A tempest in a tubule. [On-line]. Available: gopher://somecomputer.princeton.edu/pub/harnad/psyc.95.3.26/consciousness/11/bixley.
- **Electronic correspondence** (email messages and bulletin board conversations): cite as personal communication.

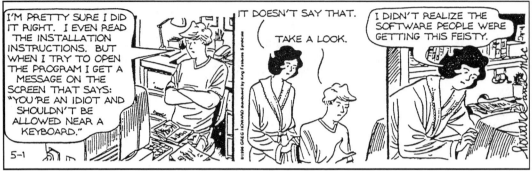

Reprinted with special permission of North America Syndicate. © 1996.

There is a place on the Web, operated by Dr. Russ Dewey, called Psych Web that has an APA Style cribsheet with how to reference on line resources.

Personal Computers, the Internet, and Health Education

Given that such revolutionary access to global information now exists, it is important to consider how this innovative tool can be effectively incorporated into the lives of health educators. Certainly all health educators should have at least a rudimentary knowledge of computer usage, as most entry-level positions require such fundamental skills. Tasks that health educators might be expected to perform using this newer technology are as follows:

Using Personal Computers
- Basic word processing functions that might range from simple reports to more complex activities such as newsletter or brochure development.
- Data collection and recording with some type of spreadsheet software.
- Presentation preparation that might include overhead transparency development, charts, graphs, and, more recently, a Powerpoint presentation (see Chapter 7).
- Utilizing health-related software, such as health risk appraisals or informational **CD-ROMS** or **DVDS**.

Using the Internet
- Researching a topic to obtain the latest data.
- Searching the Internet for Web sites that might provide differing viewpoints.
- Searching specific Web sites for archival data.
- Communicating via the Internet. This could be as basic as simple e-mail messages, talking in a chat room, posting or reading messages on a **bulletin board,** or something much more elaborate, like **distance learning** or videoconferencing.

- Reading or contributing to electronic professional journals. Many of these journals are good-quality, peer-reviewed publications that appear in an electronic format. In addition, many traditional health education journals are also accessible via the Internet, e.g., *The American Journal of Health Behavior.*

The use of computer technology has certainly created exciting learning opportunities for classroom teachers, opening up new worlds to explore in addition to enhancing the more traditional modes of learning. Peck and Dorricot (1994) offer 10 reasons why classroom teachers should use technology in the classroom, presented here with Steve Dorman's (1998) adaptation to the discipline of health education:

1. *Students learn and develop at different rates.* One tenet of health education holds that the educator must consider the individual health and learning needs of the student. Use of technology in the classroom can facilitate this goal by evaluating and assessing the health needs of the user and starting the educational activity at an appropriate level for the learner. For example, many computer-based games and learning programs are able to assess the level of competence, record the playing history, and start the user at the appropriate level of the program.

2. *Graduates must be proficient at accessing, evaluating, and communicating information.* Living in the Information Age necessitates developing skills to access and evaluate health information. The average consumer is bombarded with information. Technology makes health information ever present. However, much of the information on the Internet, for example, is not evaluated and may be subject to error. Consumers must be able to access and evaluate the quality of information. Health educators, too, must be proficient in assessing, evaluating, and communicating health information as prescribed by the competencies of the entry-level educator.

3. *Technology can foster an increase in the quantity and quality of students' thinking and writing.* Technology opens avenues for study and exploration about health, that until now would have required visiting a university campus or a major health center. The advanced information available allows the health education student to access an abundance of sources such as the Centers for Disease Control and Prevention (CDC), National Institutes of Health (NIH), and World Health Organization (WHO), which can stimulate advanced thinking about health issues and allow the student to develop more advances solutions to health issues. Access to bulletin boards and listservs allow health education students to express themselves and to critique the expressions of others. HEDIR, the student HEDIR, and HLTHPROM are listservs that stimulate discussions and writings about health education related topics.

4. *Graduates must solve complex problems.* Technology allows students to explore complex health problems that would be difficult to simulate in a classroom without technology. For example, SimHealth, a computer game developed by the Markle Foundation, enables students to explore the impact of changes in government, health manpower, funding, taxation, and politics on the health of a local community. The average individual may take years to

understand these complex relationships, yet this game presents them in a way that the user can grasp the dynamic impact they can have on health.

5. *Technology can nurture artistic expression.* Health-related graphic images such as those on the Visible Human Body Project give students access to visuals that previously were available only in the medical arena. These illustrations not only provide vital information about human anatomy but reveal the beauty of the human body in a way not seen before. In addition, with powerful software programs such as Freehand, Director 6 Multimedia Studio, and 3D Choreographer, artistically inclined students can use technology to develop health-related computer activities, animations, and videos as class projects.

6. *Graduates must be globally aware and able to use resources that exist outside the school.* The Internet, for example, allows students inexpensive and instant access to health information around the world. Whether it is information about developments in biomedicine from NIH, facts about disease transmission and epidemiology from the CDC, or late breaking news on treatment and cures from the National Library of Medicine, the Internet allows the user access to this information found outside the walls of the school.

7. *Technology creates opportunities for students to do meaningful work.* Technology provides the conduit for individuals in the health and helping professions to contact difficult-to-reach populations. Many would listen to a mass communication message on television or other media, yet would not attend a public education lecture on the same topic. Health students can use technology to assemble highly creative venues for health information, which may indeed influence health behaviors. For example, students may be involved in video production, development of a computer-assisted instruction module on a health-related topic, or assembly of a dynamic set of Web pages about a health issue.

8. *All students need access to high-level and high-interest courses.* While the teacher should not rely on technology to supplant other stimulating forms of instruction or use technological application as a placating device for bored learners, technology can provide thought-provoking and stimulating avenues of study. CD-ROMs, DVDs and laser discs, for example, provide the health education student with access to thousands of pictures of health-related issues and disorders.

9. *Students must feel comfortable with the tools of the Information Age.* The Information Age requires students to feel comfortable and proficient in ac-

---

NOTEWORTHY   **Health . . . the Internet . . . and Profit**

Former surgeon general C. Everett Koop, famous for his then radical position on HIV education and crusading attitude against the tobacco industry, recently became an Internet millionaire. Shares in the company that Dr. Koop founded were offered for public sale on Tuesday June 8, 1999, and the former surgeon general's share acquired a value of $56 million! The Web site (Drkoop.com), intended to provide medical information to the world, has over 83,000 registered users who seek understandable, reliable health information. (Washington Post, 1999a).

cessing information about health by using technology. Students must feel capable and have a high level of comfort when interfacing with computers and technology formats to access health and other information.

10. *Schools must increase their productivity and efficiency.* Technology may help schools and teachers become more productive and efficient in health instruction. For example, electronic grading devices may give teachers more time to spend with students. Currently, several computer-based grade book programs are available for free downloading to an individual's computer. Local school-based electronic bulletin boards and e-mail enable teachers to communicate easily with parents. CD-ROM technology allows teachers to implement learning stations in the health classroom, where students may engage in discovery learning at a pace on their level. Learners can be exposed to the basic facts about health by using technology, allowing the teacher to assist students with more complex tasks.

(Dorman S. 10 Reasons to Use Technology in the Classroom. *Journal of School Health* Vol. 68, No. 1, pp. 38–39. January 1998. Reprinted with permission. American School Health Association, Kent, Ohio.)

Distance Learning and Health Education

Distance learning, or *distance education,* is a term that has been with us for many years, employed whenever educators work with students over some distance. Early examples were homework help via "ham" radio in Australia and states with isolated communities like those found in Wyoming and Alaska. Later regular phone lines were used, sometimes one-on-one and at

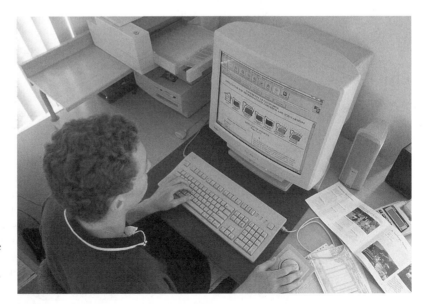

The abundance of personal computers and the Internet have made distance education a popular medium.

other times at designated centers, sometimes in groups with a speaker phone. Educational television programming was often part of the package.

The state of Wisconsin has operated an audio network for a number of years. This two-way audio network on a wide range of topics allows groups to use teleconference equipment or to interact using a phone. There were approximately 30,000 participants as of April 22, 1999.

The addition of the computer and the Internet has opened up new and exciting avenues for meeting communication needs. Generally when we refer to distance education today we are discussing Internet use, using any combination of tools and sometimes involving an entire course or workshop. Many departments of health education and programs in public health are offering such courses or workshops today. Often they supplement traditional classroom courses with activities that require use of the Internet or offer Internet sites as sources of information.

Technological problems have limited the extensive use of the Internet for distance education by health educators—namely, slow speed of transmission, poor visual reception, bandwidth limitations on standard phone line capabilities, and high cost of quality hardware. All of these limitations are being overcome. Faster phone lines are available, and cable and other access points to homes will improve the technical quality soon.

Software is now available that handles classroom chats and even examinations well. It is still very difficult to determine who is actually taking a test, however, and many institutions require some face-to-face contact when "authenticated" evaluation is an important component of the course. Drivers education is an example of a course that will require some personal contact for some time to come. At some point in the future, though, such personal contact may not be needed even in that type of course. Go to the Web site of almost any university and you will find distance education courses. You will find it interesting to examine what they offer in health education.

Chat Rooms

Most people are aware of social email chat rooms on the Internet. Such locations allow people to "talk" on the Internet, often anonymously. You enter a "room" of people with similar interests and are free to "lurk," or participate as you choose. Many people find such opportunities enjoyable and stimulating. There are chat rooms available for almost any topic. As health educators we need to be aware of the many chat rooms that are available for health information or social support. Individuals with special interests run some of these rooms, and others are operated by vendors as part of the package they sell to consumers such as America Online. As with other Internet sites, *caveat emptor* applies: "let the buyer beware." Strong cautions are in order about ever accepting any medical advice from such sources. Clearly, competent medical practitioners are not going to give a medical diagnosis over

---

Monday

Narcotics Anonymous Discussion

6:00-8:00 a.m. ET (11:00 a.m. GMT)

Host: AARF NkenaA and Friends

Keyword:A&R> A&R Chat Center: A&R's Chat Center

---

the Internet. Many vendors find such sites a good way to sell their books or other products.

Despite these cautions, it should be recognized that chat rooms can provide valuable social support to patients and family members. This can be especially true if one is in an isolated area or has a condition that is uncommon in the local community. Chat room access can be an important aid for someone caring for a patient with a serious and demanding illness or even trying to improve their personal health. For example, stop-smoking chat rooms have proved popular and helpful to many. Chat rooms are easily accessible through most vendors and generally have posted schedules of meeting times. Health issues are common subjects for chat rooms. Many health organizations run chat rooms. Examples are Narcotics Anonymous, Alcoholics Anonymous, and Sex & Love Addicts Anonymous.

Case Study: Pat   Pat finds a chat room on cancer. He is an observer for a couple of hours and then asks for information about his colon cancer. Quickly he receives recommendations regarding treatment centers. He also gets a recommendation to stop his current chemotherapy and to begin "inversion therapy." He is referred to the impressive looking Web page of a Dr. Jacob Samm. According to Dr. Samm, "inversion therapy" is proven to eliminate many cancers, including his form of cancer. The focus of the treatment is an apparatus that allows users to hang upside down at least twice a day. Pat really is unhappy with the side effects of his current therapy and decides that the new therapy would be worth a try for a few months. What are the obvious dangers of Pat's use of the Internet? (See Case Studies Revisited page 201.)

Example: Positive Use of Chat Rooms   Thomas lives in an isolated area of Nebraska and has been caring for his grandmother who has been diagnosed with Alzheimer's disease. Day after day of working on his farm and looking after his grandmother has him tired, and concerned that he is thinking ill of this woman he loves. He wonders if he is turning into an evil person because he has feelings that he thinks of as selfish—for example, wondering why he must be the one to constantly care for this woman. He attends a workshop on care of Alzheimer's patients run by a health educator that suggests that he join a chat room of like caregivers. After joining the chat room he is surprised and relieved to hear many other

Find each site on the Internet and enter the url (complete address). Good hunting!

SITE/ADDRESS	URL/ADDRESS
Home Page of Mark Kittleson (health educator)	
MMWR	
Robin Sawyer E-Mail address (health educator)	
New York University Professional resources–job postings in Community Health Education	
Maryland Dept. of Health Education	
NCHEC–National Commission for Health Education Credentialing, Inc.	
The Youth Risk Behavior Surveillance System (YRBS)	
HEDIR list serve Directory for NC	
ECU Department of Health Education and Promotion	
SRA's Grantsweb	
Go Ask Alice–ROHPNOL	
Ann Rose's Ultimate Birth Control Links Provide a proper APA citation of some located information here:	
Largest Ph.D. Graduating class in 1995. Hint try Glen Gilbert home page under Council.	
Dr. Koop Community information on Hepatitis C	

Figure 6-6
Health Internet
Scavenger Hunt

caregivers express similar feelings. He finds the chat room helps him greatly with tips on helping his grandmother and on and improving his self-esteem. He eventually even becomes one of the contributors.

Bulletin Boards

Sites where you can post questions and later come back to read the replies, or where you post a note and ask people to respond to you directly, are called *bulletin boards.* They are often topic specific, and many deal with health issues. These are set up much like chat rooms except that you can add and review comments whenever you wish.

Finding Colleagues

The Internet has expanded our ability to locate colleagues and people of similar interests. Most search engines now have databases of phone numbers, email addresses, and postal addresses. Most are a collection of available phone directories and assorted email directories. Find the option with the search engine usually labeled something like "people find" or "white pages," and enter the name and any other information you have on the individual. It will provide a list of possible matches. It is fun to look for a long-lost friend or colleague. You may need to use several different search engines. One of the authors recently looked up his own address and found that most directories listed where he had lived and worked two years ago. Only by using the fourth search engine did he find the correct information.

Technology Pioneers in Health Education

 Health educators have a great resource thanks to the work of Mark Kittleson. Dr. Kittleson has set up a home page for health education with many useful features. Included at his site are the following:

1. A directory of health educators.
2. A directory of health educators by state and country.
3. A listserv (HEDIR) for practicing health educators.
4. Job openings.
5. Archived messages from the listserv.
6. An electronic journal for health educators.
7. A chat room for health educators.

If you are looking for a health educator who uses technology, this is a great place to find a current address. Indeed, Kittleson's site is a must-see for any health educator!

Another pioneer in the use of technology by health educators is Michael Pejsach. He created the Health Education Electronic Forum before most health educators were ready to use it. Dr. Pejsach did much to raise awareness of health educators to the technology possibilities, but little use was made of the original service. The new HEEF site is on the Internet and offers much potential. All health educators should review his new site.

Videoconferencing

Videoconferencing has been with us for sometime. Typically rooms are set up to handle a group of people who are linked to other sites that are similarly set up. The result is a sort of town meeting atmosphere where you can see and

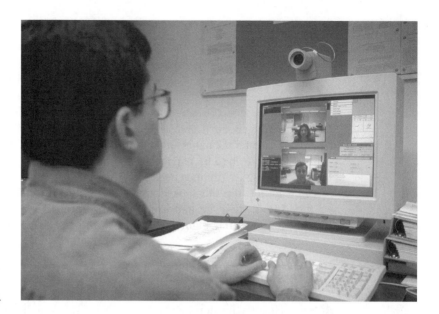

With the right equipment, video conferencing can save the time and money of traveling.

talk with others. Such sites are common at universities, community colleges, businesses, and many hotels. In addition, vendors often set up a site on a temporary basis for a special topic. Videoconferencing has become a common mode of operation to cut down on the costs and time required for travel.

A new twist on videoconferencing has come with the lowering of costs for hardware. Small digital cameras can now be purchased for as little as $75 (black-and-white) that will allow see-you-see-me conversations at any workstation so equipped. Compatible software is required and, of course, an Internet provider. Often this communication involves no long-distance charges since it uses the Internet. This holds true if it is involves the next state or a distant country. The quality varies greatly depending on the speed of connection and the quality of the camera and other hardware. The reliability is still questionable, especially for low-end systems, but future advances will no doubt improve quality.

 For more information and tools related to this chapter visit www.jbpub.com/healtheducation.

EXERCISES

1. Select any health topic and perform *two* searches using different search engines (e.g. Yahoo, Lycos, Alta Vista, Webcrawler, etc.). See how different the results of your search are, based on the first 20 sites listed by each search engine.

2. Using the evaluation criteria described in this chapter, access and evaluate five Web sites of your choice.

3. Select a health topic that might be deemed by some people to be controversial. Conduct a search on this topic, and try to identify two sites that offer opposite viewpoints. In your opinion, which site appears to be the most credible, and why?

4. Access an electronic health-related journal, then read and critique in writing any article that you choose from the journal. Do you notice any differences between the electronic article and its more traditional paper relative?

5. Select a health topic of interest, and use the Internet to see if you can obtain the most recent incidence or prevalence data for that particular topic. What is the source for your data, and would you consider it reliable?

6. Locate the email addresses and Web sites of the authors of the textbook.

7. Locate chat rooms for prostate cancer and breast cancer.

8. Find the Web site for HEDIR, and determine what role students can play in the listserv.

9. Examine the distance education offerings of your campus. Find a health education course similar to this one on the Internet. What do you see as the strengths and weaknesses of such courses?

10. Complete the Health Internet Scavenger Hunt found at www.jbpub.com/healtheducation.

CASE STUDIES REVISITED

Case Study Revisited: Robyn

Robyn clearly felt overextended and preoccupied as she prepared materials for her workshop. This may have just been a bad day for her, or it may have been indicative of a chronic problem with leaving things until the last moment. Robyn's dilemma cannot be blamed on the Internet; however, this case provides an excellent example of the dangers of collecting information from a Web site without evaluating the source. Following the evaluative steps discussed in this chapter cannot guarantee that information gleaned from the Web will always be absolutely correct, but had Robyn performed even a cursory evaluation of the Web sites, she might have avoided what must have been total humiliation and loss of face. The mere existence of a Web site is in no way indicative of legitimacy . . . check the source! (See page 177.)

Case Study Revisited: Pat

After a month of "inversion therapy," Pat is not feeling well. He returns to his physician, who says the cancer has progressed far more than expected. Probing, she learns of Pat's self-treatment. She encourages him to go back to his chemotherapy and warns him of the dangers of self-treatment. The physician also discusses the proper use of the Internet and even encourages such use and sharing of information. She also says Pat can use "inversion therapy" if he wants to as long as it does no harm but explains that she is ethically bound to inform him that she knows of no study that supports the claims of the treatment. She seems relieved when he says he will stay with chemotherapy and drop the "inversion therapy." Later Pat learns that Dr. Samm has a Ph.D. in geology and makes "inversion therapy" equipment in his basement. (See page 197.)

SUMMARY

1. The information explosion that occurred mostly in the 1990s has created an "age of information," and health educators need to be proficient and comfortable using this new medium to their best advantage.

2. The Internet offers a wealth of information sources that represent a great opportunity for all users. However, unlike written resources, most materials placed on the Internet are virtually unregulated in any way, and users need to develop evaluative skills to protect themselves from erroneous, misleading, and biased information.

3. Through the use of technology, teachers, presenters, and workshop facilitators have an outstanding opportunity to expand the world of their students/participants. Health educational professionals need to become familiar with as many facets of this technology as possible.

4. When using the Internet for research purposes, health educators should be able to effectively assess the legitimacy of the information and correctly cite the source of information.

REFERENCES

American Psychological Association. (1998). How to cite information from the Internet and the World Wide Web. Retrieved March 18, 1999 from the World Wide Web: http//www.apa.org

Bertot, J.C., McClure, C.R., Fletcher, P.D. (1997). The 1997 National Survey of US Public Libraries and the Internet, [Online]. Available: http://www.ala.org/oitp/programs.html

Dorman, S.M. (1998). 10 reasons to use technology in the classroom. *Journal of School Health 68*(1), 38–39.

Dorman, S.M. (1999) Technology briefs: Cookies—Tricks or treats? *Journal of School Health, 69*(2), 82.

Eng, T., Maxfield, A., Patrick, K., Deering, M., et al. (1998). Access to health information and support: A public highway or a private road? *Journal of the American Medical Association, 280*, 1371–1375.

Federal Trade Commission (1999). Beware false marketing techniques. Retrieved July 1, 1999 from the World Wide Web: http//www.ftc.gov.

Gilbert, G.G., Sawyer, R., & Mardon, B.F. (1997). Using the Internet in health and physical education in Maryland. *Maryland Journal of Health, Physical Education, Recreation and Dance.*

Kirk, E.E. (1996). Evaluating information found on the Internet. Retrieved March 15, 1999 from the World Wide Web: http//milton.mse.jhu.edu:8001/research/education/net.html

Kirk, E.E. (1997). Understanding and decoding URLs. Retrieved March 15, 1999 from the World Wide Web: http/milton.mse.jhu.edu:8001/research/education/net.html

Peck, K.L. and Dorricot, D. (1994). Why use technology? *Education Leader 51*(7), 11–14.

Richmond, B. (1996). 10 Cs for evaluating Internet resources. Retrieved March 15, 1999 from the World Wide Web: http//www.uwec.edu/Admin/Library/10cs.html.

Washington Post (1999a). Web site makes Koop an IPO millionaire. Business section, p. 1.

Washington Post (1999b). U.S. aims to help e-buyers beware. Health section, p. 7.

Using Media and Common Audiovisual Equipment

Entry-Level and Graduate-Level Health Educator Competencies Addressed In This Chapter

Responsibility III: Implementing Health Education Programs
Competency A: Exhibit competence in carrying out planned educational programs.
Competency C: Select methods and media best suited to implement program plans for specific learners.

Responsibility VI: Acting as a Resource Person in Health Education
Competency A: Utilize computerized health information retrieval systems effectively.
Competency D: Select effective resource materials for dissemination.

Responsibility VII: Communicating Health and Health Education Needs, Concerns and Resources
Competency C: Select a variety of communication methods and techniques in providing health information.

Note: The competencies listed above, which are addressed in this chapter, are considered to be both entry-level and graduate-level competencies by the National Commission for Health Education Credentialing, Inc. They are taken from *A Framework for the Development of Competency Based Curricula for Entry Level Health Educators* by the National Task Force for the Preparation and Practice of Health Education, 1985; and *A Competency-Based Framework for Graduate Level Health Educators,* by the National Task Force for the Preparation and Practice of Health Education, 1999.

Method Selection in Health Education

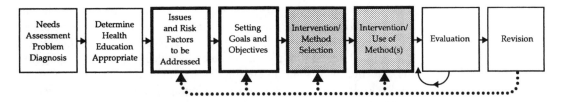

Needs Assessment Problem Diagnosis → Determine Health Education Appropriate → Issues and Risk Factors to be Addressed → Setting Goals and Objectives → Intervention/ Method Selection → Intervention/ Use of Method(s) → Evaluation → Revision

Heavy-bordered boxes indicate subjects addressed in this text; shaded boxes indicate subjects(s) of current chapter.

OBJECTIVES
After studying the chapter the reader will be able to

- Describe the major advantages and disadvantages of using each media method.
- Present a rationale for using a particular form of media, including how that medium complements the overall learning objectives.
- Develop a personal checklist for media evaluation.
- Describe the major steps involved in media development.

KEY ISSUES

Major types of media	CD-ROM and photo-CD
Films	Personal computers
Videotapes	Overhead projectors
Videodiscs	Selecting and evaluating media
Slide projectors	Media development
Filmstrips	Presentation software
Media literacy	

Case Study: Jason   The room was hot and dark. Jason was trying to count the number of dust motes as they slowly passed in front of the projector's rays of light. At a subconscious level, he could hear the narrator's voice droning on interminably about the effects of alcohol on the liver, but even a pictorial switch from talking head to a grossly abused and swollen liver was insufficient to disturb Jason's reverie. Sure, he saw the offending organ, glistening on the marble slab . . . sure, he could hear the narrator listing the dangers of an intemperate lifestyle . . . but Jason wasn't actually in the room. The warmth and darkness had transported him to a far more interesting place . . . his imagination. The football game this weekend . . . the party at Scott's place . . . catching that new movie . . . much more interesting than the talking head who had just returned to the screen. The visual switch was enough to make Jason briefly wonder why all talking heads wore white coats and sported haircuts from the 1960s . . . not that it really mattered; it was back to the party for him! Boy, the party was crowded—was everyone in the room counting dust motes and partying? . . . an alarming prospect! (See Case Studies Revisited page 228.)

Community health, school health, small groups, large groups, school children, or senior citizens—no matter what the setting or clientele, the health educator will usually use some form of audiovisual equipment or media. Devices aimed at optimizing the effectiveness of presentations are numerous, and the past decade has seen incredible technological advances, providing the presenter with some interesting choices. The following section is intended to describe the available types of equipment and help the potential user grasp some of the advantages and disadvantages of each one.

Major Types of Media

Videotapes The most common form of videotapes used today are one-half-inch VHS. Three-quarter-inch VHS tapes are more frequently used in high quality professional settings where production values are essential, and beta-type tapes are rarely used anywhere today. If you are using a videotape in a presentation or class, always check ahead of time to ensure that you will be using the correct type of machine.

Videotape usage enjoyed an incredible expansion during the 1980s and early 1990s. Videotapes are widely used in school and community health settings, and many private households now also have VCRs. The medium of videotape has clearly supplanted the 16 mm film as the most common audiovisual aid in education today. The advent of the videodisc might ultimately lead to the videotape's demise, but until the equipment necessary to play the discs becomes more commonplace, the videotape will remain an integral part of educational presentations. Its advantages and disadvantages are as follows:

Advantages
1. Videotapes are very easy to use, and because many individuals use videotapes at home, professional use has become simplified.
2. Videotape prices are cheaper than 16 mm film, usually costing from $125 to $350 for a 20 or 30 minute tape.
3. If a videotape has actually been shot in a 16 mm film format and then transferred to videotape, the videotape will have most of the quality of film without the expense.
4. Health education videotapes are becoming more plentiful, so the information depicted is more likely to be current.
5. Video cameras are now becoming more affordable, and when such technology is available in health education settings, the potential for incorporating self-generated videotapes is immeasurable (e.g. videotaping presentation styles, modeling the behavior of saying "no" to drugs, negotiating safer sex).

Disadvantages
1. Unless a video projector is available, showing videotapes to large groups is very difficult. Multiple monitors can be used, but setting up the machines becomes complicated, time-consuming, and often results in a less than satisfactory performance.
2. Videotape players and television monitors are not very portable, so the health educator is dependant on such equipment being available at the site of the presentation. Such equipment is *not* always available . . . and when it is, it sometimes doesn't work!

Videodiscs The most recent technological advance that has tremendous potential in enhancing health education delivery is the videodisc, the latest, most sophisticated type being the digitized version (**DVD**). Although current use is some-

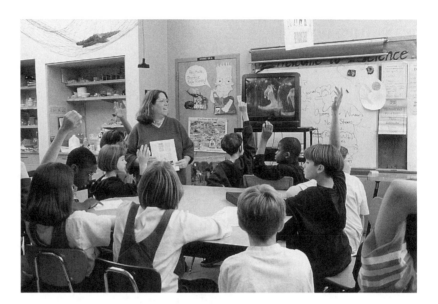

Videotapes are a cheap and easy method to bring new information into your classroom.

what limited, this form of media may eventually supersede the videotape as the most commonly used audiovisual instructional aid. Its advantages and disadvantages are as follows:

Advantages

1. Instructors have more options of how to use a videodisc than they would have with a regular videotape. For example, the disc can be stopped and then restarted at any point the instructor selects. Fast-forwarding or reversing a videotape to find a certain spot can be a lengthy and often frustrating experience.

2. Quite often, the videodiscs are designed to encourage frequent pauses to allow for discussion. This is particularly useful for reinforcing cognitive information and permitting processing of affective ideas. It is also a major advantage for instructors dealing with groups who have short attention spans!

3. Perhaps the greatest advantage of the videodisc is its interactive nature. This allows learning to be less of a spectator sport and more of a mutual endeavor. Groups can interact with the program in a community or classroom setting, or programs can be utilized that focus on the individual. The individual focus is particularly useful when dealing with sensitive, personal issues such as human sexuality and drug abuse.

4. Increasingly, videodiscs are being produced with two soundtracks, one in English and another in a second language, usually Spanish.

5. Because this technology is relatively new, the programs that exist tend to be more current than some of the other forms of instructional materials.

6. The sound and picture quality of the DVD is outstanding and far surpasses the quality a videotape can offer.

Disadvantages

1. Like most new technology, the cost of the equipment can be quite expensive. However, as this medium becomes more commonly used, the cost of purchase is likely to decrease.
2. Some individuals may be a little intimidated at first about operating the videodisc player. However, most instructors report few problems with using videodiscs after becoming familiar with the equipment and materials.
3. As with the videotape player and television monitor, this equipment is not very portable. However, videodiscs can be played on many laptop computers and used in conjunction with the most recent videoprojectors, which are both small and relatively light, so portability is fast becoming less of an issue.

Overhead Projector

The overhead projector has been used for many years in both the school and community setting. As a means to display both text and graphic information, this instructional media has proved both effective and enduring. Its advantages and disadvantages are as follows:

Advantages

1. Overhead projectors allow the instructor to display detailed information to relatively large groups.
2. Information being displayed can be changed or modified while audience is watching.
3. Overhead projectors are very easy to use.
4. Overhead transparencies are easy and inexpensive to prepare and can even be made on most photocopying machines.
5. The newer overhead projectors are quite compact and easy to transport and maintain.

Disadvantages

1. Along with an overhead projector the instructor will need to use some type of screen or find a very white wall.
2. Use of the projector necessitates semi-darkness. This has the potential for cutting off the speaker from the audience and in the classroom setting can initiate disruption.
3. Although overhead transparencies are easy to prepare, the preparation is somewhat of an art. Often individuals will try to place too much information on a single overhead or use print that is too small and difficult to read.
4. Poor transparencies and too much factual data produce boredom. To many students or workshop participants, overhead projectors and boredom are synonymous!

Presentation Software

Imagine a really slick, colorful, sophisticated, personalized, easily operated set of overhead transparencies and you will have the sense of what presentation software can provide. To continue the media analogy, presentation software is to the overhead what the DVD is to the videotape. . . more sophisticated, professional, and definitely more impressive. There are different types of available presentation software, but Microsoft's Powerpoint is by far the most used and has become the accepted standard. Powerpoint allows the user to basically custom-create a set of slides or transparencies for use in a presentation. The program provides a set of templates with many different features, including subtle backgrounds, interesting title styles, and organizational choices. The ideal use of such a program is to store the presentation materials on a disc or hard drive, then connect a computer to a video/computer projector to display the materials with the click of a mouse. If a computer/projector setup is not available, with the use of a color printer, Powerpoint materials can be used to develop overhead transparencies. Simply print the materials directly onto transparencies. Although your presentation may not look quite as polished as the computer/projector version, you will still have a set of very professional-looking overhead transparencies. Advantages and disadvantages of presentation software are as follows:

Advantages

1. Presentation software allows the instructor to custom-develop his or her own materials.
2. Using either the computer/projector or overhead projector, the instructor will be able to easily show materials to small or large groups.
3. Materials developed with Powerpoint look very professional.
4. Overhead transparencies are relatively inexpensive to prepare.
5. The computer/projector setup is becoming more feasible as both the price and size of computers and projectors become smaller.

Disadvantages

1. Using either a computer or an overhead projector, the instructor will need to use some type of screen or find a very white wall.
2. Use of either form of projector necessitates semi-darkness. This has the potential for cutting off the speaker from the audience and in the classroom setting can initiate disruption.
3. The development of Powerpoint presentations necessitates access to both a computer and available software, in addition to a reasonable amount of computer experience.
4. Although laptop computers are readily available and projectors are becoming more portable, the inconvenience of transporting expensive and sometimes awkward equipment should still be considered a disadvantage.
5. Again, although the cost of computer equipment has steadily fallen into the relatively affordable range, the initial outlay for both hardware and software could, in some cases, be prohibitive.
6. Despite advertising to the contrary, learning to use Powerpoint will take some time and effort, which is sometimes too great a barrier for many individuals.

Slide Projector

Slide projectors have been around for quite some time and continue to be an extremely useful way to disseminate information. To a major extent, this particular medium has taken the place of the film strip. Slides can be produced for use with presentation software like Powerpoint, and most photo shops will produce slides from a computer disc. Advantages and disadvantages of slide projectors are as follows:

Advantages

1. Perhaps the greatest advantage of the slide projector is that you can develop your own slides to suit your particular purposes. This allows you to tailor presentations specifically to your goals, rather than adapting less suitable material.
2. Written material and tables can be displayed on a large screen, making visibility for the audience very easy.
3. The order of presentation can be easily changed, and previous slides can be revisited with little difficulty.
4. Slides of just about anything can be made, so information from books, magazine advertisements, newspaper headlines, and so forth, can all be used in a very creative manner.
5. Slide projector use is very common, so there are many pre-prepared slide programs available.
6. Slide projectors are usually fairly light and therefore extremely portable. . . an obvious advantage for moving from classroom to classroom or traveling to a community presentation.

Disadvantages

1. Although slide projectors are usually fairly reliable, maintenance and repair costs can be quite high.
2. Although preparing your own slides has great potential value, the cost of slide preparation can be very high, particularly if slides are being made from magazine advertisements or other graphics.
3. Some people find using a slide projector fairly difficult, particularly in getting the image to be the right way up! Ideally, you should load your slides and test that you have them correctly positioned in the slide carousel *before* beginning the lesson/presentation. This will also allow you to appropriately focus the projector.
4. Slides do have the potential of being very boring, and with the lights necessarily being lowered, the potential exists for behavior problems in a classroom setting or lack of interest in a community setting.
5. The need for a screen is an added complication.

Personal Computers

Personal computer technology has advanced at an incredible rate over the past 20 years, and the computer has become a legitimate health education instructional tool in both the school and community settings. Computer applications are diverse, including small-group or individualized usage and spanning a full range of interest areas from health assessments, health education games and puzzles, to statistical analysis. Portable projector systems are also becoming more available through purchase or rental to complement the computer and increase its utility. (For more complete information on the computer, see Chapter 6.)

Gold and Duncan (1980) stress the usefulness of the personal computer as a motivational device:

> One of the most basic ways in which the computer may serve as a motivational device is through the use of self-assessment programs. Widely used among such approaches are the computerized dietary analysis models. These programs allow the student to input information concerning what they eat (on a single day or combination of days) and receive in return some output which identifies how well they have met some set of dietary standards. Such programs can provide an excellent introduction to the study of nutrition by developing and focusing student interest. We have made similar use of a life stress measurement program to introduce a unit on stress and life expectancy prediction.

Advantages and disadvantages of personal computers are as follows:

Advantages
1. Computers offer an incredibly diverse set of possibilities for use in health education, ranging from complicated statistical analysis to elementary school level health education games.
2. Many modern personal computers are now much easier to use than previous models, allowing access to children and fearful adults.
3. Computers can be fun to use and of particular value in the classroom as a motivational tool.
4. Computers can allow individual usage that permits working on personal programs where privacy might be a concern.

Disadvantages
1. Although greatly reduced in price compared to a few years ago, computers are still relatively expensive, and therefore accessibility will be limited.
2. The format of one computer per person is unlikely to be possible, and having three or four individuals crowded around one terminal can become frustrating and disruptive.
3. Computer equipment can be vary greatly from one machine or piece of software to the next. Some individuals may be expert on one type of machine yet total novices on another type. Learning can be difficult with such differing levels of skill and experience.
4. Some health educators rely on the technology to accomplish health education instead of viewing it as an additional tool in their repertoire.

The Dinosaur Section

The rapid pace of technological change inevitably consigns some of the older forms of media to the proverbial scrap heap. However, in the rare likelihood that some hapless health educator finds him or herself confronted by such dinosaurs, we have not completely obliterated from this text the existence of these "not so new" forms of media!

Film

Before the rapid development of the videotape, film usage (usually 16 mm) with the standard film projector was perhaps the most common form of audiovisual aid used in both school and community health education. Since the advent of the videotape, the use of the film projector has become much less common. It is important to realize, however, that although fewer films and projectors are being used today, many instructional materials are still being filmed in 16 mm before being transferred to the videotape format for distribution. If you have a high-quality film not available as a video, explore the possibility of having the film converted to a videotape. Advantages and disadvantages of film are as follows:

Advantages

1. Film is easy to show to relatively large audiences.
2. Film tends to be a more emotive medium than videotape.
3. Film projectors tend to be somewhat more portable than a VCR and television monitor.

Disadvantages

1. Films tend to be very expensive, often nearly double the price of videotapes.
2. Fewer and fewer films are available in a 16 mm film format; consequently, many existing materials are out of date.
3. Many individuals find loading a projector somewhat intimidating, and a projector is usually more difficult to use than a VCR.
4. Projector maintenance can be very expensive, particularly on older machines, which are more prone to mechanical failure.
5. The use of film necessitates finding an available screen or very white wall.

Film Strips

Film strips were commonly used in the school setting until more sophisticated media like the slide projector became more readily available. They are now used sparingly and are most likely to be found in the elementary school setting. Advantages and disadvantages of film strips are as follows:

Advantages

1. Film strips usually come complete with teaching guides and often include accompanying audiotapes that provide a narration.
2. Film strip projectors are small, light, and very portable.
3. Film strip projectors are usually very simple to use.
4. Film strips are generally, very low in cost.

Disadvantages

1. Many of the film strips available today are out of date.
2. Many of the film strip projectors in use are very old and do not provide projection of a very high quality.

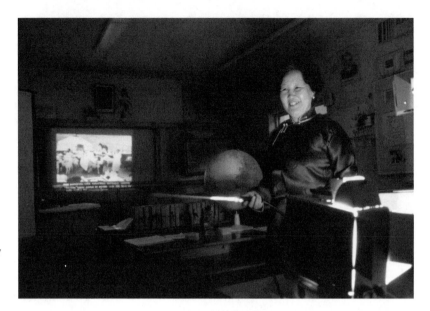

Film strip use is almost extinct, but occasionally they are still found in elementary school settings.

3. As with the slide projector, the static nature of the film strip and surrounding darkness of the room can have a high potential for boredom, particularly if the film strip is old and not very inspiring.
4. Again, the need for a screen is an added complication.

Preparing Visual Materials

Seven specific problems to avoid when preparing visual materials follow (Figures 7-1 and 7-2 illustrate a poor use of graphics and good use respectively):

1. Beware of using a tiny font size. Many presenters simply copy their notes onto a transparency for use with groups, thus importing a size 12 font that may look fine on a printed page but proves unrecognizable from the back of a large room! Always increase font size to at least 16 or 18, particularly when using smaller fonts like Times.
2. If you ever hear yourself saying, "You probably can't read this, but . . ." you probably shouldn't be showing the transparency. If people can't read what you have provided, you either need to redo the transparency, making it legible, or think of another way of presentation without the fairly useless visual.
3. The rainbow effect is undesirable. Some presenters equate lots of color with high-quality visuals, but instead of being impressive, overly colorful materials are distracting and difficult to read. The rule of thumb is to keep things simple and clear. Color can be very effective . . . just don't overdo it!

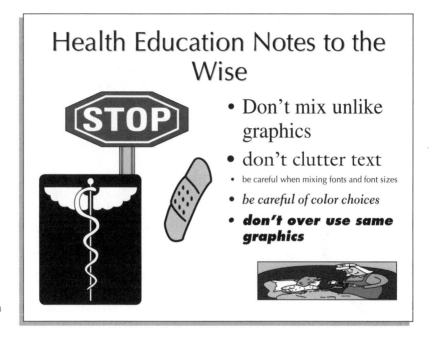

Figure 7-1
Disorganized Clutter.
Poor use of graphics can
confuse the viewer.

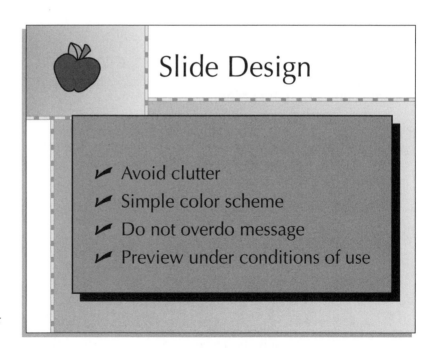

Figure 7-2
An Organized Design.
An organized use of
graphics can help the
viewer understand your
message.

4. Busy, busy, busy . . . some transparencies have way too much material on them and are so crammed with information that they become overwhelming and ultimately confusing. Rather than trying to put literally everything on the screen, limit the type of material you put on any transparency to core issues and essentials, adding to and expanding information from your narrative. Most people are easily bored and do not want to look at the same transparency for very long, so have more, shorter transparencies rather than fewer, complex images.

5. More busy, busy, busy . . . in addition to too much material, some presenters tend to confuse the inclusion of a logo or background image common to all the transparencies, with sophistication and quality. Logos or icons can prove to be very distracting and detract from the message. Keep things simple and clear.

6. Avoid using too many font changes. Some transparencies look like a ransom note—as if the presenter couldn't decide which font to use, so decided to use them all! Unless you need to change font types to make a specific point, be consistent with the appearance of the transparency, again to avoid detracting from the material itself.

7. Keep it simple. The visual aids that you develop should be just that, aids to complement your presentation, not a colorful extravaganza to advertise the fact that you've just got a new computer! Develop and use only what will enhance your presentation, and avoid bombarding the audience with too much material that ultimately may swallow up the point of your presentation.

Selecting and Evaluating Media

The selection of films, videotapes and other media forms is crucially important, particularly in health education. All too often, audiovisual materials are used for the wrong reasons. For example:

- Because the film has *always* been used for a certain topic.
- To fill a blank space on the schedule.
- Because a particular videotape is the only one available.
- Because a film is the only one that can be afforded.
- Because the topic is applicable, even though the level of the material is inappropriate.

Although these reasons for using audiovisual materials may seem obviously inappropriate, they occur frequently. Historically, very little systematic thought has been given to the selection and evaluation of media. Campeau (1974), in a review of research on the uses of audiovisual materials, bemoaned the rather dubious criteria for selecting such programs:

> All indications are that decisions as to which audiovisual devices to purchase, install, and use have been based on administrative and organizational requirements and on considerations of costs, availability, and user preference, not on evidence of instructional effectiveness (p.31).

There have been some early attempts to somehow objectively evaluate media, particularly in the area of drug education. The Audiovisual Group of the Addiction Research Foundation (ARF) provided a rating of films based on the following nine criteria (Fejer et al., 1972):

1. The scientific accuracy of information presented.
2. Its merits as a teaching aid.
3. Whether or not it was contemporary.
4. The clarity of the message.
5. Whether or not it could influence attitudes.
6. Its believability.
7. Its technical merits.
8. Whether or not it maintained interest.
9. Whether or not it was applicable to individuals from different social strata.

Although this early effort at least provided some basic guidelines for audiovisual material selection, the ambiguity of its components are obvious. It is not within the scope of this text to document further specific audiovisual research in health education, but a review of the literature clearly denotes a paucity of meaningful evaluation . . . a sad commentary, particularly in the light of how frequently such materials are used today.

To aid the health educator in choosing the most appropriate media materials, a helpful evaluation checklist has been designed:

1. Media objectives
2. Level
3. Language
4. Content
5. Culture
6. Time/duration of media
7. Cost
8. Interest level
9. Production quality
10. Evaluation
11. Availability
12. Format
13. Approval

MEDIA EVALUATION CHECKLIST

Media Objectives	___
Level of Media	___
Language	___
Content	___
Culture/Ethnicity	___
Time/Duration of Media	___
Cost	___
Interest Level	___
Production Qualities	___
Evaluation of Media	___
Availability	___
Format	___
Approved Material	___
Others	

Figure 7-3 Media evaluation checklist.

This checklist is by no means exhaustive, and additional categories could be added, but those included here are some basic principles to consider when selecting media materials. Let us examine each of these in detail, bearing in mind that the order of the items implies no ranking. For a more comprehensive and complicated media rating system, health educators should examine a scale called "An Analysis Checklist for Audiovisuals" developed by Martin and Stainbrook (1986).

Media Objectives

Will the materials used fulfill or facilitate achieving the objective(s) of the presentation? All too often materials are chosen because they are topic appropriate, and yet they may do little to achieve objectives. For example, in AIDS education, films depicting factual information about the disease or showing interviews of people with AIDS have traditionally been shown in school and community settings in an attempt to elicit attitude and sexual behavior change. Using cognitive information may well improve knowledge levels, but such an approach does little to influence attitude or behavior. If attitude change is an objective—perhaps in this case, in dealing with AIDS education, the objective might be to increase perceived susceptibility to HIV—then the film selected should be affective in nature and not didactic. If a simple increase in knowledge is the objective, then the factual film is appropriate. Clearly, an awareness of specific objectives is crucial to media selection.

One condition that has exacerbated this problem is that until relatively recently the vast majority of available media materials has been of the factual variety, thus perpetuating the axiom of "if that's all there is, then we'll have to use it!" On many occasions using nothing is more appropriate than using ineffective, inappropriate materials! Since factual information can be addressed through many different methods, using media to address affective or other more difficult objectives can often be a useful strategy.

Level   Is the level of the material suitable for the audience? It is important to consider the learning styles and levels of the audience when considering media materials. If the material is either too complex and difficult or too simplistic, the audience may become, respectively, frustrated or uninterested. Again, the availability of level-appropriate materials might be limited, so the health educator must make a decision as to the material's potential utility. As stated earlier, inappropriate materials may well do more harm than good.

Language   Is the language used in the materials appropriate for the audience? This question can be posed on two levels: Is the language used offensive in any way, and possibly inappropriate, particularly in school settings? Perhaps more important, is the language intelligible to the audience? For example, can you use a film in English in a predominantly Hispanic setting? There are no easy answers to these questions, and solutions may be different in each case. For example, if the only film available on a certain topic is in English, showing such a film to an Asian or Hispanic group is not necessarily out of the question. The group's level of English may be quite sufficient to understand the meaning of the film. Health educators should consider both the language capabilities of the group, and the language complexity of the media materials.

Content   Is the content of the materials accurate and up to date? Here is where the "we've always used this film!" doctrine can be dangerous. Many health issues change so quickly that as new information transposes the old, media materials can become outdated and, even worse, inaccurate in relatively short periods of time. The high cost of some materials makes updating media libraries a difficult task, and, again, the health educator may be faced with the decision of not using media materials rather than risking the dissemination of inaccurate information. It is perhaps useful to note that affective materials less concerned with cognitive information probably have a longer "shelf life" than their more factual counterparts.

Culture   Are the media materials culturally sensitive? That is, are they appropriate for a specific audience? This question is probably one of the most difficult to address in a satisfactory manner. In an ideal situation the health educator would be able to choose media materials that are both topic specific and completely culturally appropriate. For example, when considering a drug education film, the health educator should ideally be able to choose from affective to factual films, with alternative versions for each different ethnic group, whether black, Hispanic, Asian, white, and so on. But wouldn't we then also have to have even more versions, not only for race but for socioeconomic status? It would certainly seem insensitive to assume that individuals within races are all the same! To that end, achieving this Utopia would necessitate the development of literally hundreds of new media materials, each culturally specific and appropriate. Given the cost of media development, this situation will never exist, and the health educator is again left with making some type of compromise. The search for media materials that will satisfy the needs of *every* group is both futile and unreasonable. The health educator must make every effort to obtain materials that are as inclusive as possible and will not patently offend groups or individuals. A decision that no useful or appropriate materials are available to be used in certain contexts would not be unusual.

Time/Duration of Media   Just how long does it take to show specific materials? Is it reasonable to take up the entire 50-minute classroom period to show a film? In the community setting while facilitating a 90-minute workshop, what length of videotape would be reasonable to show? Is it reasonable to show a film in two parts because the film is too long to complete in one session? Again, each situation must be evaluated individually, with both the context of the presentation and the objectives of using specific media materials being of paramount importance in making a decision. What should be avoided is the selection of media materials because they happen to fit the presentation time frame. If some materials are deemed to be valuable but too lengthy, perhaps with careful preparation crucial pieces can be substituted for the whole.

Cost   No matter how useful some educational materials may be, there will always be the question of cost. As with anything related to consumerism, you tend to get what you pay for. High-quality, well-produced, interesting, educationally sound media materials are usually expensive. As production costs continue to rise, the price of the finished media products also increases. As mentioned earlier, the average cost of a high-quality 20-minute videotape will range from $150 to $400. With ever diminishing budgets in both the school and community settings, media selection must be made very carefully, and made with an eye to longevity and maximized usefulness of the materials. It is perhaps sad to note that with all the important factors incorporated in media selection in an effort to maximize the educational experience, the single greatest factor determining the final decision may well be the issue of cost.

Interest Level   How interesting are the materials? Will students in the classroom find the materials so dull that they mentally absent themselves from the experience, making the time and expense of using such materials futile? Will the community health smoking-cessation group find the videotape "talking head" to be so technical and boring that they begin to question continuing their involvement in the program? Perhaps the single most common criticism of health education materials has been their dull, lifeless, uninspiring format. No matter how important and useful the health information may be, if individuals have "tuned out," then the whole experience has achieved nothing. One useful tip when seeking media materials is to look for something the audience can *closely* relate to. For example, some of the best health education films for middle and high school audiences have been the ABC network's *After School Specials.* But would this material be applicable to college students, or would they dismiss the information as irrelevant because of the age difference? Is it effective to show a predominantly young, heterosexual, non-drug-using college population a film depicting middle-aged drug abusers or homosexual men describing how they contracted AIDS? Parker Palmer (1990) believes that such strategies ensure low interest levels and decreased potential for learning: "When students do not see the connection between subject and self, the inducement to learn is very low" (p. 14). Health education materials have certainly improved over the past few years, but in selecting such products, health educators should never underestimate the importance of interest levels in making their final decision.

Production Quality   How good are the production levels of health education materials? Historically, health education materials, particularly films, have been of poor quality. Over a decade ago, health education leaders were complaining about the appalling quality of educational materials. These materials were being produced to combat the much more sophisticated and glossy materials originating on Madison Avenue to promote unhealthy products. The criticism of the health education productions was that they tended to be boring, preachy, and unimaginative and that by making such films, health educators were wasting the most powerful medium of all. Today's youth in particular has become accustomed to the high-tech, high-quality level of media typically found in contemporary television. To present health education materials in a form any less sophisticated is to risk a total loss of credibility and usefulness. High-quality, interesting health education materials are now becoming more common, but as mentioned earlier, they come at a significant cost. Health educators may well be faced with deciding between using materials of poor quality, or using nothing at all . . . and it would not be unreasonable to choose the latter.

Evaluation   One factor to consider is, have the materials under review ever been evaluated in any way? It would probably be safe to say that the vast majority of media materials have never been evaluated. Films and videotapes may have been reviewed by other health educators, but often these reviews are very subjective and are prey to the vagaries of personal opinion. Little or no quantitative evaluation exists that examines the effects of specific forms of media (Sawyer and Beck, 1991). Most evaluation tends to center around the effects of specific programs or courses of study, giving scant attention to the individual component of media. With such little objective data available, the health educator should take great care to always preview new materials prior to use, and if necessary seek additional opinions from colleagues.

Availability   In selecting educational materials, the health educator needs to be concerned with the issue of availability. Do companies provide preview copies of materials? How long can you keep the materials? Is renting expensive products an option? If so, how much notice is needed for reservations? If you want to purchase something, how long will it take to receive the material? Although these questions appear to be fairly obvious concerns, the importance of planning ahead and gaining all possible relevant information cannot be overemphasized. If, for example, a film is a crucial part of a presentation, then the presenter should begin planning to obtain the film well in advance of the presentation. All types of complications are possible, and the simple process of determining the availability of materials can prevent many problems.

Format   Format is a particular concern in the area of film, videotape, and computer usage. As discussed earlier, film is used much less frequently than videotape. To that end, many productions are no longer available on film, or have become prohibitively expensive. The vast majority of videotapes are one-half-inch VHS format, but three-quarter-inch VHS, and beta tapes are also available. Health educators need to establish what type of format they can use before ordering. Ordering software for computer usage also presents some choices. Most software is still not compatible with other types, so if educators see software programs that they want to order, they must make sure that the program is available in the correct format.

Approval   Being able to use specific media materials in an educational setting may well be determined not by the individual health educator as by outside agencies. For example, in most public school settings any materials used in the classroom must be preapproved by a board or committee in the school system. This is particularly common when teaching "sensitive" topics such as human sexuality. A school health educator would obviously be well advised to ensure that materials he or she intends to use are "approved." Individual teachers may not always agree with a committee's opinions on which materials are acceptable, yet ignoring this approval process invites professional sanctions. The community health educator is less likely to confront such formal approval procedures. Nevertheless, the educator should take every precaution to ensure that he or she selects materials that will be deemed appropriate by the community. Consultation with professional peers and community leaders would certainly reduce the possibility of embarrassment.

Case Study: Amy   Amy has some end-of-the-year funds in her budget and decides to spend the money on some educational videotapes that look very good in the catalogue. Later she is disappointed when her staff give the videotapes poor reviews and most refuse to use them. It appears that Amy has wasted valuable resources. What steps could Amy have taken to prevent this situation? (See Case Studies Revisited page 228.)

Media Development

One of the major problems of applying rigorous evaluation standards to media materials is that given the limitations of many of the products currently available, the health educator may be unable to find anything suitable. Some individuals may be able to compromise and use the materials despite their obvious limitations. Others may decide that the price of compromise is too high, and the media materials are simply not used. Finally, some very few individuals may decide in the absence of useful materials that they will develop their own!

Historically, health education materials, particularly film and videotape, have been designed by media production companies, not health educators, and health educators have used them because the subject matter has been health-related . . . a sort of marriage of convenience. This situation has often resulted in high-quality production levels but less effective health education messages than desired. Conversely, many of the productions designed by health educators have adhered more closely to principles of health education but because of low production qualities were viewed as boring, amateurish, and ineffectual. The development of high-quality, credible health education materials that can compete with glossy and sophisticated commercial productions is of paramount importance. Health educators know better than anyone else the types of materials that would be effective. Unfortunately, their lack of technical expertise makes them reluctant to embark on media development. Although the development of new, exciting, high-quality materials is not easy, the process is well within the grasp of many educators. Some important points to consider when contemplating media development follow:

1. Objectives
2. Present resources
3. Format
4. Expertise
5. Cost
6. Financing
7. Marketing
8. Production quality
9. Evaluation

Once again, this list is not exhaustive, but it provides some useful fundamental questions that you, the health educator, should consider. Let us examine each in detail.

Objectives What do you specifically want to accomplish? The development of specific objectives or learning outcomes is the first crucial step in material development. From which domains are the objectives derived: cognitive, affective or psychomotor? Do the objectives include components from more than one domain? Before even deciding what type of media to produce, think through and commit to paper no more than three behavioral objectives. A common mistake is expecting to be able to accomplish multiple objectives from one production . . . an incredibly difficult task irrespective of the elaborate nature of the materials. You may well find yourself concentrating on and limiting yourself to one major objective.

Present Resources Does a vehicle already exist that will meet your desired objective(s)? Before embarking on what is usually a very time-consuming and often expensive venture, you need to be absolutely certain that such materials have not already been developed. This is of particular importance if you intend to market your materials in an effort to recoup production costs.

Format What will be the most effective format for the new materials—slides, overhead transparencies, videotape? Unfortunately, the most effective format is not necessarily the most practical. For example, a film might be considered the most effective manner to lessen the fears of adolescents before experiencing their first pelvic examination. However, the production of a good-quality film can be quite involved and very expensive. The health educator might decide that the development of a high-quality set of slides accompanied by a well-written script would be a more practical strategy. The sequence of brainstorming here is important. Begin by thinking through *the* most effective format, regardless of cost and impracticality, and do not compromise until you have explored every possibility to develop your first choice. Talk to others in your field or individuals who have expertise in media development—you may be surprised at what is possible!

Expertise Do you have the knowledge and level of expertise necessary to develop your own materials? For most of us in health education the answer to this question will be a resounding "No!" . . . and that's all right. You may be an expert in health education, but probably your skills and knowledge concerning the intricacies of media production are limited. Finding individuals who are skilled in production is an absolutely vital component in the successful development of quality materials. Such individuals exist in many settings, not only the expensive, professional film production company but also the university where talented students are studying film and television, graphics, art, journalism, and other related fields. Develop your ideas for media materials, shape them into a preliminary proposal and then seek out some individuals who can react to your ideas. Many individuals in the university setting would be delighted to be involved in media development. Some will be looking for payment, but not necessarily exorbitant payment. Students might be interested in course credit. Other individuals might simply be interested in the experience. The key point here is to pursue your ideas with enthusiasm. You won't know what is possible unless you try!

Cost How much will the development and production of your materials cost? The answer is nearly always "too much!" In most cases the cost of production will be the critical determining factor in deciding on the media format. Once again, as a health educator, you might have little idea as to production costs, so the necessity of consulting the media professional becomes obvious. For example, if your initial objective is to produce a videotape, in order to obtain a fairly accurate estimate of cost, you would need to develop a rough script and outline. If money is no problem, a production company could do this for you, but a more likely scenario is to collaborate with someone who has an interest in this area. The film/video producer can then give you a fairly accurate estimate of cost, given your project requirements.

The sequence of events is fairly similar for all media formats—think through your ideas, focus on specific objectives, develop an outline and proposal, and then research cost. Obviously, selecting a less involved format of materials means that you can do more of the production yourself and be less concerned with cost. Once you feel that you have a fairly accurate estimate, the next step is to seek financing.

Financing Can you access sufficient sources of funding to develop your materials? Now that you know what you would like to produce and how much it is going to cost, you need to work out if you can fund the materials. If you feel that your intended materials might fill a need shared by others, then with some persistent searching you may be able to find some financial help. Collaboration with several groups, organizations, or departments will certainly reduce individual burdens. Investigate the possibility of funding through grant writing. Many federal, state, and private organizations offer grants for health-related issues, and the development of educational materials is certainly a legitimate avenue. Again, consulting with individuals who are knowledgeable in obtaining grants would be very useful.

Also, approach private companies who manufacture products relevant to your topic. Although you would need to tread carefully in the area of sponsorship, the development of useful new educational materials can sometimes be facilitated by collaboration with the private sector. Media distributors who produce their own materials may be receptive to a proposal, leading to their producing the educational materials. Often the key to confronting the cost of media development is a combination of creativity and sheer persistence. Before you decide that the cost of developing your materials is too prohibitive, make sure that you have solicited every source!

Marketing   Do you intend to develop your materials for personal use, or would you consider marketing your product at the local or national level? One important point to consider is that if you are developing materials because a void exists in what is currently available, there is a good chance that other health educators are experiencing the same problem and may be interested in what you produce. This whole issue is integrally linked to obtaining initial funding. If you can provide a very strong proposal that includes evidence of a widespread universal need for your materials, the chance of winning some type of funding is greatly enhanced. If individuals or groups are likely to recoup their initial investment and even perhaps make a profit, they are far more likely to help finance a project than if they perceive their support as a donation. Health educators could certainly distribute their own materials, but without any real expertise in this area, their success would be limited.

Professional organizations could be helpful in this process, either in distributing the actual materials or providing mailing lists of fellow professionals (at a cost!). Examples of such organizations are the American College Health Association (ACHA); American Alliance for Health, Physical Education, Recreation and Dance (AAHPERD); American School Health Association (ASHA); and American Public Health Association (APHA). In addition to professional organizations, commercial media distribution companies are only too glad to distribute high quality products, but at a large cost to the developer. For example, commercial distributors of videotapes will customarily take 70–75 percent of the selling price of each tape sold, leaving the producer with a much lower 25–30 percent of the share. Although the rates might seem unreasonable, a good, aggressive distribution company can potentially sell many more videotapes than could the producer, thus compensating for offering a smaller share of the profits. As with sponsorship discussed in the previous section, association with commercial distribution companies should be thoroughly investigated, often with legal advice, before any commitment is made.

Finally, be advised that publishing companies that previously concentrated only on printed materials have begun to broaden their horizons. In the light of diminishing book sales these companies are becoming more progressive and are demonstrating a firm interest in alternative or supplementary educational materials, in particular videotapes, interactive videodiscs, and computer software programs.

Production Quality   What level of production quality do you anticipate developing? A good part of this question will have already been answered by considering the factors of cost and marketing previously mentioned. These factors are inextricably linked and probably should be considered simultaneously. Obviously, if national marketing is anticipated, then production qualities must be of the highest order. This in turn will ensure that production costs are fairly high. On the other hand, there is absolutely nothing wrong with setting your sights lower, keeping production costs to a minimum, and confining the use of the materials to yourself and local colleagues.

Evaluation   Although the vast majority of media materials has not been exposed to rigorous outcome evaluation, many of the products currently available have at least been developed through some type of professional and/or student validation. When developing media materials it is often useful to involve the intended target audience in the production. Small focus groups to test various components of the materials can provide invaluable feedback, as can input by fellow professionals. Changes and alterations can easily be made along the way, whereas attempting to change completed materials can be expensive, time-consuming and sometimes impossible.

Media Literacy

The powerful nature of the media and its influences on young people's lives is well documented. In fact, some individuals might go so far as to suggest that the media has become so pervasive that it should be recognized as the biggest educator in today's society (Davies, 1993). "By age 18 a young person will have seen 350,000 commercials and spent more time being entertained by the media than any other activity except sleeping" (p. S–28). So concerned was the federal government with the role that the media plays in shaping lives, particularly within the context of health information, that the Office of Disease Prevention and Health Promotion, the National Cancer Institute, and the Office for Substance Abuse Prevention joined forces to examine how the mass media and health agencies could better work together (U.S. Department of Health and Human Services, 1988). Some of the major recommendations from this study included improving the communication skills of public health professionals, using all types of media to develop health messages, and teaching individuals how to interpret messages disseminated by the mass media (U.S. Department of Health and Human Services, 1988). Yates (1999) argues strongly for the need to increase **media literacy** instruction, particularly in the lower grade levels, in order to assist students in combating mixed and often confusing health messages so often found in the media.

The concept of media literacy emerged during the 1980s and continues to receive much attention. Media literacy is based on the premise that much of what people see and believe is based on contact with various forms of media, which would not represent a problem if what the media provided was consistently accurate, honest, unbiased, and neutral information. Many writers and researchers have suggested that media is more interested in ratings and sales than in presenting an undistorted reality (Considine, 1990; Melamed, 1989); therefore, in order to protect individuals from falling prey to the vagaries of media messages, media education should become a necessary part of existing educational programs (Kahn and Master, 1993; Sneed, Wulfmeyer, and Van Ommeren, 1989).

Early definitions of media literacy were based on the idea of helping young people develop an informed and critical understanding of the nature

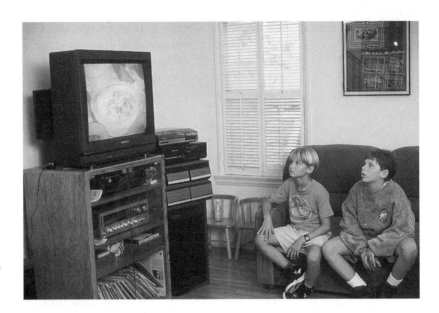

The media, especially television, is one of the biggest educators in today's society.

of mass media, the techniques utilized by various media, and how these techniques influence each individual's perceived reality (Ontario Ministry of Education, 1989). As the interest in media literacy grew, basic definitions broadened to include all populations. For example, the National Leadership Conference on Media Literacy proposed that a media literate person is someone who "can decode, evaluate, analyze and produce both print and electronic media." It furthermore stated, "The fundamental objective of media literacy is critical autonomy in relationship to all media. Emphases in media literacy training range widely, including informed citizenship, aesthetic appreciation and expression, social advocacy, self-esteem, and consumer competence" (Aufderheide, 1993, p. 1). The Media Literacy Project (1999) proposes a simpler, three-part definition: "Media literacy is (1) the process of asking questions about what you watch, see, and read; (2) literary skill applied to mass media culture and technology information messages; and (3) a necessary skill for life in a media-saturated society."

Clearly, if the mass media plays some type of role, either intentionally or unwittingly, in distributing material that somehow contributes to the negative health status of the public, then a logical preventive measure would be to better educate the public on how to be more critically aware of the messages they are receiving. Expecting the producers of mass media to take a more open and perhaps honest approach to programming is unrealistic in that the driving force of private media is a sound profit margin. Given this stark reality, media literacy becomes an important concept to consider in the realm of health education. A greater understanding of how mass media can shape people's perceptions can only help to make individuals more critical and selective when receiving health-related messages.

Resources An abundance of available information exists regarding media literacy, and much of it can be found on the Internet. Here are four selected Web sites that will provide some excellent resources in addition to a wealth of links to other related sites:

- *The Media Literacy OnLine Project:* This Web site, maintained by the University of Oregon, has a wealth of information on this topic in addition to a large number of links to related web sites.
- *Media Literacy Project:* This Web site, maintained by Babson College, also provides some great links to other sites, in addition to project ideas, curriculum materials, teacher education, and research articles.
- *Center for Media Education:* This is the home page for a national, nonprofit organization "dedicated to improving the quality of the electronic media." Information on research, advocacy, policy making and public education.
- *Center for Media Literacy:* This nonprofit organization, established in 1989, develops and distributes educational materials and programs that "promote critical thinking about the media." This Web site has a large amount of resources on this topic including books, videotapes, and teaching materials and also provides a free email bulletin, a listserv discussion group, and a calendar of events describing upcoming conferences and training.

 For more information and tools related to this chapter visit www.jbpub.com/healtheducation.

EXERCISES

1. You are a high school health teacher and have just been told by a friend about a new videotape on HIV/AIDS. You are scheduled to teach a unit on AIDS in a few weeks and would potentially like to use the videotape. Carefully describe all the steps you would take to achieve this goal.

2. You are a school or community health educator who has received a $1,000 grant to purchase media materials related to heart health. Make a detailed budget list of the materials you will purchase. (Do not make up a fictitious list! Do some research and consult some audiovisual catalogues, film, videotape, and audiotape libraries, bookstores, health professionals, etc.) You must reference all items, for example, the name of the videotape, its dis-

tributor, address, cost, and so on. You may be surprised how little you get for $1,000!

3. You are a school or community health educator who is interested in media materials. Thinking of your particular area of interest or expertise (if you do not have one, just select a health topic), what sort of media materials could be developed that would really enhance education in this area? Where do you consider the gaps to be in available media when related to your area of particular interest? Do some initial research to ensure that the materials do not already exist, and then write a descriptive outline of *your* proposed new media materials. Be creative! Do not worry about budget or lack of previous experience. What do you think would really enhance your teaching or presentations? What type of media would you develop? What would be your goals and objectives? What type of approach would you use? Give it a try!

4. Select two films or videotapes from the same subject area, and, utilizing Figure 7-3 (or, if you prefer, a similar instrument), evaluate the films/videotapes. Include in your eval-

uation what you would consider the goals and objectives of each film/videotape and whether or not you would use either of them in your work.

5. Select any health topic, and, using Powerpoint or other presentation software, create a brief presentation, perhaps no more than two to three slides/transparencies.

CASE STUDIES REVISITED

Case Study Revisited: Jason

This case presents an alarming prospect indeed, but unfortunately an all too common one. As modern technology has become more sophisticated and available, the use of educational media has increased in both the school and community setting. This increased usage, however, has not always proved beneficial to program participants. Too often the materials used are outdated, of poor technical quality, too heavily laden with facts, inappropriate for the audience, or, perhaps the greatest sin of all, they are often excruciatingly boring! Modern-day individuals like Jason, who have been nurtured on extremely high production-quality shows on television (like MTV) and movie theaters have developed the uncanny ability of being able to identify poor quality in health education media within a matter of seconds. The classic clues on a film or videotape might include an extremely dated soundtrack, characters wearing flared pants and giving the "peace" sign, no sign of any automobiles built since 1978, and the talking head in the form of a physician wearing the ubiquitous white coat and pointing to a list of written information. Any or all of these attributes are guaranteed to encourage Jason and his peers to leave their bodies in search of greater stimulation! (See page 204.)

Case Study Revisited: Amy

Amy should probably have consulted her staff initially to see whether or not they had seen the videotapes that she was about to order and also to ask them if they had any suggestions. Also, to purchase a videotape without previewing it is a very risky if not foolhardy practice. Most media companies will allow the customer to preview prior to purchase. Amy would have been wise to do just that, in addition to asking her staff members to preview the materials with her to obtain some additional input. (See page 221.)

SUMMARY

1. The use of media materials in health education has become extremely common. Unfortunately, much of the material produced in earlier years is of poor production quality and low interest and generally does little to enhance health education programming.

2. A recent trend in media materials is a move away from the fact-filled production to a more affective, process-oriented approach.

3. There is an obvious need for health educators to use materials that match the quality of shows produced by commercial agencies that often promote unhealthy lifestyles.

4. Health educators need to be aware of the advantages and disadvantages of the various forms of media.

5. Health educators would be well advised to develop a basic operating knowledge of media equipment.

6. Selecting media materials should be based on more than cost, availability, and personal preference. Selection should be based on the goal of achieving behavioral objectives formulated before the review process.

7. Media selection is a multifaceted process that should be based on a combination of sound principles described in this chapter.

8. The decision to use no media material rather than something of dubious quality will usually be the right decision. Poor-quality, outdated, or boring materials will usually have a detrimental effect on the presentation.

9. Media materials should be viewed as vehicles to enhance learning, not products that stand alone. Processing materials is an essential part of using educational resources.

10. New media development should always be considered an option when existing materials are deemed to be insufficient. The production of media should be based on the sound principles of development discussed in this chapter.

11. Media literacy is a field that advocates the critical analysis of mass media messages to enable the individual to more accurately distinguish between reality and the media's version of the truth.

REFERENCES

Aufderheide, P. (1993). Media literacy: A report of the national leadership conference on media literacy. ERIC Document Reproduction Service No. ED 365 294.

Campeau, P.L. (1974). Selective review of the results of research on the use of audiovisual media to teach adults. *Audio-Visual Communications Review 22,* 5–40.

Considine, D.M. (1990). Can we get there from here? *Educational Technology* 30(12), 27–32.

Davies, J. (1993). The impact of the mass media upon the health of early adolescents. *Journal of Health Education* 24(6), S28–S25.

Fejer. D., Hawley, P., Kuchar, E., Lucitis, D., & Webster, C. (1972). Assessing audiovisual aids for drug education: Preliminary study. Addiction Research Foundation of Ontario, Toronto, Canada.

Gold, S., & Duncan, D. (1980). Computers and health education. *Journal of School Health, 50,* 503–505.

Kahn, T.M., & Master, D. (1992). Multimedia literacy at Rowland: A good story well told. *Technological Horizons in Education Journal* 19(7), 77–83.

Martin, C., & Stainbrook, G.L. (1986). An analysis checklist for audiovisuals when used as educational resources. *Health Education,* 17(4), 31–33.

Media Literacy Project (1999). Definition of media literacy. http://www.babson.edu/medialiteracyproject) Retrieved from the World Wide Web, June 3, 1999.

Melamed, L. (1989). Sleuthing media "truths." *History and Social Science Teacher* 24(4), 189–193.

Ontario Ministry of Education (1989). *Media Literacy*, p. 225. Ontario: Ministry of Education.

Palmer, P. (1990). Critical Thinking. *Change*, Jan/Feb, 14.

Sawyer, R.G., & Beck, K.H. (1991). The effects of videotapes on the perceived susceptibility to HIV/AIDS among university freshmen. *Health Values*, *15*(2), 31–40.

Sneed, D., Wulfmeyer, K.T., Van Ommeren, R., & Riffe, D. (1989). Media literacy ignored: A qualitative call for the introduction of media studies across the high school social science curriculum. Paper presented at the annual meeting of the Association for Education in Journalism and Mass Communication, Washington DC.

U.S. Department of Health and Human Services. (1988). *Mass Media and Health: Opportunities for Improving the Nation's Health*. A report to the Office of Disease Prevention and Health Promotion, and the Office for Substance Abuse Prevention. Washington DC: U.S. Department of Health and Human Services, Public Health Service.

Yates, B.L. (1999). Media literacy: A health education perspective. *Journal of Health Education* 30(3), 180–184.

Minority Health

Entry-Level and Graduate-Level Health Educator Competencies Addressed in This Chapter

Responsibility I: Assessing Individual and Community Needs for Health Education
  Competency A: Obtain health related data about social and cultural environments, growth and development factors, needs, and interests.
  Competency C: Infer needs for health education on the basis of obtained data.

Responsibility III: Implementing Health Education Programs
  Competency B: Infer enabling objectives as needed to implement instructional program in specified settings.
  Competency C: Select methods and media best suited to implement program plans for specific learners.

Responsibility VII: Communicating Health and Health Education Needs, Concerns and Resources
  Competency A: Interpret concepts, purposes, and theories of health education.
  Competency B: Predict the impact of societal value systems on health education programs.

> Note: The competencies listed above, which are addressed in this chapter, are considered to be both entry-level and graduate-level competencies by the National Commission for Health Education Credentialing, Inc. They are taken from *A Framework for the Development of Competency Based Curricula for Entry Level Health Educators* by the National Task Force for the Preparation and Practice of Health Education, 1985; and *A Competency-Based Framework for Graduate Level Health Educators,* by the National Task Force for the Preparation and Practice of Health Education. 1999.

Method Selection in Health Education

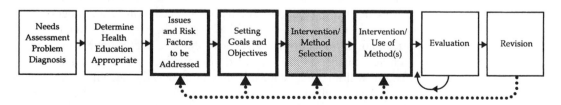

Heavy-bordered boxes indicate subjects addressed in this text; shaded boxes indicate subjects(s) of current chapter.

OBJECTIVES   After studying this chapter the reader should be able to:

- List some populations that might require the health educator to prepare material differently for presentation.
- Describe ethnic and racial disparities in selected areas of health.
- Describe the extent of research related to health and minority populations.
- Explain the research concerns and difficulties in studying minority health.
- Describe the legacy of suspicion and concern among ethnic and racial minorities in the wake of the Tuskegee study.

KEY TOPICS   Race   Cultural competence
Ethnicity   Health knowledge levels
Culture   Sources of health information
Literacy levels   Political awareness
Language   Community gatekeepers

Proportionately, most health educators today are both white and middle class. As opportunities for ethnic minorities increase, the discipline will become more multicultural, and sensitivity to the specific needs of others will be heightened. However, health educators currently practicing in the United States need to make great efforts to gain information about the individuals or groups with whom they will be working. Sometimes that information will make little difference to how a presentation is made, but in other situations radical change will be seen to be necessary. The key to successful teaching and presentations in any discipline is preparation, and learning about the lives of different populations is essential to preparation. This chapter presents suggestions for facilitating this learning process, but, as the reader will discover, for some minority populations little research has been performed to identify specific health needs and in these cases, documented methodologies for health education interventions are scarce.

Case Study: Susan   Susan is a community health educator who has recently been planning and implementing presentations related to increasing the number of women receiving pelvic examinations. She has been asked to present a program to a women's group on the east side of the city. Having performed several of these presentations before, Susan gives little thought to preparation and arrives with her materials at the appointed time and place. Susan quickly realizes that this will not be a "standard" presentation as the audience is predominantly Asian, with almost no grasp of English. The group leader graciously offers to translate, and the presentation moves laboriously along despite the translator obviously being troubled at having to translate graphic informa-

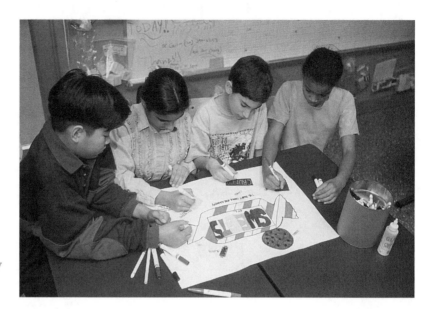

Health educators must consider ethnic diversity when planning programs and strategies.

tion related to sexuality. The presentation finally concludes with both audience and presenter feeling uncomfortable and dissatisfied. How could Susan have reduced the likelihood of this situation occurring? (See Case Studies Revisited page 254.)

Changing Demographics in the United States

The United States of America has often been described as a "melting pot" in reference to the diverse ethnic backgrounds of its population. This country is indeed heterogeneous, and along with the richness and vitality that such diversity brings comes an intriguing complexity. Here are some important questions to consider:

- Are all ethnic groups affected in the same way by specific health problems?
- Do we even have data that will enable us to generalize about health problems of certain ethnic groups?
- Will an educational intervention that seems to be successful with one group work with another?
- Can only health educators who are themselves from an ethnic group work successfully with that particular group?
- Do ethnic groups trust "outside" sources of information?
- Is ethnicity the real "key" to planning health behavior interventions, or is socioeconomic status a more powerful factor?

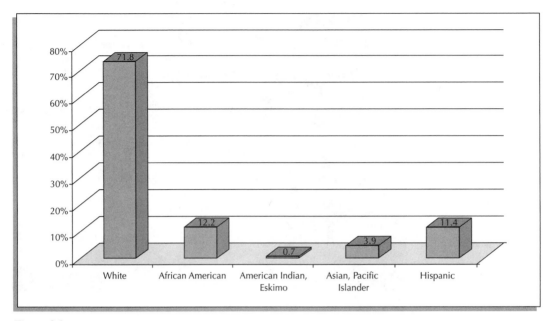

Figure 8-1
U.S. Population by Ethnicity 2000.

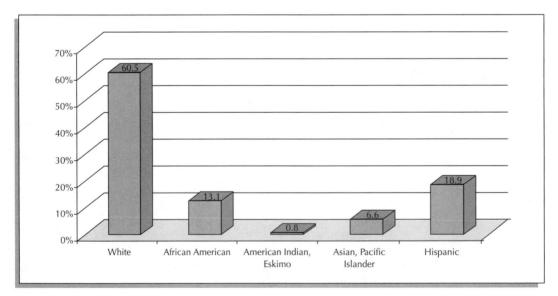

Figure 8-2
U.S. Population by Ethnicity 2030.

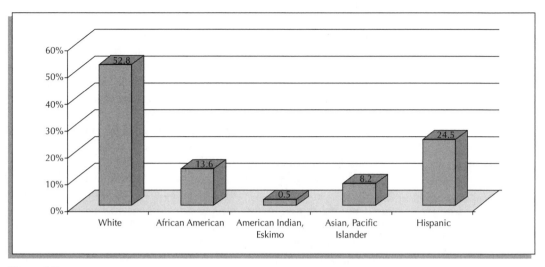

Figure 8-3
U.S. Population by Ethnicity 2050.

These are important questions to consider, particularly in the light of the rapidly changing demographic face of America. The charts in Figures 8-1 through 8-3 vividly demonstrate the projected population changes the United States will experience over the next 50 years. Such a shift in populations will inevitably affect the health care system and, specifically, how health educators develop and implement successful programming with the ever increasing diversity of communities. The charts were developed using 1998 data from Census Bureau.

Should We Study Minority Health?

Although to many health professionals studying minority health as a separate entity is a reasonable strategy, an opposing viewpoint certainly exists. Some researchers argue that separating health issues out by race, and examining race as a unique variable, encourages misinterpretation of the data and potentially increases racism. The argument continues that because race is not considered a scientifically valid biological concept, discrepancies in race data serve only to perpetuate racist stereotypes about biological differences and genetic inferiority (Osborne and Feit, 1992; Leslie, 1990). However, other health professionals argue that we need more, not less, research on minority health and, to avoid encouraging racism, that we simply need to do a better job of performing the research (LaVeist, 1996).

One criticism of using race as a variable in health studies is that the term *race* is poorly defined. All too often, researchers assume that there is no variance within ethnicity, nationality, or culture, lumping individuals together because they speak the same language (Spanish–Hispanic) or because they originate from approximately the same part of the world (Asian). Two individuals, one from Mississippi and one from Haiti, may both be black, but they come from cultures worlds apart and may engage in completely different patterns of health behavior. Hispanic Americans originate from many different countries and continents, such as Mexico, Puerto Rico, South America, Central America, and Cuba (see Figure 8-4). Additionally, many Dominicans and some Puerto Ricans consider themselves racially black but ethnically Hispanic, while Hispanics from some Central American countries are racially Indian (Nickens, 1995).

Similar ranges of diversity are also found in what is known as the "Asian" population. Such a blanket term actually tells us very little with regard to specific ethnicity or culture in groups of individuals originating from countries such as China, Vietnam, Japan, Korea, or the Philippines. In addition, such broad categories result in missing many differences *within* groups or categories. For example, Americans of Vietnamese and Mexican origin tend to have low mean family incomes and low median age, whereas Japanese Americans and Cuban Americans have relatively high mean incomes and high median age (Bureau of the Census, 1991). In fact, one could argue further that although the white majority population in the United States today is also all categorized as one entity, the health behaviors of Irish, Italian, Swedish, and German Americans are not necessarily the same.

The authors of this text believe that health issues as they relate to minority populations should indeed be discussed, with the condition that such top-

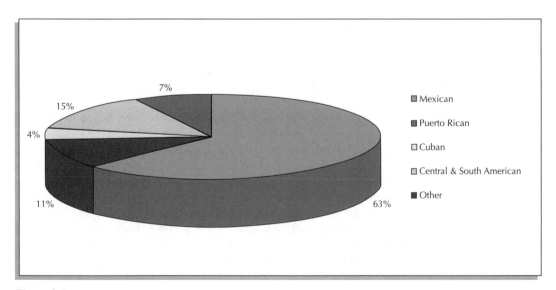

Figure 8-4
Hispanic Americans in the U.S. 1997.

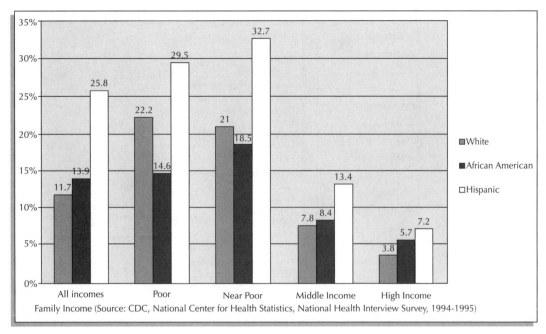

Figure 8-5
Children Under Age 18 with No Health Insurance: 1994–1995.

ics be viewed not through the narrow lens of race alone, but rather within a fuller context that more accurately reflects the complexity involved. There is a clear need to look beyond the obvious markers of race such as skin color or language and examine the additional factors of culture, country of origin, and socioeconomic status. For example, an obvious influence on health status is access to health care, and as Figure 8-5 clearly shows, access is by no means equal and is affected by, among other things, ethnicity and income levels. Additionally, there are numerous intervening factors that shape the connection of race and health outcomes, as illustrated in Figure 8-6. Health educators need to understand that looking at race or ethnicity as a single descriptor is too simplistic; additional factors should also be considered.

Racial and Ethnic Disparities in Health

Rather than develop an exhaustive list of health problems, laboriously broken down by ethnicity, the reader might be better served by examining a selected number of important contemporary health issues that provide telling examples of discrepancies by ethnicity. The following section describes six health problems that have been targeted by the federal government in an at-

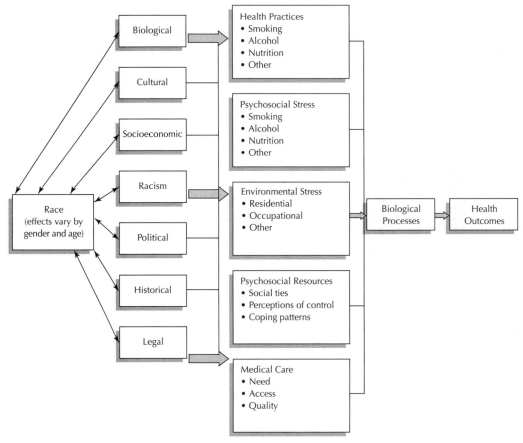

Figure 8-6
A Framework for Understanding the Relationship Between Race and Health.

tempt to eliminate such discrepancies and is taken from an initiative overview developed by the Office of Minority Health (1999).

The Initiative to Eliminate Racial and Ethnic Disparities in Health

In a radio address on February 21, 1998, President Clinton declared that by the year 2010 the United States would eliminate the disparities in six health areas experienced by racial and ethnic minority populations. The Department of Health and Human Services (HHS) is leading the effort to eliminate disparities in health access and outcomes in the following areas:

Goal 1. Infant Mortality Rates

Infant mortality is often cited as a measure of a country's health status. Although infant mortality has been decreasing over the past few decades, and in 1996 was at a record low of 7.2 deaths per 1,000 live births, the United States still ranks 24th in infant mortality compared to other western industrialized nations.

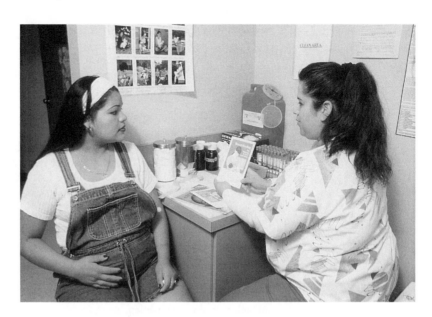

Prenatal care is an important factor in the effort to reduce infant mortality.

Rates of infant mortality vary greatly between and within racial and ethnic groups. Infant death rates among many minority groups (African American, American Indians, Alaska natives and Hispanics) were well above the national average of 7.2 deaths per 1,000 live births in 1996. The infant death rate among African Americans was 14.2 per 1,000 live births, more than double that of white Americans (6.0 per 1,000 live births in 1996). Although the overall American Indian rate (9.0 per 1,000 live births) does not appear to be alarmingly high, this number does not reflect the diversity among Indian communities, some of whom report infant death rates that are nearly twice the national average.

One well established predictor of improved pregnancy outcome is involvement in prenatal care, particularly in the first trimester of pregnancy. The likelihood of delivering a very low birth weight (VLBW) baby (less than 3lb 4oz) is estimated to be 40% higher among women who receive late or no prenatal care compared to women entering prenatal care during the first trimester. Approximately 95% of VLBW babies are born early (less than 37 weeks) and the risk of death for VLBW babies is about 65 times that of infants who weigh at least 3lb 4oz.

In 1996 the proportion of pregnant women in the U.S. receiving prenatal care in the first trimester was 81.8%, a proportion that reflects a consistent improvement from the 1989 figure of 75.5%. However, the sad fact remains that one in five pregnant women, nearly three quarters of a million women, did not receive timely prenatal care, and nearly 47,000 pregnant women received absolutely *no* prenatal care. There are substantial racial disparities in the receipt of prenatal care. Although 84% of white pregnant women received timely prenatal care in 1996, that proportion was only 71% for black and Hispanic pregnant women.

When examining specific causes of infant deaths, racial and ethnic disparities seem to be particularly acute in preterm or premature birth (PTB) and sudden infant death syndrome (SIDS). A much higher incidence of PTBs occurs among black mothers than among white mothers (17.7 versus 9.7), while SIDS, which accounts for approximately 10% of all first year infant deaths, is also more common in minority populations, with some American Indian and Alaskan Native groups experiencing a rate three to four times higher than white mothers.

Higher rates of infant mortality in minority groups are influenced by many factors, such as, socioeconomic and demographic factors, medical conditions, quality of and access to health care. The near-term goal to reduce infant mortality in African Americans (the group with the greatest disparity in terms of infant death rates) is by at least 22% from the 1996 rate by the year 2000—or from 14.2 per 1,000 to 11.0 per 1,000 live births.

Near-Term Goal: Reduce infant mortality among African Americans by 22%.

Goal 2. Cancer Screening and Management

Cancer is the second leading cause of death in the United States, resulting in more than 544,000 deaths each year. The chances of developing cancer in a lifetime are nearly 50% for men and nearly 40% for women. Disparities exist in both mortality and incidence rates.

Major Mortality Discrepancies:

- For men and women combined, African Americans have a cancer death rate about 35% higher than that of whites (171.6 vs. 127.0 per 100,000).
- The African American male cancer death rate is about 50% higher than it is for white men (226.8 vs. 151.8 per 100,000).
- The death rate for lung cancer is about 27% higher for African Americans than for whites (49.9 vs. 39.3 per 100,000).
- The prostate cancer mortality rate for African American men is more than twice that of white men (55.5 vs. 23.8 per 100,000).

Major Incidence Discrepancies:

- The incidence of lung cancer in African American men is about 50% higher than in white men (110.7 vs. 72.6 per 100,000).
- Native Hawaiian men have elevated rates of lung cancer compared with white men.
- Alaska Native men and women suffer disproportionately higher rates of cancers of the colon and rectum than do whites.
- Vietnamese women in the United States have a cervical cancer incidence rate more than five times greater than white women (47.3 vs. 8.7 per 100,000). Hispanic women also suffer elevated rates of cervical cancer.

The incidence of certain forms of cancer could be greatly reduced through various types of prevention. For example, tobacco use is responsible for nearly one-third of all cancer deaths, while evidence suggests that diet and nutrition are probably associated with another 30%–40% of cancer deaths. For the forms of cancer we do not know how to prevent, early detection can reduce the risk of death. Regular mammography screening and follow-up can reduce deaths from breast cancer by about 30% for women 50 years of age and older,

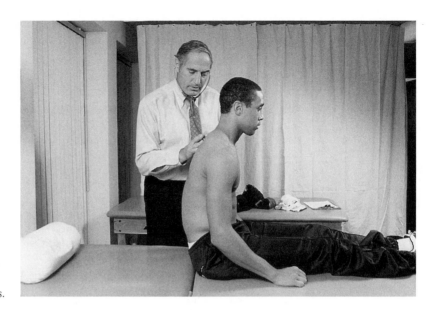

Equal access to health care screening is essential to reduce cancer mortalities in minorities.

while regular Pap tests for cervical cancer along with follow-up care can virtually eliminate the risk of developing this disease. Despite the gains in screening in the African American community, the mortality rate from breast cancer for black women is greater than that for white women. Some possible reasons for this might include irregular screening, limited follow-up opportunities, and lack of access to treatment services. Hispanic, American Indian, Alaska Native and Asian and Pacific Islander women also experience similar barriers related to screening, access to treatment and follow-up, often compounded by problems such as culture differences, language, and in some cases, negative provider attitudes.

This HHS initiative hopes to decrease the existing discrepancies in this category by eliminating these barriers to prevention and screening practices.

Cervical cancer—the goal for the year 2000 is to increase to at least 85% the proportion of all women aged 18 and older who have received a Pap test within the preceding 3 years.

Near-Term Goal: Increase to at least 60% those women of all racial or ethnic groups, aged 50 and older, who have received a clinical breast exam and a mammogram within the preceding two years.

Goal 3. Cardiovascular Disease

Cardiovascular disease, primarily coronary heart disease and stroke, kills nearly as many Americans as all other diseases combined. The annual national economic impact of cardiovascular disease is estimated at $259 billion as measured in health care expenditures, medications and lost productivity due to disability and death. The major modifiable risk factors for cardiovascular disease are *high blood pressure, high blood cholesterol, cigarette smoking, excessive body weight, and physical activity.*

Major disparities exist among minority groups, with a disproportionate burden of death and disability from cardiovascular disease existing in minority and low-income populations.

- The age-adjusted death rate for coronary heart disease for the total population declined by 20% from 1987 to 1995; for African Americans, the overall decrease was only 13%.
- Compared with rates for whites, coronary heart disease mortality was 40% lower for Asian Americans but 40% higher for African Americans in 1995. Stroke is the only leading cause of death for which mortality is higher for Asian-American males than for white males.
- Racial and ethnic minorities have higher rates of hypertension, tend to develop hypertension at an earlier age, and are less likely to undergo treatment to control their high blood pressure.
- From 1988 to 1994, 35% of African American males ages 20 to 74 had hypertension compared with 25% of all men.
- When age differences are controlled, Mexican-American men and women also have elevated blood pressure rates.
- Among adult women, the age-adjusted prevalence of overweight continues to be higher for African American women (53%) and Mexican-American women (52%) than for white women (34%).
- Only 50% of American Indians/Alaska Natives, 44% of Asian Americans, and 38% of Mexican Americans have had their cholesterol checked within the past 2 years.

Near-Term Goals

- Reduce the heart disease mortality rate among African Americans by 25%.
- Reduce the stroke mortality rate among African Americans by 40%.

Goal 4. Diabetes

Diabetes is the seventh leading cause of death in the United States and is a serious public health problem, affecting nearly 16 million Americans. The estimated direct and indirect costs of diabetes to the nation was estimated to be $98 billion in 1993.

- The prevalence of diabetes in African Americans is approximately 70% higher than in whites and the prevalence in Hispanics is nearly double that of whites.
- The prevalence rates among American Indians and Alaska Natives is more than twice that for the total population and at least one tribe, the Pimas of Arizona, have the highest known prevalence of diabetes of any population in the world.

Cardiovascular disease is the leading cause of death among people with diabetes, and achieving mortality reduction among high-risk populations will require an effort to reduce cardiovascular risk factors among these groups. Individuals with diabetes not only face a reduced life span but the possibility of many acute and chronic complications, including end-stage renal disease

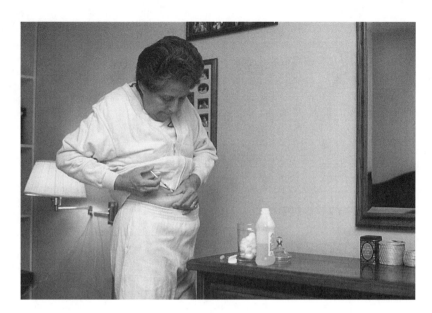

Diabetes is a serious health problem disproportionately affecting minorities.

(ESRD), blindness, and lower extremity amputations. All of these complications have the potential to be prevented:

- If uncontrolled hypertension among people with diabetes were reduced by half, about 25% of ESRD due to diabetes could be prevented.
- Diabetic retinopathy is the leading cause of new cases of blindness among people 20-44 years of age. Clinical trials have demonstrated that approximately 60% of diabetes-related blindness can be prevented with good blood glucose control or by early detection and laser photocoagulation treatment, which is widely available but underused.
- One half of all lower extremity amputations can be prevented through proper foot care and by reducing risk factors such as hyperglycemia (abnormally high blood sugar), cigarette smoking, and high blood pressure.

Preventive interventions should target high-risk groups. African Americans and American Indians, for example, are more likely than white populations to experience diabetes-related complications such as ESRD and amputations. Even among similarly insured populations, such as Medicare recipients, African Americans are more likely than whites to be hospitalized with septicemia, debridement, and amputations—signs of poor diabetic control. Although diabetes is a serious problem, recent studies have shown that careful control of blood glucose levels is a strategy that can be successful for preventing complications of diabetes. The challenge is to make proper diabetes management part of daily clinical and public health practice.

Near-Term Goals

- Reduce the rate of ESRD from diabetes among African Americans and American Indians/Alaska Natives by 65%.

- Reduce lower extremity amputation rates from diabetes among African Americans by 40%

Goal 5. HIV Infection/AIDS

In 1998, HIV infection/AIDS was the leading cause of death for all persons 25 to 44 years of age. Between 650,000 and 900,000 Americans were estimated to be living with HIV infection, while by June 1998, over 400,000 of the 665,357 adults and adolescents reported with AIDS in the United States had died from the disease (CDC, 1999).

AIDS has clearly disproportionately affected minority populations.

- Racial and ethnic minorities constitute about 25% of the total U.S. population, and yet they account for nearly 54% of all AIDS cases.
- While the epidemic is decreasing in some populations, the *number* of new AIDS cases among African Americans is now greater than the number of new AIDS cases among whites.
- Although the number of AIDS diagnoses among gay and bisexual white men has decreased dramatically since 1989, the number of AIDS diagnoses among African American men having same-gender sex has increased.
- New cases of AIDS where the identifiable route of transmission is injecting drug use, are increasingly concentrated in minorities; of these cases almost 75% are among minority groups (56% African American and 20% Hispanic).
- Of AIDS cases reported among women and children, more than 75% are among racial and ethnic minorities.

In addition to disproportionate rates of AIDS, minority groups have not kept pace with reduced death rates reported in majority populations. For example, during the years 1995 and 1996, AIDS death rates declined 23% for the total U.S. population, but only 13% for African Americans and 20% for Hispanics.

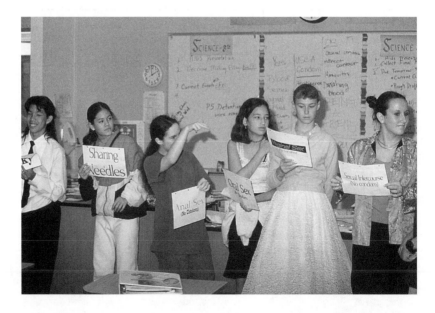

Innovative methods of education can help to reduce high risk behaviors.

Major contributing factors to this discrepancy include late identification of disease and lack of health insurance to pay for drug therapies and treatment that can cost between $10,000 and $12,000 per patient per year.

Inadequate recognition of risk, detection of infection, and referral to follow-up care are major issues for high-risk populations. It is estimated that about one-third of persons who are at risk of HIV/AIDS have never been tested. More effective prevention strategies are needed that are acceptable to the target audience (i.e., they must be culturally and linguistically appropriate), and the capability of organizations serving at-risk populations to develop, implement, evaluate, and fund prevention and treatment programs must be improved.

Inadequate recognition of risk, detection of infection, and referral to follow-up care are major issues for high-risk populations. It is estimated that about one-third of persons who are at risk of HIV/AIDS have never been tested. More effective prevention strategies are needed that are acceptable to the target audience (i.e., they must be culturally and linguistically appropriate), and the capability of organizations serving at-risk populations to develop, implement, knowing ones's serostatus, access to counseling and testing, and referral and access to medical services, including efficacious therapies, will continue to guide the development and administration of Federal initiatives to prevent HIV transmission and improve access to care for individuals living with HIV/AIDS.

Near-Term Goals: Ensure early and equal access to life-enhancing health care and appropriate drug therapies for at least 75% of low-income persons living with HIV/AIDS.

Goal 6. Child and Adult Immunization

The reduction in incidence of vaccine-preventable diseases is one of the most significant public health achievements of the past century. This success is best illustrated by the global eradication of smallpox in 1977. The major factor in this success is the development and widespread use of vaccines, which are among the safest and most effective preventive measures.

Childhood immunization rates are at an all-time high, with the most critical vaccine doses reflecting coverage rates of over 90%. The 1996 immunization targets for all five vaccines (measles, mumps, and rubella [MMR]; polio; diphtheria, tetanus, and pertussis [DPT]; *Haemophilus influenza* typeB [Hib]; and hepatitis b [Hep B] were exceeded. Although immunization rates have been lower in minority populations compared with the white population, minority rates have been increasing at a more rapid rate, thus significantly narrowing the gap. However, efforts must be made to achieve and maintain at least 90% coverage for all recommended vaccines in all populations. Particular areas of concern are pockets of need within each state and major city where numbers of under-immunized children reside. These areas are of great concern because, particularly in large, urban areas with traditionally underserved populations, there is a potential for outbreaks of vaccine-preventable diseases.

In addition to the very young, older adults are also at increased risk for many vaccine-preventable diseases. Approximately 90% of all influenza-associated deaths in the United States occur in people aged 65 and older, the fastest growing age group of the population. Reduction of deaths in this age group has been hindered in part by relatively low vaccine utilization. Each year, an

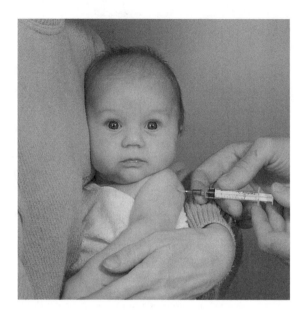

Immunization continues to be one of the most effective methods of controlling infectious diseases.

estimated 45,000 adults die of infections related to influenza, pneumococcal infections, and hepatitis B despite the availability of safe and effective vaccines to prevent these conditions and their complications. There is a disproportionate burden of these diseases in minority and underserved populations. Although vaccination levels against pneumococcal infections and influenza among people 65 years and over have increased slightly for African Americans and Hispanics, the coverage in these groups remains substantially below the general population and the year 2000 targets.

Childhood Immunization

Near-Term Goals: Achieve and maintain at least 90% coverage for all recommended childhood vaccines in all populations.

Adult Immunization

In order to achieve this near-term goal, the 1994 influenza immunization rates among African Americans, Hispanics, and Asians and Pacific Islanders will need to nearly double, and among these same groups, the 1994 pneumococcal immunization rates will need to quadruple.

Near-Term Goals: Increase pneumococcal and influenza immunizations among all adults aged 65 years and older to 60%.

Cultural Competency

A relatively recent concept aimed at improving health outcomes for traditionally underserved populations is that of **cultural competency.** This concept developed from the premise that not all individuals within the health care system are treated equally, particularly those with cultural mores outside the "mainstream." Cultural competency is intended to optimize the likelihood that individuals from all cultures, ethnicities, and races will receive appropriate and sensitive care. Chen (1998) suggests that cultural competency comprises three components: purpose, attitude, and skills. The inherent *purpose* is to achieve improved health outcomes; *attitude* is the willingness to adapt oneself to others' needs; and *skills* refers to those behaviors that exemplify correctness of technique in interactions between the professional and the patient. Chen believes that health professionals who are minorities themselves are the most likely people to be able to empower communities to improve their health status. The logical need, then, would be an increase in the number of trained minority health professionals. Chen also gives some additional practical recommendations for achieving cultural competency:

- Develop better access to services by hiring bilingual and bicultural staff members.
- Tailor interventions by learning about other cultures.
- Modify services by integrating traditional medicine with Western medicine.
- Develop a specialized program model, such as the Native Hawaiian health care system.

Obviously, the development of effective cultural competence in the health professions could have a profound effect on potential or existing clients, particularly those who have felt marginalized by the system. Health care should acknowledge the client's health-related beliefs and cultural mores, as well as consider the community from which the person has come.

Case Study: Denise   Denise, a community health educator, has been asked to speak with representatives from several local Hispanic women's groups to explore their perceived needs concerning preventive health services. Eager to be prepared for the encounter, Denise thoroughly researches health issues relevant to Mexican Americans. On learning that fluency in English among the women is very limited, she persuades a good friend visiting from Madrid to accompany her in the role of translator. Denise's confidence that she is well prepared is short-lived as the workshop begins! Denise had made the seriously wrong assumption that all Hispanic people are alike and come from the same culture. The women at the workshop represent group members from Mexico, South America, Central America, Cuba, and Puerto Rica. Although the women had some similar concerns, they were offended that Denise was making broad assumptions based on information that was foreign to their particular cultures. To make matters worse, Denise's interpreter friend was experiencing major difficulties understanding and being understood! This exploratory session was rather less than effective. What type of impact did

Denise's assumptions have on her workshop, and how could she avoid making that same mistake again? (See Case Studies Revisited page 255.)

Tuskegee—A Legacy of Doubt

One of the major issues discussed in this chapter is the difficulty experienced by health educators attempting to plan and effectively implement programs when viewed as an "outsider." Although most young health education students will probably be unaware of research begun in the 1930s, the Tuskegee Syphilis Study provides an excellent example of why a community, in this case the African American community, might exhibit a pervasive sense of distrust of public health agencies.

In the late 1920s the Public Health Service (PHS) was completing a study of the prevalence of syphilis in the black population in Mississippi. In order to expand syphilis research in the rural south, the PHS was awarded a grant from the Julius Rosenwald Foundation, a philanthropic organization located in Chicago. The research was to study the testing and treatment of syphilis in five rural counties in the south: Albemarle county, Virginia; Glynn County, Georgia; Pitt County, North Carolina; Macon County, Alabama; and Tipton County, Tennessee. (Parran, 1937)

The Depression, beginning in 1929, played havoc with the research funding, and the treatment phase of the study was never completed. In Macon County, Alabama, the prevalence of syphilis had been reported as high as 35–40 percent of all age groups tested. It was this community in Alabama that was to serve as the proving ground for the effects of untreated syphilis. A PHS physician, T. Clark, stated simply, "The Alabama community offered an unparalleled opportunity for the study of the effect of untreated syphilis." (Jones, 1981)

One of the great ironies of this study was the astonishingly thorough and textbook approach taken by the PHS in implementing the program. Prestigous black institutions were persuaded to cooperate, several black churches added their credibility, and individual black community leaders ensured participation (Thomas and Quinn, 1991) The research continued, and little concern was voiced that anything questionable was taking place. However, in addition to not treating the infected individuals, the PHS team also chose not to provide any education about syphilis (Jones, 1981) No mention was made of the disease by name. It was simply referred to as "bad blood," a rural, southern term descriptive of many health problems at that time. Individuals were not told that the disease could be sexually transmitted, or that infants could be born infected (Thomas and Quinn, 1991).

America's involvement in World War II began in 1941, and so desperate was the PHS not lose their subjects to the war that they pressured the draft board into not drafting these men. In 1943 the recently developed "miracle drug" penicillin was being widely used, including in the treatment of people infected with syphilis. This effective form of treatment was withheld from the men in the study. Clearly, treatment of the infected individuals would end the study and future research, something the PHS did not want to occur. The study and the withholding of treatment continued until 1972 when the Washington Star's front-page exposé created enormous public outcry, finally stirring health officials into ending the study.

What are the implications of the Tuskegee study for health educators? What can we learn from this obviously inhumane and unethical research? Thomas and Quinn (1991) draw a powerful connection between the Tuskegee study and the current AIDS epidemic. The authors point out that the legacy of Tuskegee is a legitimate and understandable fear and distrust of the "health establishment." They cite the fears of some African Americans who believe that AIDS is an agent of white forces developed as a form of genocide. Mark Smith from Johns Hopkins University described the African American community as "already alienated from the health care system . . . and somewhat cynical about the motives of those who arrive in their communities to help them" (p.19). (National Commission on AIDS, 1990) A health educator from Dallas, testifying before the National Commission on AIDS, commented, "So many African American people that I work with do not trust hospitals or any of the other community health care service providers because of that Tuskegee experiment. It is like . . . if they did it then, they will do it again" (p.43).(National Commission on AIDS, 1990)

As health educators we must not underestimate the importance and power of past events. Twenty years after the study ended, and over 60 years since it began, the effects of the Tuskegee study are still with us. It would be easy to dismiss as preposterous the notion that AIDS is a deliberate attempt at genocide. Yet, in the light of Tuskegee, is that type of fear so far-fetched? Thomas and Quinn make a forceful point when they describe the necessary ingredients for a successful community-based HIV education program that is ethnically acceptable and culturally sensitive: (1) the use of program staff indigenous to the community, (2) the use of incentives, and (3) the delivery of health services within the target community. The authors comment, though, that these were the exact methods used in the Tuskegee study and that health educators will have to work hard to ensure that these sound strategies are not diminished by their association with this fateful study. (Thomas and Quinn, 1991)

Tuskegee Postscript

In a White House ceremony on May 16, 1997, nearly 65 years after the advent of the now notorious Tuskegee study, President William Clinton apologized for the 40-year government study. In 1997 there were only eight survivors of the Tuskegee experiment still alive, and five of them, accompanied

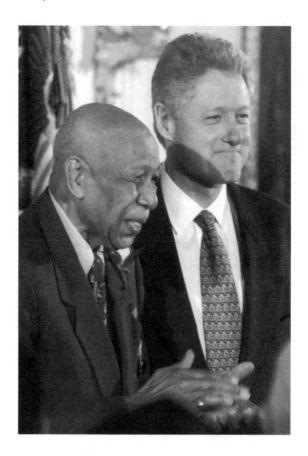

Sixty-five years after the Tuskegee study began, President Clinton apoligized to the survivors.

by family members of some of the deceased, attended the ceremony. The president remarked,

> The legacy of the study at Tuskegee has reached far and deep, in ways that hurt our progress and divide our nation. We cannot be one America when a whole segment of our nation has no trust in America. What was done cannot be undone, but we can end the silence, we can stop turning our heads away, we can look at you, in the eye, and finally say, on behalf of the American people, what the United States Government did was shameful, and I am sorry. (White House, 1997).

President Clinton also announced that he was awarding a $200,000 grant to Alabama's Tuskegee University to help build a center on bioethics and research and that he had directed Donna Shalala, secretary for Health and Human Services, to report back to him in 180 days with recommendations for how to more effectively include minority populations in health care research (Washington Post, 1997a).

NOTEWORTHY   Tuskegee Revisited?

President Clinton's words were prophetic in that in September 1997 the media and popular press had picked up a controversy surrounding the Centers for Disease Control and Prevention (CDC) and National Institutes of Health (NIH) sponsored drug treatment trials in Third World areas. One trial under scrutiny was a project that sought to test the efficacy of reduced dosage treatment of an AIDS drug, AZT, in a population of more than 12,000 HIV-positive pregnant women. The study design included one group that was to receive the full dose, another that was to receive a half dosage, and a control group that would receive a placebo. The purpose of the study was pragmatic in that most developing countries could not afford expensive medications such as AZT, and researchers were trying to see whether or not a lower, less expensive dose would still be effective. The withholding of an effective treatment regimen certainly reminded some ethicists of the Tuskegee situation. Writing in the *Washington Post*, William Raspberry described how Marcia Angell, the executive editor of the *New England Journal of Medicine*, had written an editorial fiercely criticizing such studies, calling them unethical and akin to the Tuskegee study (Washington Post, 1997b). Dr. Angell asserted, "Some of the same arguments that were made in favor of the Tuskegee study many years ago are emerging in a new form in the AZT studies in the third world." Raspberry had also talked to two ethics professors about the issue, both of whom thought that the removal of the control group would eliminate any ethical problems.

Elizabeth Kiss of Duke University stated, "The inarguable point is that it is totally unethical to withhold a known effective treatment," while Arthur Kaplan of the University of Pennsylvania remarked that the Tuskegee comparison was rash. He stated, "Tuskegee was clearly in the inexcusable zone, because it didn't have the interest of the subjects at heart. The AIDS research, on the other hand, is undertaken by people who are seriously trying to do something to help poor people who otherwise might get no effective treatment at all." Responding to the criticism of the studies, Dr. Helene Gayle, director of CDC's National Center for HIV, STD, and TB prevention, stated that the tests had not been carried out "behind closed doors" and noted that "this was done with a lot of discussion from the international community." (New York Times, 1997).

Whether or not this latter day example of medical research could be construed as "another Tuskegee" is a matter for discussion. What is perhaps a positive legacy of Tuskegee is the fact that individuals are now more sensitized to the obvious unethical and inexcusable treatment of individuals in a government sponsored research project, and future studies will be scrutinized far more carefully in the light of the shameful events that have become known simply as "the Tuskegee study."

Suggested Health Promotion Strategies
for Diverse Cultures

The Task Force on Black and Minority Health (1985) offers the following suggestions for programs aimed at diverse cultures:

- Channel efforts for minority communities through local leaders who could represent a powerful force for promoting acceptance and reinforcement of the central themes of health promotion messages.
- Data suggest that health messages are more readily accepted if they do not conflict with existing cultural beliefs. Where appropriate, messages should acknowledge existing cultural beliefs.
- Involve family, churches, employers and community organizations as a support system to facilitate and sustain behavior change to a more healthful lifestyle. For example, although hypertension controls in African Americans depend on appropriate medical therapy, blood pressure control can be improved and maintained by family and community support of activities such as proper diet and exercise.
- Language barriers, cultural differences, and lack of adequate information on access to care can complicate health maintenance and treatment. Health educators must ensure that culturally sensitive information is available in many forms within a specific community. This information should not only be subject-specific, but also include basic explanations of *how* to access services.
- Assess suitability of existing information and materials and/or develop new, culturally sensitive materials. Enlist the participation of professional and lay members of each minority group to assess the suitability of the materials.
- Encourage private organizations, such as religious and community organizations, clubs, and schools, to participate in developing minority support networks and other incentive techniques to facilitate the acceptance of health information and education.

Important points to consider before teaching and/or presenting to diverse populations follow:

- What is the precise ethnic mix of the class or audience? A description of *Hispanic* or *Asian* is probably not precise enough. Obtain as much specific information as possible.
- Find out more about the demographics of the group. Where do they live—in an urban, suburban, or rural setting? Do you have any information about educational levels or socioeconomic status.
- Consider the language proficiency of classes or groups. Is there a high proportion of recent immigrants who speak little English? Is a translator necessary, and, if so, can you find one?
- Are there any health problems unique to this group of which you should be aware? Research the health status of the group.

- Identify and consult individuals, perhaps school and community leaders, who are from, or at least familiar with, a specific race or culture.
- Adopt teaching or presentation strategies that will be culturally sensitive to specific groups. Your presentations will be much more effective and accepted better if the students/audience can closely relate to your style and content.
- Be aware of strong cultural influences within specific cultures, such as the family and the church. Gaining support and even cooperation from both these areas will add much credibility to the learning experience.

Case Study: Monica Monica is a young and inexperienced community health educator presenting a workshop to a group of middle-aged Hispanic (Mexican American) women. The topic of the workshop is the importance of having a regular pelvic examination. Monica has been told that Hispanic women tend to report low rates of Pap smear screening, and Monica's main objective is to increase compliance with this important test. Monica believes that many women feel uncomfortable with their own bodies and has decided to begin the workshop with an exercise designed to reduce this discomfort. To the amazement of the group of Hispanic women, Monica lies down on the table at the front of the room, lifts up her dress, pulls off her underwear, and proceeds to identify her cervix with the aid of a mirror. Meanwhile, an assistant moves around the audience slowly, handing out similar mirrors to the stunned and silent group. Once the audience realizes the intention of the instructor, there is a mass exodus toward the nearest exit . . . the workshop is over. Was this an appropriate strategy to use with any group? If not, why not? How else could Monica have accomplished her objective? (See Case Studies Revisited page 255.)

Ethnicity and the Health Educator

One question that is often raised with regard to health education and race is whether the race of the health educator need always be the same as the race of the intended audience. This often becomes a moot point in that there are simply insufficient numbers of minority health educators to serve all populations. However, all things being equal, the consensus seems to be that a presenter/teacher of similar culture to the audience is preferable. Obviously, familiarity with a culture would avoid some major pitfalls in sensitivity, as, for example, were committed by the over-zealous Monica in the case study. The issue of trust must also be considered. The Tuskegee study is an excellent illustration of why some cultures are suspicious of "external" interference. A more recent study seems to confirm the continuing suspicion of certain populations toward "outside influences." In a study of African American women attending a public health clinic, the researcher found that 21 percent of the women did not trust the federal government's reports on

AIDS, and 54 percent were uncertain about them. In addition, when questioned as to whether they considered AIDS to be an act of genocide against the black race, only 52 percent disagreed with the notion (Sharon, 1992). Given this issue of mistrust, a same-race health educator would seem to be optimal. Ironically, among the women in the previously mentioned study, 70 percent, when asked if the race of the information "messenger" was of any consequence, responded that it was not.

 For more information and tools related to this chapter visit www.jbpub.com/healtheducation.

EXERCISES

1. Consider the case study where Monica's presentation to the Mexican American women went so poorly. You have been asked to perform the same one-hour workshop for middle-aged Mexican American women on the importance of having a pelvic exam. Taking into account the features of this population, design a presentation plan (including behavioral objectives) that you think would be appropriate.

2. You have been asked to present a program on HIV/AIDS to an African American youth group (approximately 20 boys and girls aged 14–16 years). Write two objectives that you feel would be appropriate in this situation, then select two strategies/methods that you feel might be successful (keeping in mind what your objectives are). Justify your objective selection and choice of strategies.

3. In the light of what you know about the Tuskegee study and the more recent controversy concerning AIDS treatment studies in the third world, describe another contemporary minority health issue that might have the potential to cause some concern or suspicion within ethnic or racial minorities.

4. Selecting one of the areas of health targeted by the *Initiative to Eliminate Racial and Ethnic Disparities in Health,* briefly describe what you perceive to be the major barriers to effectively reducing discrepancies in the chosen area.

5. Define the term *cultural competency,* and briefly describe some practical measures that might increase the likelihood that cultural competency could be achieved.

CASE STUDIES REVISITED

Case Study Revisited: Susan

Susan had been presenting her important information to very homogenous groups and had not stopped to consider the culture of this latest group. Had she discovered the ethnic background of the participants beforehand, Susan could have identified levels of language, knowledge, and specific perceived needs of this population. Although advanced planning would not have removed the language issue, Susan could have taken steps to alleviate the problem. For example, she might have been able to identify a nurse or other health professional who was from that particular community and would have been willing to assist with the presentation, providing invaluable translation skills. (See page 232.)

Case Study Revisited: Denise Although Denise's motives were laudable, she made some obvious mistakes based on erroneous assumptions. If a health educator has any doubts at all about a group or population with which he or she is unfamiliar, questions should be directed whenever possible to individuals within the group in question. Denise could have contacted some of the women leaders beforehand to familiarize herself with the groups and assess what would be required to make the workshop successful. If this is not possible, perhaps there are fellow educators who have worked with these individuals or groups before who could provide information and advice. Working with diverse populations is not a simple matter, and we should all definitely avoid making assumptions based on what may not be true. (See page 247.)

Case Study Revisited: Monica Monica's rather radical introduction to the workshop is great example of poor method selection! This type of activity might have been problematic in many settings, and had Monica carried out the necessary research on this particular target population she would have realized that such a strategy was entirely inappropriate. Although Monica's intention was understandable, this type of overt and direct activity could not be successful with a population that is generally modest and self-conscious about sexuality. This rather disastrous workshop illustrates the necessity for thoroughly researching the characteristics of specific populations before designing intervention strategies. (See page 253.)

SUMMARY

1. Health educators need to have a good working knowledge of non-majority populations, including important information such as basic demographics and health disparities.

2. All individuals within minority populations are not the same. Appropriate methods of presentation must be considered to optimize the effectiveness of the program. Health educators can consult community members to help in developing potentially effective strategies.

3. Cultural competency is a concept designed to optimize the service and treatment received by racial and ethnic minorities within the health care system.

4. Health educators need to be aware of the influence of history on the receptiveness of racial and ethnic minorities to "outside" interventions.

REFERENCES

Centers for Disease Control and Prevention (1992). HIV/AIDS Surveillance, U.S. Department of Health & Human Services, Public Health Service, Atlanta, GA.

Centers for Disease Control and Prevention (1999). HIV/AIDS Surveillance Report 10(1). Atlanta, GA.

Cheng, M. (1998). Cultural competency. Closing the gap. *Office of Minority Health Newsletter*, March, 6. Washington DC: U.S. Department of Health & Human Services.

Ellerbrock, J.V., Bush, T.J., Chamberland, Me.E., & Oxtoby, M.J. (1991). The epidemiology of women with AIDS in the U.S. 1980–90. *Journal of the American Medical Association, 265*(22), 2971–2975.

Harris, J., & Fletcher, M. (1997a). Six decades later, an apology, *Washington Post,* September 17, AO1.

Jones, J. (1981). Bad blood: The Tuskegee syphilis experiment—A tragedy of race and medicine. New York: Free Press.

LaVeist, T.A. (1996). Why we should continue to study race . . . but do a better job: an essay on race, racism and health. *Ethnicity and Disease, 6,* 21–29.

Leslie, C. (1990). Scientific racism: Reflections on peer review, science and ideology. *Social Science Medicine, 31*(8), 891–912.

National Commission on AIDS. (1990). Hearings on HIV disease in the African American Communities.

Stolberg, S. (1997). U.S. AIDS research in poor nations raises outcry on ethics. *The New York Times,* September 18, A.33.

Nickens, H.W. (1995). The role of race/ethnicity and social class in minority health status. *Health Services Research, 30*(1):151–162.

Osborne, N.G., & Feit, M.D. (1992). The use of race in medical research. *Journal of the American Medical Association, 267,* 275–279.

Parran, T. (1937). *Shadow on the Land: Syphilis.* New York: Reynal and Hitchcock.

Raspberry, W. (1997b). Shades of Tuskegee, *Washington Post,* September 22, A.19;

Sharon, L.M. (1992). Assessing the AIDS education needs of black women in an urban epicenter for HIV infection: A descriptive analysis. Unpublished master's thesis, University of Maryland.

Thomas, S.B., & Quinn, S.C. (1991). The Tuskegee syphilis study, 1932–1972: Implications for HIV education and AIDS risk education programs in the black community. *American Journal of Public Health, 81*(11), 1498–1505.

U.S. Census, Department of Commerce (1999). "Resident Population of the United States: Middle Series Projections 2000–2050." Retrieved April 7, 1999, from the World Wide Web: http//www.census.gov.

U.S. Census, Department of Commerce (1998). "Selected Social Characteristics of All Persons and Hispanic Persons, by Type of Origin: March 1997." Internet release date: August 7, 1998. Retrieved April 16, 1999, from the World Wide Web: http//www.census.gov.

U.S. Office of Minority Health. (1999). *The Initiative to Eliminate Racial and Ethnic Disparities in Health.* Department of Health and Human Services. Retrieved April 15, 1999 from the World Wide Web: http//www.omhrc.gov.

U.S. Task Force on Black and Minority Health (1985). Secretary's Report. Washington DC: U.S. Department of Health and Human Services.

White House (1997) Remarks by President Clinton in apology for study done in Tuskegee. Press release, Office of the Press Secretary, May 16.

Williams, D.R. (1993). A framework for understanding the relationship between race and health. From "Race in the Health of America: Problems, Issues and Directions." *MMWR, 42,* (RR-10), 9.

Special Challenges

Entry-Level and Graduate-Level Health Educator Competencies Addressed in This Chapter

Responsibility I: Assessing Individual and Community Needs for Health Education

Competency A: Obtain health related data about social and cultural environments, growth and development factors, needs, and interests.

Competency C: Infer needs for health education on the basis of obtained data.

Responsibility III: Implementing Health Education Programs

Competency B: Infer enabling objectives as needed to implement instructional program in specified settings.

Competency C: Select methods and media best suited to implement program plans for specific learners.

Responsibility VII: Communicating Health and Health Education Needs, Concerns and Resources

Competency A: Interpret concepts, purposes, and theories of health education.

Competency B: Predict the impact of societal value systems on health education programs.

> Note: The competencies listed above, which are addressed in this chapter, are considered to be both entry-level and graduate-level competencies by the National Commission for Health Education Credentialing, Inc. They are taken from *A Framework for the Development of Competency Based Curricula for Entry Level Health Educators* by the National Task Force for the Preparation and Practice of Health Education, 1985, and *A Competency-Based Framework for Graduate Level Health Educators* by the National Task Force for the Preparation and Practice of Health Education, 1999.

Method Selection in Health Education

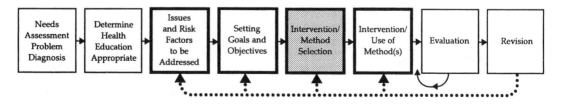

Heavy-bordered boxes indicate subjects addressed in this text; shaded boxes indicate subjects(s) of current chapter.

OBJECTIVES   After studying the chapter the reader should be able to

- List some populations that might require the health educator to prepare material differently for presentation.
- Describe health concerns unique to certain populations.
- Define terms related to disability and exceptionality.
- List some common mistakes when working with special populations.
- Describe strategies to enhance presentations for special populations.

KEY TOPICS

Culture	Disability
Literacy levels	Health knowledge levels
Language	Sources of health information
Political awareness	Presentation preparation

Just as health educators have to adapt their presentations to accommodate the needs of ethnically diverse populations, so must they do the same for groups or individuals who have particular special needs. Becoming an expert in all the subsets of populations that might utilize health education services is an unlikely and unrealistic proposition, yet health educators need to consider some of the challenges inherent in working in diverse settings. Simply considering and finding out about populations would be a solid first step in preparing more effective interventions. In some instances, unique factors that exist in certain populations may make little difference in how a presentation is made, yet the health educator needs to at least consider these factors in his or her preparation. It is beyond the scope of this text to focus in great depth on all different populations with special needs, so the intent of this chapter is simply to give health educators a glimpse into the worlds of individuals with whom they may at some point be working.

Case Study: Kareem   Kareem, a community health educator, has been asked to make a presentation on contraception to students at a school for special students. He has made many such presentations to students in the local high schools on this topic but has never worked with an exceptional population. Kareem is surprised at the request, believing that such a population doesn't really need this type of education; after all, aren't they supervised most of the time? Maybe he could wait until next year, when many of the students will be placed in regular schools. Kareem really doesn't understand the point of covering such material with them. What do you think of Kareem's reaction? (See Case Studies Revisited page 282.)

Exceptional Populations

A much underserved and underconsidered population with regard to health education is one often labeled as **exceptional.** Mainstream health education students may be justifiably confused by descriptive labels related to this area, so some definition is necessary. Mandell and Fiscus (1981) offer three fairly straightforward clarifications of often used labels:

> **Exceptional**—atypical; a performance which deviates from what is expected, either a higher or lower performance.
>
> **Disability**—total or partial behavioral, mental, physical, or sensorial loss of functioning. All disabled people are exceptional, but the reverse is not necessarily true.
>
> **Handicap**—environmental restrictions placed on a person's life as a result of a disability or exceptionality (p. 3).

Beware, for the most sacred cow may become the tiger's breakfast.
—Mohan Singh

To illustrate the endless possibility of variations of exceptionality, the same authors describe a case study of a six-year-old boy named James who was born with spina bifida, a condition where the spinal column fails to close and where the extent of disability can be extremely varied. James has limited use of his legs and has no bowel or bladder control. With regard to academic potential, he has been identified as gifted, and he attends a regular first-grade class. Table 9-1 shows how James would fit into the preceding definitions.

This profile clearly illustrates how labeling can be applied to specific conditions. However, although labeling serves a useful purpose in identifying the type of educational interventions that might prove optimal for individual development, the procedure is not without criticism. Meyen (1978), for example, believes that labeling, or classifying an individual, can be problematic for the following reasons:

1. All too often the label emphasizes the negative instead of stressing the positive. This stresses the individual's limitations not strengths . . . what the person *cannot* do rather than *can*. This may become a self-fulfilling prophecy.

Table 9-1
Definitions of Three
Common Terms

Label	Corresponding Behaviors
Exceptional	James deviates from the norm (below average) with regard to physical performance and exceeds the norm in intellectual performance.
Disabled	James is unable to walk or control bowel and bladder functions.
Handicapped	James cannot move physically through his environment without assistance. In addition, he requires educational programs for the academically talented. (Although giftedness is not considered by most to be a **handicap,** it is the authors' opinion that the gifted are handicapped in that their superior abilities, for the most part, are not developed in most traditional educational programs.)

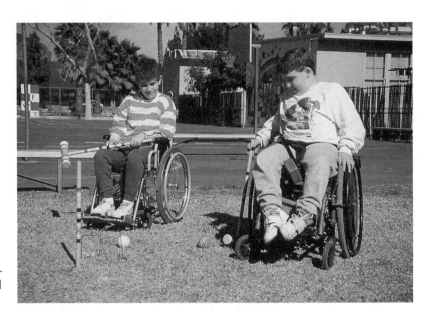

Health educators can expect to work with individuals from exceptional populations.

2. The accuracy of the label may be questionable. Often labels are simplistically given on the basis of single factors and thus may conceal a more complex causation.
3. Labeling does not accurately account for differences within individual classifications. A broad range of disability can be found within any classification, a good example of this being hearing loss (discussed in this chapter).
4. Conditions of individuals rarely remain static, and classifications do a poor job of including this temporal concept. Individuals tend to change over time, as will their educational needs. Specific labeling, therefore, may no longer be accurate after a period of time.

As a result of these concerns about labeling, some propose abandoning the practice completely. In its place, educators would substitute a more precise description of each individual, with a focus on the implications for learning strategies (Goldstein et al., 1975).

Categories of Exceptional Children

The passage of Public Law 94-142 (PL 94-142) in 1975 codified the rights of all exceptional children and youth to a free, appropriate education. Exceptional children who are eligible by law for services through special educational placements are categorized as follows: mentally retarded, deaf and hard of hearing, speech impaired, visually impaired, emotionally disturbed, orthopedically and other health impaired, and learning disabled. These descriptors, or labels, are very broad, and to fully describe the population served by this law, a more precise definition is needed. The *Federal Register* of August 1977 contains the rules and regulations of PL 94-142 and defines its labels as follows:

Sec. 121a.5 Handicapped Children

Deaf means a hearing impairment which is so severe that the child is impaired in processing linguistic information through hearing, with or without amplification, which adversely affects educational performance.

Deaf-blind means concomitant hearing and visual impairments, the combination of which causes such severe communication and other developmental and educational problems that they cannot be accommodated in special education programs solely for deaf or blind children.

Hard of hearing means a hearing impairment, whether permanent or fluctuating, which adversely affects a child's educational performance but which is not included under the definition of "deaf" in this section.

Mentally retarded means significantly sub-average general intellectual functioning existing concurrently with deficits in adaptive behavior and manifested during the developmental period, which adversely affects a child's educational performance.

Multihandicapped means concomitant impairments (such as mentally retarded-blind, mentally retarded-orthopedically impaired, etc.), the combination of which causes severe educational problems that they cannot be accommodated in special education programs solely for one of the impairments. The term does not include deaf-blind children.

Orthopedically impaired means a severe orthopedic impairment which adversely affects a child's educational performance. The term includes impairments caused by congenital anomaly (e.g., clubfoot, absence of of some member, etc.), impairments caused by disease (e.g., poliomyelitis, bone tuberculosis, etc.), and impairments from other causes (e.g., cerebral palsy, amputations, and fractures or burns which cause contractures).

Other health impaired means limited strength, vitality or alertness, due to chronic or acute health problems such as heart condition, tuberculosis, rheumatic fever, nephritis, asthma, sickle cell anemia, hemophilia, epilepsy, lead poisoning, leukemia, or diabetes which adversely affects a child's educational performance.

Seriously emotionally disturbed is defined as follows:
(i) The term means a condition exhibiting one or more of the following characteristics over a long period of time and to a marked degree, which adversely affects educational performance:

A. An inability to learn which cannot be explained by intellectual, sensory, or health factors.
B. An inability to build or maintain satisfactory interpersonal relationships with peers and teachers.
C. Inappropriate types of behavior or feelings under normal circumstances.
D. A general pervasive mood of unhappiness or depression or;
E. A tendency to develop physical symptoms or fears associated with personal or school problems.

(ii) The term includes children who are schizophrenic or autistic. The term does not include children who are socially maladjusted, unless it is determined that they are seriously emotionally disturbed. Special learning disability means a disorder in one or more of the basic psychological processes involved in understanding or in using language, spoken or written, which may manifest itself in an imperfect ability to listen, think, speak, read, write, spell, or to do mathematical calculations. The term includes such definitions as perceptual handicaps, brain injury, minimal brain dysfunction, dyslexia, and developmental aphasia. The term does not include children who have learning problems that are primarily the result of visual, hearing, or motor handicaps, of mental retardation, or of environmental, cultural or economic disadvantage.

Speech impaired means a communication disorder, such as stuttering, impaired articulation, a language impairment, or a voice impairment, which adversely affects a child's educational performance.

Visually handicapped means a visual performance which, even with correction, adversely affects a child's educational performance. The term includes both partially seeing and blind children. (20 U.S.C.1401(1),(15).)

It is not practical, nor is it within the scope of this text, to describe in great detail all these categories of "exceptionality." The majority of mainstream health educators will have extremely limited contact with individuals included in some of these categories. Consequently, the remainder of this chapter will focus on the categories of exceptionality with which school and community health educators are likely to have the most frequent contact.

Visually Impaired

The term *visually impaired* is used to describe individuals who have defective or impaired vision. Definitions of impairment or blindness can be either legally or educationally based. Legal definitions are based on a technical evaluation, whereas educational definitions tend to be more pragmatic and simplified, stating that the visually impaired are those people whose visual condition is such that special provisions are necessary for successful education (Meyen, 1978). This is an important population for the health educator to be familiar with, as many individuals with visual impairments are being mainstreamed in both the school and community settings.

As with the deaf population, the effects of health education for visually impaired people depend to a great extent on the age of onset of visual impairment, the degree of any accompanying disability, and the availability of developmental opportunities. Identifying the extent of visual impairment is reasonably straightforward, but measuring secondary effects of impairment on such things as language development and cognition skills is more difficult, simply because most available instruments and standardized tests are written and are not available in braille. Even if they were available in braille, many participants could not use them, as not all visually impaired people know braille.

Lowenfeld (1962) describes the primary effects of visual impairment as restrictions imposed on the individual in

1. Range and variety of possible experiences.
2. Ability to move about the environment.
3. Control of the environment and of the self in relation to it.

The ability to move about the environment is particularly important, as it is this freedom that provides the sighted individual the opportunity for observation and experience. The absence of this opportunity will obviously affect the development of any individual. A concrete example of restricted experience is in the development of language. As most children develop, they take notice of what is happening around them. Children can then question a parent or other person about what they see . . . sometimes in an endless string of questions that only children can ask! A child who does not see a small animal or large gray raincloud has a compromised ability to ask questions and learn about the world. Vocabulary may then become limited, as will comprehension of the environment.

Case Study: Robert Robert is preparing to present a workshop on nutrition and fitness for college students. He has ascertained that approximately 35 students will attend. In anticipation of a workshop filled with a great deal of information, he has prepared a large number of overhead transparencies to facilitate teaching. As Robert is adjusting the focus on the overhead projector, he notices two students with canes carefully entering the classroom. They are obviously significantly visually impaired. Robert has a sinking feeling as he stares at his pile of overhead transparencies and wonders what to do next. What would you do next? (See Case Studies Revisited page 282.)

In its initial stages, motor development is dependent on vision. Seeing objects in the immediate environment stimulates an infant to raise a head or reach out a hand. If an infant is blind, the motivation to move may well be inhibited, and subsequently the visually impaired child cannot develop the experience of being able to move through his or her environment. The obvious lack of visual stimulation can lead some blind individuals to resort to *blindisms*, or primitive movements—perhaps a rocking back and forth motion, or excessive rubbing of the eyes. If an environment is provided that stimulates a child and encourages physical response, the visually impaired child's motor development will probably progress within the typical chronologic range (Cratty, 1971).

Meyen (1978) suggests four important principles that the teacher of any subject should consider when instructing visually impaired people:

1. Because all visually impaired people are not the same, instruction should be *individualized* as much as possible.

2. Teachers should stress as much as possible, relationships between things in the environment which are not discernible to the blind.
3. Stimulation of all types must be provided to attract and maintain attention.
4. Some visually impaired children must be taught to actively engage in the learning process. Children devoid of stimulae might tend to be somewhat passive and need to be taught how to become more involved.

Mandell and Fiscus (1981) also offer some valuable suggestions to individuals who might be teaching visually impaired people:

- Explain about, and allow individuals to explore their physical environment—classroom, meeting room etc.
- Maximize the remaining vision of the visually impaired—consider adequate levels of light, classroom seating, using larger writing, etc.
- In the school setting, give non-visually impaired children the opportunity to discuss blindness with the students who have vision problems.
- Provide learning opportunities that will actively include people who are blind.
- Ask other involved professionals, or in the case of children, ask parents, "What works?" Don't be afraid to ask for advice.
- In the classroom setting, be sure to orally repeat anything that is written on the blackboard.
- Verbally clarify any predominantly visual materials that you may be using, e.g. maps, charts, and graphs.
- If an individual is utilizing braille, allow additional time.
- Encourage individuals to utilize any alternative techniques and or technology that might facilitate learning.

Learning Aids and Material for Visually Impaired

Learning aids can basically be divided into two categories: optical and nonoptical. Examples of optical aids might be glasses, magnifiers, etc., while an example of a nonoptical aid would be the use of braille. Simply stated, braille consists of a series of raised dot patterns that represent elements of

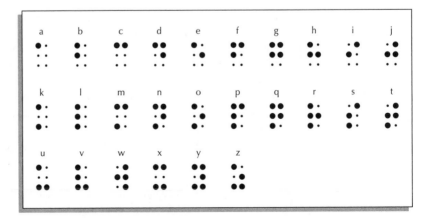

Figure 9-1
Braille: a Nonoptical Reading Aid.

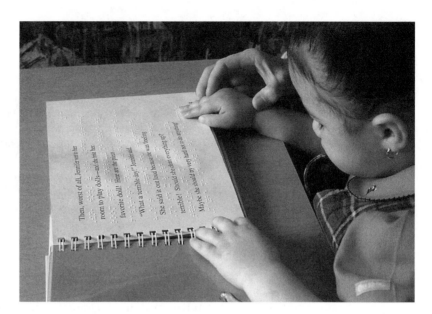

A person reading with braille might require a little extra time.

language. The dot patterns are placed within a six-dot cell to denote letters of the alphabet, numbers, and punctuation. (See Figure 9-1.) The braille characters are "read" by a person's fingertips.

An important point for educators to remember is that braille is more ambiguous than the printed word. Children who are blind and utilizing braille might take longer to read material than seeing children who are reading print. This discrepancy in reading speed is often continued into adulthood. For example, in a study comparing the reading speeds of blind and seeing high school seniors, the blind students using braille averaged 90 words per minute versus 250 words per minute by students reading print (Myers et al., 1958). This time discrepancy needs to be acknowledged and included when planning presentations or lessons.

Individuals who are blind may also write in braille. The two major options for doing this are a braillewriter, a machine somewhat similar to a typewriter in appearance that embosses paper with the braille code, and a slate and stylus. The latter device consists of a hinged frame between which paper is clamped. The writer presses down with the stylus, pushing the paper on to the back of the frame, which contains six depressions arranged like dots in the braille cell. The writer thus creates the braille cells by hand as opposed to using a machine, the braillewriter, which performs this function more easily.

An additional and frequently utilized nonoptical aid is the audiotape. Cassette audiotapes are relatively inexpensive and easy to record with and can provide the opportunity for the visually impaired to listen to a lecture, take a test from a tape, or even listen to a best-selling novel that has been transposed onto tape.

**Assisting the
Partially Sighted**

Many individuals who are not blind nevertheless have a vision impairment. Thus, they are able to only partially see. These individuals might be helped by taking the following simple steps, proposed by Mandell and Fiscus (1981), to facilitate learning:

- Use specially adapted books with larger print (Figure 9-2).
- Carefully consider background colors when preparing presentation materials. Ensure that print and graphics are clearly defined against the background.
- Seating an individual at the front of the room might be helpful.
- Ensure that good levels of lighting are available.
- Allow extra time for completion of work.
- For some individuals, listening might be a more effective learning device than reading. To that end, ensure that a quiet atmosphere exists that might be more conducive to learning.

One of the primary agencies providing resources for the visually impaired, is the American Printing House for the Blind in Louisville, Kentucky. For additional information, see the appendix.

Figure 9-2
Font size can be
enlarged to help the
visually impaired.

This is the type of font size that is often used in books and other written resources specifically developed for people with visual impairment.

Notice how different the above font size is to this example (Times 12), a font typically used for individuals without any form of visual impairment.

Learning Disabled

The label of **learning disabled** has become a somewhat amorphous term, often applied to any students who do not succeed in school. Some definitions include "slow learners" or "mentally retarded," and others incorporate "emotionally unstable" and even blindness. Other experts in this field believe that the label of "learning disabled" should be much more specific than failing to succeed in school. There are obviously many reasons why children might fail in school that would hardly be designated as a learning disability—lack of motivation, inappropriate or mediocre teaching methods, difficulties in the home life, poor nutrition, lack of sleep, and so on. Mandell and Fiscus (1981) suggest this yardstick: if learning difficulties can be overcome by a different type of instruction, then the child should not be considered learning disabled.

A national definition of learning disabled was established in 1977 as a result of PL 94-142 (*Federal Register*, 1977):

> Specific learning disability means a disorder in one or more of the basic psychological processes involved in understanding or in using language spoken or written which may manifest itself in an imperfect ability to listen, think, speak, read, write, spell or to do mathematical calculations. The term includes such conditions as perceptual handicaps, brain injury, minimum brain dysfunction, dyslexial and developmental aphasia. The term does not include children who have learning problems which are primarily the result of visual, hearing or motor handicaps, of mental retardation, of emotional disturbance, or of environmental, cultural or economic disadvantage.

The *Federal Register* (1977) goes on to identify seven areas where a major discrepancy may exist between ability and achievement:

1. Oral expression
2. Listening comprehension
3. Written expression
4. Basic reading skill
5. Reading comprehension
6. Mathematics calculation
7. Mathematics reasoning

In order for a child to be eligible for special educational services, an evaluation team must agree that

- The child must exhibit learning difficulties in at least one of the seven areas just listed.
- The child has a severe learning achievement problem.
- The major reason for the discrepancy between achievement and ability is not other handicapping conditions or sociological factors.

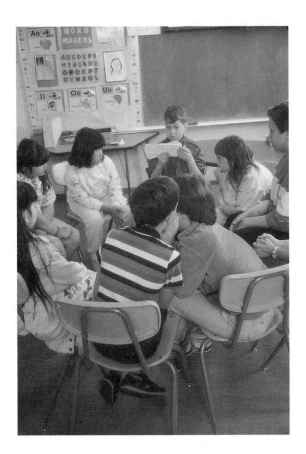

Learning disabilities can sometimes be difficult to detect.

In 1966 the Easter Seal Research Foundation, a federally sponsored task force, published a report that listed the ten most frequently cited characteristics of learning disabled children (Clements, 1966). Being aware of these more prevalent characteristics might be useful to the health educator in considering health education methodology:

1. **Hyperactivity**—a problem with remaining seated; constant movement from one point of the room to another.
2. **Perceptual-motor impairments**—experiencing difficulty reproducing information received through the senses. Difficulty with copying, problems with written information, identifying letters of the alphabet, reading from left to right, and reproducing basic shapes. One of the better known learning disabilities in this category is **dyslexia.**
3. **Attention**—a problem with focus and holding attention for any length of time. Individuals might experience difficulty in completing tasks, are easily distracted, and often cannot remain seated for long periods of time.
4. **Memory**—difficulty in memorizing information over long and short periods of time. Indicators might include an inability to remember basic in-

formation like the family's address and telephone number or being unable to remember things learned the day before.

5. **Speech and hearing**—some children who have a form of communication disorder might have a problem with using correct grammar, and articulating words and thoughts. Another indicator might be a repetition of the same phrases, over and over, resulting from restricted language development.

6. **Emotional lability**—some children might not have developed emotionally and socially to an age-appropriate level. This may result in a low threshold for frustration, difficulty with social interaction, and on occasion a temper tantrum.

7. **Coordination defecits**—these deficits might become identifiable as awkward or clumsy physical movements or problems with fine motor skills such as using scissors or pencil and paper.

8. **Impulsivity**—these children rush into reactions or responses without any thought for the consequences. This characteristic could be manifested by writing down the first answer that comes to mind in a test, or running out into the street after a ball without regard for traffic.

9. **Learning deficits in basic academic subjects**—these students may demonstrate a wide discrepancy in achievement between subjects. For example, a student might be a full grade level ahead in reading ability but two years below in math. Relevant terms in this section are

   Dyslexia—problems in reading (also *reading disability*)
   Dysgraphia—problems in writing
   Dyscalcula—problems with arithmetic
   Word blindness

10. **Equivocal neurological signs**—*equivocal* means questionable or uncertain. For children in this category, there is no direct evidence of neurological damage, yet the individuals demonstrate characteristics such as hyperactivity, poor attention, problems with concentration, easily distracted, impulsivity, hyperactivity, or poor motor functioning.

Attention Deficit Disorder (ADD) and Attention Deficit Hyperactivity Disorder (ADHD)

On March 12, 1999, the federal government released the final regulations to the Individuals with Disabilities Education Act (IDEA). These regulations were an attempt to more tightly define and operationalize already established rules and regulations for ensuring educational access to all people and were intended to be incorporated into each state's existing standards. Prior to these new regulations, children with **attention deficit disorder (ADD)** or attention deficit hyperactivity disorder (ADHD) were eligible for special educational services only if their difficulties were accompanied by an additional qualifying disorder. Now ADD or ADHD alone can make a child eligible for special educational services. Some surveys estimate that 3–5 percent of U.S. schoolchildren (1.5 million to 2.5 million) have been diagnosed with either ADD or ADHD. Although a small percentage of ADD/ADHD students are taught in self-contained classrooms, the vast majority will spend at least part of a day in a regular setting. Thus, health educators are very likely to encounter children with ADD/ADHD in both the school and community settings. Here are some tips that might be helpful when working with these students.

K–12
- *Promote high self-esteem:* be friendly, respect opinions, provide immediate feedback, give reinforcement.
- *Establish control:* be consistent, follow definite rules, offer explanations for any rule that was broken.
- *Maximize academic improvement:* allow for flexibility in amount of time needed to complete a project, offer alternatives to writing (e.g. word processing).
- *Schedule activities to accommodate student's fluctuating energy levels:* mix high and low energy activities.
- *Provide organizational tools:* create checklists, develop a routine, use labels on articles.
- *Reward success:* use stickers, charts, shake hands, high five, smile, verbal praise.
- *Use group work:* encourage problem solving, teamwork, and cooperation.
- *Grab the student's attention:* give short, clear instructions, and ask students to repeat the information (Hogan, 1997).

K–6
- Have the student sit close to the teacher.
- Surround the ADHD student with good student role models.
- Put extra materials away to minimize distractions.
- Enhance listening skills by making good eye contact before giving instructions, and make directions clear and concise.
- Establish very specific rules and implement them.
- Respond immediately when disruptive behavior occurs.
- Establish an incentive program based on points or tokens.
- Assist with developing self-esteem by smiling, praising, or otherwise recognizing achievement.
- Establish realistic and achievable goals (McFarland, 1995).

With such a wide variety of potential problems, designing methods of instruction for this population can be extremely complicated, and there are no simple solutions for planning presentations. Hammel and Bartel (1978) believe that when constructing materials for teaching learning disabled students, instructors must consider three areas: design, methods, and practicality. The *design* component speaks to the basic organization of the material that the authors believe should be presented in logical, sequential building blocks. The *method* component considers whether the material should be used individually or in groups. Because of the variety of existing learning levels, a diversity of presentation methods is necessary, with a willingness to be flexible toward varying student responses. *Practicality* dictates that materials be "durable" (able to stand the test of time) and that they can be usable both independently and with supervision (Hammill and Bartel, 1978).

In an examination of instruction styles that seemed to produce better than expected results, Westwood (1993) suggests that the most effective teachers/presenters

- Were more specific about presentation/lesson objectives.
- Were better able to judge accurately the time needed to accomplish the objectives.
- Successfully divided the presentation/lesson into a manageable and logical sequence.
- Anticipated problems and made successful accommodations for them.
- More often modified instruction based on participant responses.
- Used vocabulary and materials that were age and ability appropriate.
- More often provided an opportunity for learner success.
- Spent time and effort in creating an atmosphere of concern about the importance of the presentation/lesson.

Westwood (1993) discusses the phenomenon of the *failure cycle,* experienced by all children but more acutely by the learning disabled child. The child attempts to master a specific skill but fails. Because other children seem able to perform this skill, the child loses confidence, leading to a deliberate avoidance of the activity. This avoidance then assures that no skill practice occurs, guaranteeing, in turn, that competency and proficiency are never attained. Constant failure leads to decreased self-esteem and a generalization of failure to nearly all activities. The basic message of this cycle is, "If at first you don't succeed, you don't succeed!" The implications of this concept are twofold. In order to avoid the possibility of early failure, presenters/teachers must plan and develop new activities with great clarity and provide enough assistance to the learners to make success extremely likely. Second, the only means of breaking the failure cycle is to develop ways in which participants can be successful and ultimately feel that they are improving. Rather than dwelling on the negatives of the child, on what he or she cannot do, educators are encouraged to focus on ways to allow the child to feel successful, using those gains as a springboard for future development and achievement (Westwood, 1993).

Some health educators believe that it is particularly important for learning disabled students to receive sound information related to sex education. Gordon (1973) explains that people with learning disabilities need sex education for three major reasons: for the most part, they have the same desires as other people for companionship, love, and sexual activity; the passage from adolescence to adulthood is often intensified for this population; and learning disabled individuals may have difficulty processing information and therefore remain dangerously uninformed. In the context of human sexuality, Haight and Fachting (1986) suggest the following principles for teaching learning disabled students:

- Use printed materials that have a fairly low reading level.
- Use materials that have a mature theme. Many learning disabled students are of average or higher intelligence and will be bored and feel patronized by immature content and approach.
- Use interactive teaching methods to actively involve students in the learning process (role play, games, skits, etc.).
- Make material as relevant as possible to real-life situations.
- With written materials, use simplified syntax, short sentences, and also short paragraphs with the main subject first.

Deafness

The deaf and hard of hearing are included in this chapter because they are truly minority populations in regard to language and culture. Many individuals might believe that people who are deaf or hard of hearing are exactly like hearing individuals, with the one obvious exception that they cannot hear. But this is a simplistic notion. The impairment in hearing has repercussions in various areas. Here are some important questions that health educators should consider in planning a presentation:

- Are the health needs of the deaf identical to the health needs of the hearing?
- Are the health knowledge levels of the deaf similar to the knowledge levels of the hearing?
- Is there any difference in health behavior between the deaf and hearing populations?
- How do knowledge levels, attitudes, and behaviors differ within the deaf and hard-of-hearing communities?
- Can health educators use the same methods of health education with deaf people as they do with hearing people?
- Can materials originally developed for hearing audiences be used effectively by deaf or hard-of-hearing audiences?

Case Study: Jill   Jill was a community health educator who had been asked to present a one-hour workshop on safer sex to a group of 30 new students at a local community college. The organizer had mentioned the possibility that one or two students who were either deaf or hard of hearing might attend the workshop. Jill gave the matter little further consideration, feeling that if the students did attend they could be seated at the front of the room and that she would attempt to speak louder and enunciate more clearly. Two deaf students did indeed attend, and after seating them in the front row Jill proceeded with the workshop, taking great care to speak loudly and clearly, facing the deaf students as much as possible. Part of the workshop included a short videotape on safer sex practices, and when the two deaf students left the room five minutes into the film, Jill supposed that the students had been offended by the explicit nature of what they had seen. Jill completed the workshop oblivious to her mistaken assumptions and beliefs. What do you think the real problem was, and what steps could Jill take should this issue arise again? (See Case Studies Revisited page 283.)

Before attempting to address some of these questions, it is essential for the health educator to understand some basic information related to deafness.

Deaf Culture   Like any true subculture or minority group, people who are deaf adhere to certain cultural norms that are passed on from one generation to the next. Most cultures pass on their culture within the family unit. However, the deaf community is unique in the way that its culture is perpetuated. Because 90 percent of deaf children have two hearing parents, only a minority of deaf individuals acquire their cultural identity and social skills in the home. The majority of deaf people learn about their culture in schools for the deaf, from other children, and from teachers and houseparents (Gallaudet University, 1990).

Study about the deaf culture has isolated and defined the following characteristics and values, as presented by The National Academy, Gallaudet University, 1990:

1. Membership is based on deafness. Members have little or no hearing, and define themselves as deaf.
2. There is a heavy emphasis on vision. **American Sign Language,** a visual mode of communication, is the language used within the deaf community. Members gain the vast majority of their information through their eyes and make a point of observing closely what is happening around them.
3. There is a specific set of social norms. Members follow certain social habits that are somewhat different from those of general society. Among these are the following:
   a. Members do not generally use their voices with deaf friends even if they do so with hearing friends. Some members of the deaf community purposely refrain from using their voices in order to dissociate themselves from speech.
   b. Members will wave, tap, or throw a small piece of paper to attract a person's attention.
   c. Members use a variety of devices to replace ordinary alarm clocks, door bells, telephones, fire alarms, etc.
4. Members place a strong emphasis on fostering and maintaining social ties within the community.

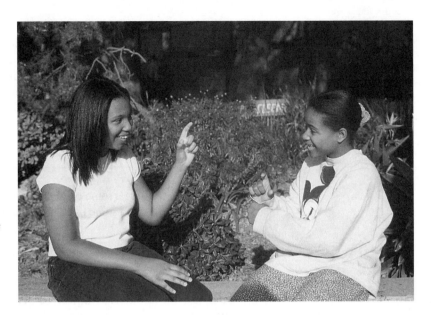

American sign language is the most commonly used form of communication in the deaf and hard of hearing community.

Social etiquette within the deaf community can be slightly different from that of the hearing community. For example, although the hearing culture generally considers staring to be rude, deaf culture has no prohibition against this, as staring is necessary for effective sign communication.

The two most common descriptors related to individuals who have a hearing loss are *deaf* (cannot make use of residual hearing for the purposes of communication) and *hard of hearing* (can use residual hearing to assist in communication). The term *hearing impaired* is often avoided for two reasons. First, as with many other contemporary issues, deafness is influenced by its own political agendas, and for some deaf individuals the word "impaired" suggests that something is "broken." This descriptor, therefore, is viewed as inaccurate and undesirable by many in the deaf community. Second, this terminology does not usefully distinguish between "deaf" and "hard of hearing" and so has limited practical use. Keeping up with terms that are constantly changing is not easy, particularly when individual health educators live outside many of the cultures in which they are asked to work. However, the educators should make every possible attempt to remain current in order to prevent offending individuals and to maintain crucial credibility.

Deafness can be divided into two types: *congenital* (deaf from birth) and *acquired* (becoming deaf after birth because of illness or accident). Acquired deafness can then be divided into *prelingual* (becoming deaf before spoken language skills had been developed) and *postlingual* (becoming deaf after spoken language had been developed) categories. (See Figure 9-3.)

Although at first glance these distinctions might seem subtle, they carry important implications for health educators as they approach program and

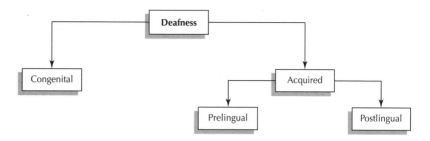

Figure 9-3
Forms of Deafness.

material development. Those individuals who are congenitally or prelingually deaf will not have been exposed to the more typical methods of language development—repetition of the spoken word, constantly hearing words and sounds, and learning to read by hearing written words spoken aloud. As a result, congenitally or prelingually deaf individuals may struggle with written and spoken English. Studies have shown that many deaf and hard-of-hearing students read at lower than the norm grade levels for their age. One study estimated that approximately half of those individuals with hearing loss aged 18 and below read on less than a fourth-grade reading level and only 10 percent read at above an eighth-grade level (Trybus and Karchmer, 1977).

Unfortunately, many individuals mistakenly equate reading levels with intelligence, and health educators must be careful not to make this assumption. Although deaf and hard of hearing individuals might indeed read at lower grade levels, their I.Q. scores do not differ greatly from the hearing population. However, because of this lack of comprehension of both written and spoken language, communication can become a major barrier between deaf and hearing people. . . a barrier of which the health educator must be aware. Consideration must be given as to how to overcome the barrier in effectively educating the deaf and hard-of-hearing communities about important health issues.

Here are some examples of questions addressed to the health educator of a college for the deaf via the computer/mail system (Morrone-Joseph, 1992). Take note of the wide range of linguistic ability among students.

Example 1   *Hi . . I want to know and curious. Suppose I did period on the end of the month at Feb . . later in the two weeks and the sperm did in the vagina. But the period will come on the end of march . . is it possible to be pregnant or not . . please let me know this week so I can aware that . . .*

Example 2   *There are two questions I need to know . . . I am 20 years old female. Am I suppose to take pap-smear and breast check up? Or is it too early for me to test? Can you tell me the difference between the pap-smear and breast check up?*

Example 3   *Which days are safe to have sex without getting pregnant, without using any method of birth control? I was told that the time before ovulation is safe.*

These three examples above clearly represent a cross-section of written-English levels. Although the writing levels are very different, it is interesting to note that all of these excerpts do effectively communicate their questions. It is often necessary to read for content and not be put off by "strange" English. The health educator must be aware that all deaf individuals are *not* the same, nor do they operate at identical levels of communication. This factor must be taken into account when developing and planning programs.

If I speak in a clear manner, can't they read lips? The foregoing is a common misconception about communicating with the deaf. Remember, in the case study, Jill assumed that speaking in a loud voice with clear enunciation was sufficient accommodation for her deaf and hard-of-hearing students. But the notion that a good way to communicate with the deaf is for them to read lips is a myth. There are many reasons why reading lips is fraught with problems, not the least of which is that the English language has many words that look the same on the lips. One estimate places the proportion of words in the English language that are considered *homophonous* (look alike on the lips) to be 40–60 percent (Fitzgerald and Fitzgerald, 1980). Here are some examples of words with very different meanings but identical appearances on the lips:

MAIL	MALE
BAIL	BALE
PAIL	PALE
SAIL	SALE

In addition, factors such as distance from the speaker, people in between, poor lighting, head movements, and poor speech patterns all contribute to making lipreading an ineffective mode of communication. It is perhaps ironic to note that because they have developed speech and language through hearing, the best lip-readers are in fact hearing individuals (Lowell, 1958).

Couldn't I take a quick course in sign language? The idea that a hearing person could take a brief course in sign language and then effectively communicate with a deaf person is, unfortunately, as common as it is absurd! Imagine that in one month you will be expected to present a one-hour workshop on stress management to a group of 30 Russian immigrants who speak no English. In preparation for this, you will polish your presentation material and then take a short course in Russian! As absurd as this example might appear, the comparison is not inaccurate. Many people believe that deaf individuals communicate in a language that is essentially English transformed into signs. This is not the case. *American Sign Language (ASL), which is the native language of most culturally deaf Americans, is not English.* This visually based language bears little relationship to English, particularly in grammar and syntax. An interpreter who is signing for a deaf person is not always signing what is being said word for word. Rather, concepts and ideas are signed.

Most cultures have a colloquial element to their language that all of us outside that specific culture find difficult to follow. People from the northern regions of the United States often find expressions unique to the south impossible to understand, and vice versa. Also, many of us who have taken French in school or college have experienced the horrors of visiting Paris or other French cities and been left wondering just what language *are* these people speaking?! This problem with understanding colloquialisms is no less important in communicating with the deaf. Here are just a few examples of idioms that hearing health educators would probably not hesitate to use under normal circumstances but that might prove to be dysfunctional in the communication process with the deaf:

"pulling my leg"	"check it out"
"really hits home"	"sink or swim"
"cut the light"	"hooking up"
"hit on her"	"a no-brainer"

Health educators must be aware that many deaf individuals are in an almost identical situation to foreigners . . . English is a *second* language to them. This does not mean that they are less intelligent or able. It simply means that efforts to communicate will be compromised unless this factor is taken into account and measures are implemented to compensate for it.

Sources of Information

Very little data exist to assist the health educator in comprehending the world of deaf people. Do deaf individuals gain most of their health information in the same manner as their hearing peers, or do they follow an alternative route? One of the few studies that even considers this issue seems to suggest that deaf individuals do indeed gather information and learn about health in a manner that is different from the typical hearing individual. Fitzgerald and Fitzgerald (1980) postulate that, at least in the area of sexuality, deaf individuals, because of their lack of hearing, are denied access to all the usual agents contributing to sexual knowledge and awareness. For example, young people in the hearing world gain information in a multitude of ways: talking with others, watching television, going to the movies, listening to the radio, attending classes in school, reading, and personal experience. The authors suggest that deaf individuals are denied these *incidental learning* opportunities that hearing individuals take for granted. Very few films are captioned, radio is not an option, limited language skills often make reading difficult, and even observations can lead to mistaken impressions.

Fitzgerald and Fitzgerald (1980) relate the story of the 11-year-old deaf boy who on entering the classroom began to share his packet of Certs with the girls in the class. It quickly became obvious that the young man was expecting to be kissed by the girls in return for the Certs! The boy had seen the televised Certs commercial without the benefit of sound, had missed the verbal communication related to breath freshness, and had come to the very reasonable conclusion that anyone who was given a Cert was expected to respond with a kiss.

It is the contention of Fitzgerald and Fitzgerald (1980) that without the benefit of incidental learning, deaf individuals might rely on personal experience more than their hearing counterparts. The pitfalls and dangers of learning through experience are obvious for most areas of health but are particularly acute in the arena of contemporary sexuality, given the threat of AIDS and other sexually transmitted diseases as well as unintended pregnancy. One of the few studies ever to compare the sexual knowledge, attitudes, and beliefs of deaf and hearing college students was performed by Grossman in 1972. This study reported that deaf individuals had less sexual knowledge, were more accepting of myths, and were more sexually active than their hearing peers. A later study comparing deaf and hearing college students found that although hearing students scored higher than deaf students on sexual knowledge items, both populations had low levels of sexual knowledge, and gender was a more accurate predictor than hearing status of age at first intercourse, number of sexual partners, and preventive health practices. This study also reported that a significantly higher rate of forced sexual intercourse existed in the deaf community (Sawyer, Desmond, and Joseph, 1996).

In addition to missing the benefits of incidental learning, deaf individuals are less likely to have the opportunity to attend formal sexuality education courses. Sexual knowledge for many deaf individuals, therefore, might often be derived from personal experience. There is insufficient research to demonstrate whether or not this one finding could be generalized to other populations or even other areas of health. However, it does suggest that a health education approach of assuming that deaf individuals have identical health interests, concerns, and behaviors to hearing individuals might be unwise.

Teaching Methods and Strategies

Research into the effectiveness of health education teaching methodology for the deaf is scant. Tomasetti, Beck, and Clearwater (1983) compared the effectiveness of three different types of teaching methods used in *cardiopulmonary resuscitation* (CPR) education for both the hearing and deaf populations. Three deaf groups each received a different teaching method: standard course through signed instruction; standard instruction with a captioned videotape; and standard instruction with uncaptioned videotape, signed by an interpreter. The hearing group, which received a standard course, performed the best of all groups on psychomotor skills in an immediate posttest. However, in a four-month retest, the deaf group that had received a signed videotape performed better on psychomotor skills than any of the other groups, including the hearing group. It is not clear why the signed film was more effective than the captioned. One possibility might be that poor reading levels compromised the participants' ability to comprehend the captions, or perhaps the presence of an interpreter caused the students to identify with the instructor, thus influencing retention levels.

An interesting addition to this study would have been a group instructed by a deaf health educator who was able to sign. Whether or not levels of learning are enhanced by having an educator from the same community as the group receiving the education is a subject worthy of further research. This concept would seem no less important to the deaf community as it would in the African American or Latino populations. However, the limited number of minority health educators underlines the necessity for nonminority health educators to be educated about other cultures.

Beck and Tomasetti (1984) make an important contribution to health education teaching methodology for the deaf in their description of a safety training program. The authors describe the preparation for teaching a special population and the adaptations they made to successfully complete the workshop. Many of their recommendations are included here in the methods summary.

The almost complete absence of research related to the health education needs, knowledge, attitudes, and behavior of the deaf means that health educators working with this population must really give a great deal of thought to method selection. As emphasized in this text, not all deaf or hard-of-hearing individuals are alike, and some effort by the educator should be made to discover specific information about individuals and their needs. Here are some suggestions that might facilitate working with the deaf:

- Make no assumptions! Obtain as much information you can about the hearing levels, reading levels, and so forth, of the individuals involved.
- Come to terms with the idea that most presentations will require an interpreter. Forget about depending on your audience's ability to read lips . . . get an interpreter.* Some organizations will provide them, some deaf individuals will bring their own . . . make some inquiries! Often the expense or shortage of interpreters continues to limit deaf people's access to health education.
- Do not expect a deaf person to look at printed information and the interpreter at the same time. Allow time for the participants to look over any printed information before resuming the discussion.
- If you're using an overhead or slide projector, or any method where the lights are dimmed, give some thought to the interpreter. Provide a side light for him or her, or turn the lights back on between slides or transparencies to discuss information.
- Take a "hands on" approach to learning. This move away from the lecture format necessitates less translation, and in addition may be a more effective means to facilitate comprehension.

*The Americans with Disabilities Act (ADA), initiated in 1988, provides civil rights protections to persons with disabilities and is comparable to legislation in force to protect women and minorities. The act protects individuals with disabilities from discrimination and states that physical and communication barriers must be removed. Reasonable accommodation must be made for all persons with disabilities (West, 1991). To that end, presentations performed by public agencies (e.g., state, local, and community) must provide and pay for interpreters if requested. In addition, private agencies (e.g., a Health Maintenance Organization) must also provide and fund any reasonable accommodation, including an interpreter, if requested.

Myths About Deafness

Like all minority groups, deaf people are the target of stereotyping. Some myths about deaf people follow:

MYTH: *All hearing losses are the same.*
FACT: The single term *deafness* covers a wide range of hearing losses that have very different effects on a person's ability to process sound and thus to understand speech.

MYTH: *All deaf people are mute.*
FACT: Some deaf people speak very well and clearly; others do not because their hearing loss prevented them from learning spoken language. Deafness usually has little effect on the vocal chords, and very few deaf people are truly mute.

MYTH: *People with impaired hearing are "deaf and dumb."*
FACT: The inability to hear affects neither native intelligence nor the physical ability to produce sounds. Deafness does not make people dumb in either the sense of being stupid or mute. Deaf people, understandably, find this stereotype particularly offensive.

MYTH: *All deaf people use hearing aids.*
FACT: Many deaf people benefit considerably from hearing aids. Many others do not; indeed, some find hearing aids to be annoying and choose not to use them.

MYTH: *Hearing aids restore hearing.*
FACT: Hearing aids amplify sound. They have no effect on a person's ability to process that sound. In cases where a hearing loss distorts incoming sounds, a hearing aid can do nothing to correct this and may even make the distortion worse.

MYTH: *All deaf people can read lips.*
FACT: Some deaf people are very skilled lipreaders, but many are not. This is because many speech sounds have identical mouth movements. For example, *p* and *b* look exactly alike on the lips.

MYTH: *Deaf people are not sensitive to noise.*
FACT: Some types of hearing loss actually accentuate sensitivity to noise. Loud sounds become garbled and uncomfortable. Hearing aid users often find loud sounds, which are greatly magnified by their aids, very unpleasant.

MYTH: *Deaf people are less intelligent.*
FACT: Hearing ability is unrelated to intelligence. Lack of knowledge about deafness has often limited educational and occupational opportunities for deaf people.

MYTH: *Deaf people are alike in abilities, tastes, ideas, and outlooks.*
FACT: Deaf people are as diverse in their abilities, tastes, ideas, habits, and outlooks as any other large group of people.

- Practical demonstrations rather than descriptions and handouts can facilitate learning when poor reading comprehension levels exist. Use models and pictures.
- Films should be captioned or an interpreter used. Here again, the absence of good, captioned materials continues to be a major problem in program delivery.
- The use of games as a teaching method can be an effective way to involve participants in an interactive manner.
- Be aware that programs might take more time with a deaf audience, and allow for this difference. The extra time allows individuals to feel less pressure and permits the educator to reiterate and consolidate important points. Issues requiring more complex levels of comprehension can be covered more than once.
- Never ask, "Do you understand?" The likely response will be an affirmative nod of the head. Always use the "check back" technique, asking for a review of information understood.

Communication Tips Following are some tips for communicating with deaf and hard-of-hearing people that were developed for use by health professionals by The National Academy, Gallaudet University, 1991.

Helpful Tips for Speaking

- Face the deaf person.
- Maintain eye contact with the deaf person.
- Be sure that there is a light source in front of you.
- Speak slowly and clearly.
- Do not exaggerate your mouth movements.
- Keep objects/hands away from your mouth.
- Isolate or emphasize key words when appropriate.
- Give the deaf person as many visual cues as possible.
- Consider your choice of words carefully.

Helpful Tips for Communicating through Writing/Drawing

- Keep your writing brief and to the point.
- Look for meaning in the deaf person's message; ignore any grammatical errors.
- When appropriate, use a drawing in addition to your written message.
- Use open-ended questions.
- Face the deaf person after you have written your messages, and ask for a communication check.
- Often, requesting that the deaf person rephrase what he/she has understood is the best way to identify and prevent potential misunderstandings.

Helpful Tips for Working with an Interpreter

- Stand or sit close to the interpreter.
- Place graphics or models near you and the interpreter.
- Speak at a reasonable pace.
- Look at deaf person(s).

- Address deaf person(s) directly. Do not say to the interpreter, "Tell her. . . . ."
- Leave time for the interpreter to finish.
- Adjust lighting appropriately.
- Allow time for the deaf person(s) to ask and respond to questions.
- Say only what you want interpreted; remember that it is the interpreter's job to interpret *everything* you say and *everything* the deaf person signs.

 For more information and tools related to this chapter visit www.jbpub.com/healtheducation.

EXERCISES

1. A group of deaf college students (approximately 15 male and female students, aged 19–23 years) has requested a speaker on birth control. You have been given the assignment. With your newfound knowledge of people who are hearing impaired or deaf, describe the steps you would take to plan for this presentation. Then list some presentation methods related to contraception education that might be appropriate with this group.

2. You are teaching a combination ninth/tenth-grade high school health education course. You have been informed that 3 of the 25 students are special education students. Describe the steps you would take to accommodate these students in your course, both in preparation for teaching and during individual classes. (You can either respond in general terms or select specific learning disabilities.)

3. Jennifer, one of the students in your seventh-grade health education classes, is visually impaired. Describe the steps you would take to discover the extent of the impairment, and make some suggestions as to how you would accommodate Jennifer in your classes.

CASE STUDIES REVISITED

Case Study Revisited: Kareem   Kareem is in need of some education and perhaps sensitivity training. Unfortunately, many educators when faced with special population groups make equally unfounded assumptions. No health educator can be an expert concerning every exceptional population, but even a small amount of research and investigation on the health educator's part would go a long way to reduce the likelihood of Kareem's type of aberrant thinking. (See page 258.)

Case Study Revisited: Robert   Robert could take the easy way out and just continue with his prepared lecture. But if he has some initiative, he will take steps to alleviate a possible problem. The most obvious initial step would simply be to welcome the visually impaired participants and before beginning the lecture ask them if there is anything that he can do to make the workshop more effective. Would seating arrangements make a difference—perhaps closer to the front of the room? Ask yourself whether Robert should make a greater effort to verbalize the written material to facilitate understanding. Would written materials like pamphlets be useful for participants to take home after the workshop so that someone could read them to the visually impaired participants or perhaps even translate them into braille? Obviously, there is a limit to what Robert can do at such short notice, but these simple steps would be reasonable in an attempt to accommodate all his workshop participants. (See page 263.)

**Case Study
Revisited: Jill**

Jill was fortunate enough to have gained the information that deaf students might be attending her workshop *before* the event took place. Had she done some basic research into the deaf population, Jill could have avoided some very basic mistakes. Her first thought should have been to find out if an interpreter was needed, and if so, seek help in making such an arrangement. The presence of an interpreter could have prevented the whole problem. Jill also believed the myth that if you speak loudly and clearly enough, a deaf person will understand you. As this chapter explains, lipreading is not an easy or efficient means of comprehension for the vast majority of deaf or hearing impaired people. Jill made the assumption that the deaf students left during the videotape because of its sexually explicit nature. Although this could have been the case, a more obvious explanation would be that the students could simply not hear the narration and therefore had little understanding of what was occurring. This case study illustrates the need for a greater knowledge of special populations when planning health education interventions. (See page 272.)

SUMMARY

1. Health educators need to have a good working knowledge of special populations, including important information such as basic demographics and health problems unique to specific populations.

2. Health educators must familiarize themselves with the laws relating to the provision of services for special populations.

3. As the trend to mainstream exceptional individuals continues, the health educator is more likely to have to be prepared to devise presentation methods that will optimally include these individuals in the learning process.

4. Health educators need to familiarize themselves with available resources specifically designed to meet the needs of exceptional populations.

REFERENCES

Aukerman, R. (1972). *Reading in the Secondary Classroom*. New York: McGrawHill.

Beck, K.H., & Tomasetti, J.A. (1984). Safety training for the deaf. *Professional Safety*, May, 20–23.

Clements, S.D. (1966). *Minimal Brain Dysfunction in Children: Terminology & Identification, Phase 1 of a Three-Phase Project*. Washington DC: U.S. Department of Health, Education & Welfare, Public Health Service Bulletin No. 1415.

Cratty, B.J. (1971). *Movement & Spatial Awareness in Blind Children & Youth*. Springfield, IL: Charles Thomas.

Deaf Culture. (1990). Handout prepared by College for Continuing Education, National Academy, Gallaudet University.

Federal Register (Part III) (1977). Washington DC: Department of Health, Education & Welfare, December 29 (65083), 42.

Federal Register (Part IV) (1977). Washington DC: Department of Health, Education & Welfare, August 23 (163), 42.

Fitzgerald, D., & Fitzgerald, M. (1980). Sexuality and deafness—An American overview. *British Journal of Sexual Medicine,* September, 30–34.

Goldstein, H., Arkell, C., Ashcroft, S.C., Hurley, O.L., & Lilly, M.S. (1975). In N. Hobbs (Ed.), "Differentiating Learning Disability", *Issues in the Classification of Children,* San Francisco: Jossey-Bass.

Gordon, S. (1973). *The Sexual Adolescent,* North Scituate, MA: Duxbury Press.

Grossman, S. (1972). *Sexual Knowledge, Attitudes and Experiences of Deaf College Students.* Unpublished master's thesis, George Washington University.

Haight, S.L., & Fachting, D.D. (1986). Materials for teaching sexuality, love and maturity to high school students with learning disabilities. *Journal of Learning Disabilities, 19*(6), 344–350.

Hammill, D.D., & Bartel, N.R. (1978). *Teaching Children with Learning Disabilities and Behavior Problems.* Boston, MA: Allyn & Bacon.

Harlan, L.C., Bernstein, A.B., & Kessler, L.G. (1991). Cervical cancer screening: Who is not screened and why? *American Journal of Public Health,* 81(7), 885–890.

Hogan, D. (1997). ADHD: A travel guide to success. *Childhood Education,* 73, (3).

Lowell, E.L. (1958). *John Tracey Clinic Research Papers III-VII,* John Tracey Clinic, Los Angeles, CA.

Lowenfeld, B. (1962). Psychological foundations of special methods of teaching blind children. In P.A. Zahl (Ed.), *Blindness.* New York: Hafner.

Mandell, C.J., & Fiscus, E. (1981). *Understanding Exceptional People.* St. Paul, MN: West Publishing Co.

McFarland, D.L., Kolstad, R., & Briggs, L.D. (1995). Educating attention deficit hyperactivity disorder children. *Education 115*(4), 597–603.

Meyen, E.L. (1978). *Exceptional Children and Youth.* Denver: Love Publishing Co.

Morrone-Joseph, J. (1992). Personal files, Gallaudet University, Washington DC.

Myers, E., Ethington, D., & Ashcroft, S. (1958). Readability of braille as a function of three spacing variables. *Journal of Applied Psychology,* 42, 163–165.

Tomasetti, J.A., Bech, K.H., & Clearwater, H.E. (1983). An analysis of selected instructional methods on CPR retention competency of deaf & nondeaf college students. *American Annals of the Deaf,* August, 474–478.

Trybus, R.J., & Karchmer, M.A. (1977). School achievement scores of hearing impaired children: National data on achievement status and growth patterns. *American Annals of the Deaf Directory of Programmes and services,* 122, 62–69.

Sawyer R.G., Desmond, S.M., & Joseph, J.M. (1996). A comparison of sexual knowledge, behavior and sources of information between deaf and hard of hearing university students. *Journal of Health Education 27*(3), 144–152.

U.S. Census (1990). *U.S. Department of Commerce News Release,* June 12, 1991, CB 91-215, Washington DC.

West, J. (1991). *The Americans with Disabilities Act: From Policy to Practice,* New York: Milbank Memorial Fund.

Westwood, P. (1993). *Commonsense Methods for Children with Special Needs.* London: Routledge.

10
CHAPTER

Controversial Topics: Sexuality Education

Entry-Level and Graduate-Level Health Educator Competencies Addressed in This Chapter

Responsibility I: Assessing Individual and Community Needs for Health Education
  Competency A: Obtain health related data about social and cultural environments, growth and development factors, needs, and interests.
  Competency C: Infer needs for health education on the basis of obtained data.

Responsibility III: Implementing Health Education Programs
  Competency B: Infer enabling objectives as needed to implement instructional program in specified settings.
  Competency C: Select methods and media best suited to implement program plans for specific learners.

Responsibility IV: Evaluating Effectiveness of Health Education Programs
  Competency C: Interpret results of program evaluation.
  Competency D: Infer implications from findings for future program planning.

Responsibility VII: Communicating Health and Health Education Needs, Concerns and Resources
  Competency A: Interpret concepts, purposes, and theories of health education.
  Competency B: Predict the impact of societal value systems on health education programs.
  Competency C: Select a variety of communication methods and techniques in providing health information.

Method Selection in Health Education

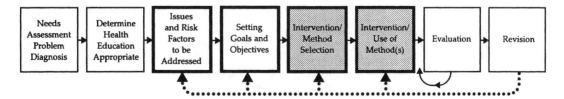

Heavy-bordered boxes indicate subjects addressed in this text; shaded boxes indicate subjects(s) of current chapter.

Note: The competencies listed on page 285, which are addressed in this chapter, are considered to be both entry-level and graduate-level competencies by the National Commission for Health Education Credentialing, Inc. They are taken from *A Framework for the Development of Competency Based Curricula for Entry Level Health Educators* by the National Task Force for the Preparation and Practice of Health Education, 1985; and *A Competency-Based Framework for Graduate Level Health Educators* by the National Task Force for the Preparation and Practice of Health Education, 1999.

OBJECTIVES

After studying the chapter the reader should be able to

- Describe the potential problems inherent in planning, implementing, and evaluating programs concerning controversial topics.
- Provide a justification, or rationale, for implementing human sexuality and drug abuse prevention programs.
- Develop meaningful, realistic goals and objectives in human sexuality and drug abuse prevention programs.
- Describe the major concerns of sexuality education opponents.
- List the most common mistakes that occur when presenting programs on sexuality education.
- Describe a diversity of approaches to sex and drug education.

KEY ISSUES

Goals and objectives   Defending a program
Educational philosophy   Effects of programming
Educational approaches   Political correctness
Opposition concerns

The **health education field** today deals with many topics and issues that are sometimes considered controversial. One obvious difficulty with this area is trying to define what exactly is meant by the term *controversial*. What might be considered sensitive, difficult, or even dangerous material by some people may be considered by others as mundane, basic, and unthreatening. Although most health educators certainly tend to subscribe to the less threatened mindset, they should not be oblivious to the fact that many **health education programs** can attract certain constituencies who will inevitably have a problem with either material or approach. Working with various types of issues on a daily basis can sometimes lead to the health educator becoming desensitized to the material, and he or she should always remember that the general public might well feel less comfortable about many areas.

Obviously, sex education/human sexuality comes immediately to mind when controversy is mentioned. The fact that many **school health education** programs and **school health services** feel the necessity to camouflage even the name "sexuality" by using the more comfortable euphemism **family life** speaks volumes for the potential difficulties surrounding this topic. A second major topic that has drawn almost as much criticism is that of alcohol and other drug education. In fact, almost any health topic can become controversial!

Case Study: Todd   Todd is a recently appointed health educator who has been asked to attend an upcoming PTA meeting to discuss the proposed implementation of a new sex education component in the school system's curriculum. . Todd is a fervent believer in the necessity of sex education and puts together an impressive set of overhead transparencies which explains the curriculum. He intends to strengthen his presentation by citing national data on the prevalence rates of adolescent STIs, HIV infection, and unintended pregnancy. Todd's initial enthusiasm as he sees large numbers of parents at the meeting quickly turns to dismay as his presentation is largely ignored and some very vocal parents barrage him with questions and comments that he is not adequately prepared to answer: "Why do we need sex education in our town . . . our community doesn't have these problems," "These programs only increase sexual activity, don't they?" "Can you say that your program will reduce pregnancy rates?" "Why don't you teach some type of moral values?" "Why don't you stay out of this . . . this type of education should happen in the home, not the school." The meeting deteriorates into a shouting match, Todd is unable to make any progress, and the evening ends without any type of resolution. Should Todd have been surprised at the meeting's outcome? How could Todd have been better prepared to face such a volatile situation? (See Case Studies Revisited page 320.)

Because of the focus of this text, this chapter will concentrate mainly on sex education as an example of how to anticipate and minimize potential controversy. Covering other controversial topics in any great depth is beyond the scope of this text as it is not intended to be a content book. However, the health educator should be aware that even the areas within health education that appear at first glance to be benign are sometimes fraught with problems. For example, nutrition, particularly when concerned with dieting, has become an area that can stir emotions, and achieving a consensus about weight management is often very difficult. The topic of death and dying is considered by many to be sufficiently sensitive that the home is the only place to deal with the issue. Also one of the most contentious recent topics to receive a great deal of attention and discussion has been violence prevention, particularly in the light of the tragic 1999 shootings at Columbine High School in Littleton, Colorado.

It is interesting to note that drug education and sex education seem to have followed a very similar evolutionary direction in regard to the development of strategies and methods of education. In the 1960s, when many of the first sexuality and drug education programs were being implemented, the focus was clearly on disseminating factual information. The rational but simplistic triad of knowledge, attitude, and behavior was being routinely utilized, the hypothesis being that if we give individuals the "facts" (knowledge), then their attitudes will change for the better, and ultimately the individuals will cease their risky and dangerous health behaviors. This type of approach then dictated that the methods of educating about these subjects would take a biological/physiological direction. It is interesting to note that as long ago as 1919 the U.S. Government Printing Office published a text titled, *A High School Course in Physiology in Which the Facts of Life Are Taught* (Means, 1992). No need to guess the method utilized in this approach to sexuality! In the drug area, nearly 20 years later, the element of fear was added to the educator's arsenal in the form of a new film intended to depict the evils of marijuana use. The now classic 1936 film titled *Reefer Madness* showed how paragons of normalcy could be transformed into crazed perpetrators of rape and murder after a single exposure to marijuana (Anderson, 1973). Although this type of hysterical approach can be viewed as ridiculous by today's more sophisticated youth, elements of this method still survive today as health educators struggle to stimulate just the right amount of anxiety (Taqui, 1972)!

In more contemporary times, health educators began to realize that facts alone would not change human behavior. Sex education in the form of "plumbing" that stressed biology and drug education that focused on pharmacology seemed to have little relevance to the lives of young people. The trend that seems to characterize contemporary methods in both drug and sex education is that of decision making. Most of the newer curricula, although still including factual information, tend to focus on the more abstract practice of decision making. For example, in drug education a plethora of school-based programs have been developed that stress skills of saying "No" to drugs and actively resist the pressures to use drugs (Botvin, 1983; Battjes, 1985).

One example of a much utilized school-based drug education is the DARE program. This program, adopted now in as many as 49 states, relies on the cooperation of specially trained uniformed police officers and combines factual information with a major emphasis on the resistance of societal and peer pressures to use drugs (Ringwalt, 1991). Students are actively encouraged to participate in the development and practice of measures of resistance. Methods and strategies with this type of program necessitate more innovative learning opportunities than the simple exchange of facts. However, despite the ubiquity of the DARE program, recent research has questioned DARE's ability to have any significant effect on the drug-related behaviors of its participants (Lynam, 1999), reinforcing the notion that curriculum programs alone are likely to be less effective than a **comprehensive school health program.**

Sexuality education has traveled a similar road to drug education in its diversion from straight facts to individual and group process, incorporating decision making. The whole field of sexuality education has taken on a broader perspective, with more organizations involved in the process, more children being exposed to education at an earlier age, and the development of programs that address the emotional as well as the physical components of the issue (Greenberg, 1981). Statistically, there does appear to have been an increase in the prevalence of sex education. In 1980 only 3 states mandated sex education, compared with 47 states in 1993 that require or *recommend* sex education (*Time*, 1993). Unfortunately, the onus is on "recommend," as a 1999 analysis of a state-by-state review of mandated sexuality education demonstrated (SIECUS, 1999). The data, originally collected by NARAL (National Abortion and Reproductive Rights Action League), indicated that in fact in 1998, only 20 states mandated sexuality education, with even fewer states (13) including contraception education in the mandate. Thirty-six states mandated HIV/STD education, suggesting perhaps that HIV/AIDS was viewed as a more acceptable and maybe a more pressing topic, the omission of which would be difficult to justify.

However, states do not mandate any minimum number of **contact hours,** nor does any state monitor carefully to ensure that existing requirements are fully implemented. Specifically, these data cannot report how much of the recommended sexuality education actually occurs, or describe the quality or amount of teaching in this area. In an era of educational accountability through testing, a major problem for health and sexuality education is the absence of standardized tests. As health and sexuality education are not part of the testing process, there exists little or no incentive for principals and administrators to fully **implement** such programs. Table 10-1 shows the states that are required to provide sexuality or HIV/AIDS education.

Table 10-1
State Policy Requirements for Sexuality, STD, and HIV/AIDS Education, 1998

Schools Required to Provide Both Sexuality Education and STD or HIV/AIDS Education

Alabama	Minnesota
Arkansas	Nevada
Delaware	New Jersey
District of Columbia	North Carolina
Georgia	Rhode Island
Hawaii	South Carolina
Illinois	Tennessee
Iowa	Utah
Kansas	Vermont
Maryland	West Virginia

Schools Not Required to Provide Either Sexuality Education or STD or HIV/AIDS Education

Alaska	Mississippi
Arizona	Montana
Colorado	Nebraska
Idaho	North Dakota
Kentucky	South Dakota
Louisiana	Texas
Maine	Virginia
Massachusetts	Wyoming

Source: NARAL, 1998.

This increase in exposure to sexuality education remains well below the levels that most sexuality experts believe is needed to achieve minimally effective educational levels. For example, Popham (1993) suggests that for an AIDS education unit to have the slightest possible chance of influencing behavior, it must consist of a number of 3–5 hour instructional activities in early grades, 10–15 hours of education in grades 9 or 10, followed by one or more 3–5 hour booster sessions after the main AIDS unit has been concluded . . . all, by the way, taught by the most talented, first-rate teachers. How do these minimal standards compare with common AIDS education practices in our public schools?

The AIDS epidemic is undoubtedly responsible for allowing sexuality educators to gain access to hitherto unreachable audiences, and most states and regions have mandated some compulsory AIDS education programming. Despite this temporary acceptance of the need for increased awareness, sexuality education continues to meet much opposition from individuals and groups who either are opposed to the approach taken by educators or to the idea that such education should even exist. Health educators involved with human sexuality, **sex educators,** should at least acknowledge the strong possibility of individual and community opposition to such programming.

Justification of Program Development

Developing a rationale for program development is a crucial factor in gaining support and acceptance for new or continuing programs. Even a cursory glance at the scope of problems related to sexuality and drug abuse reveals little argument against the necessity for program development. During the past decade, although there is evidence of a reduction in the use of illicit drugs, the following data concerning drug and alcohol use among *high school students*, summarized from the *1997 Youth Risk Behavior Survey* (Centers for Disease Control and Prevention, 1997), should still be of major concern:

- 79.1 percent of students have had at least one alcoholic drink during their life.
- 50.8 percent of students had at least one drink in the 30 days preceding the survey.
- 33.4 percent of students had five or more drinks on a single occasion in the 30 days preceding the survey.
- 47.1 percent of students have used marijuana at least once in their lifetime.
- 26.2 percent of students had used marijuana in the 30 days preceding the survey.
- 17.0 percent of students have used "other" drugs ("PCP," amphetamines, mushrooms, "ecstasy," heroin) at least once during their lifetime
- 36.4 percent of students had smoked cigarettes in the 30 days preceding the survey.

Data taken from the *National College Health Risk Behavior Survey* (Centers for Disease Control and Prevention, 1995), examining the alcohol and other drug-related behaviors of *college students* reflect continued usage into early adulthood:

- 89.9 percent of students have had at least one alcoholic drink in their lifetime.
- 68.2 percent of students had at least one drink in the 30 days preceding the survey.
- 43 percent of men and 27.0 percent of women had five or more drinks on a single occasion in the 30 days preceding the survey.
- 50 percent of men and 47.7 percent of women had used marijuana at least once in their lifetime.
- 17.1 percent of men and 11.6 percent of women had used marijuana in the 30 days preceding the survey.
- 14.8 percent of men and 14.1 percent of women had used cocaine at least once in their lifetime.

Sexual Behavior   Data chronicling the sexual behavior of young people are also difficult to ignore. The *Youth Risk Behavior Survey* (Centers for Disease Control and Prevention, 1997) paints a clear picture of the sexual behavior of *high school students*:

- 48.4 percent of students have had sexual intercourse.
- 43.2 percent of students had not used a condom at last intercourse.
- 16.0 percent of students have had four or more different sexual partners in their lifetime.

Data examining the sexual behavior of *college students* reinforces the concept that young people are both sexually active and placing themselves at risk for various sexually related problems (Centers for Disease Control and Prevention, 1995):

- 86.1 percent of students have had sexual intercourse
- 68.2 percent of students had intercourse in the 3 months preceding the study.
- 34.5 percent of students have had six or more different sexual partners in their life.
- 35 percent of students had been pregnant or had impregnated a partner.
- 13.1 percent of students had engaged in sexual activity against their will.

Obviously, substantial numbers of young people who are sexually active translates to a significant potential for increased health problems. Again, an abundance of available data reflect the problems inherent in widespread, often unsafe sexual activity.

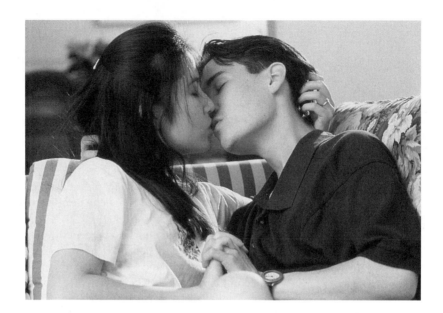

Despite recent improvement, U.S. teen pregnancy rates are the highest in any western industrialized nations.

The Bad News   **Unintended Pregnancy**

Since the early 1980s the United States has led the western world in unintended-pregnancy rates. Compare the following teen pregnancy rates for women under 20 years of age (Jones, 1986):

United States	96 per 1,000
Great Britain	45 per 1,000
Canada	44 per 1,000
France	43 per 1,000
Sweden	35 per 1,000
Holland	14 per 1,000

Although there is some evidence to suggest that teen pregnancy rates may be decreasing, in general, the problem continues, costing the United States an estimated $7 billion a year (Holmes, 1996). Consider the following statistics:

- Each year 11 percent of teens aged 15–19 years old become pregnant (Guttmacher Institute [GI], 1998).
- Each year 78 percent of all teen pregnancies are unplanned, accounting for about 25% of all unintended pregnancies annually (G.I., 1998).
- Among sexually active teens, about 8 percent of 14-year-olds, 18 percent of 15- to 17-year-olds, and 22 percent of 18- to 19-year-olds become pregnant each year (G.I., 1998).

Sexually Transmitted Infections (STIs)

Sexually active American youth is at high risk for many sexually transmitted infections and, in fact,

- Nearly 86% of all cases of STIs and AIDS occurs among persons aged 15–29 years (Centers for Disease Control and Prevention, 1992).
- Every year 3 million teens (about one in four sexually active teens) contract an STI (Guttmacher Institute, 1998).
- Chlamydia is more common among teens than older men and women (Guttmacher Institute, 1998).
- Teens have a higher rate of gonorrhea than do sexually active men and women aged 20–44 (Guttmacher Institute, 1998).
- Teenage women have a higher rate of hospitalization than older women for acute pelvic inflammatory disease (PID) (Guttmacher Institute, 1998).

The Good News A trend analysis of sexual behavior among high school students demonstrates that some small but positive changes are occurring (Centers for Disease Control and Prevention, 1998).

- "Ever had sex before"

1991	*1993*	*1995*	*1997*
54%	53%	53%	48%

- "Had intercourse with 4 or more partners"

1991	*1993*	*1995*	*1997*
18.7%	18.7%	17.8%	16%

- "Currently sexually active . . . within last 3 months"

1991	*1993*	*1995*	*1997*
37.4%	37.5%	37.9%	34.8%

- "Condom used at last intercourse"

1991	*1993*	*1995*	*1997*
46.2%	52.8%	54.4%	56.8%

- Teenage women's contraceptive use at first intercourse increased from 48 percent to 65 percent during the 1980s, almost entirely because of a doubling in condom use. By 1995 contraceptive use at first intercourse reached 78 percent, with two-thirds of it being condom use (Guttmacher Institute, 1998).
- Since 1980 abortion rates among sexually experienced teens have declined, mainly because fewer teens are becoming pregnant and, in recent years, fewer teens have elected to have an abortion (Guttmacher Institute, 1998).

Current Issue: Abstinence Versus Responsibility

Like all topics in health education, particularly controversial issues such as human sexuality or drug education, nothing remains static, and different approaches to education come and go. One of the current dilemmas in approaching sexuality education in both the school and community can be

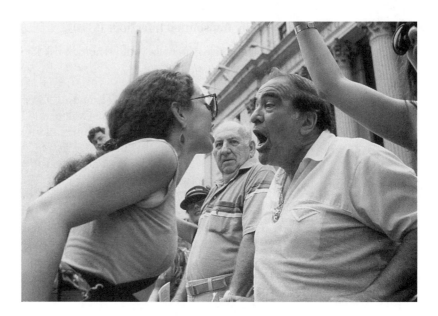

Sexually related issues can create passionate and heated disagreements.

categorized as *abstinence versus responsibility*. Should we teach young people from the perspective that if only they would remain or become sexually abstinent, then they would not have to be concerned with sexual problems? Or should we take a more pragmatic approach, acknowledge that whether adults like it or not, many young people are sexually active, and therefore we need to talk about sexual responsibility.

There is no question that much sexuality education is politically and religiously motivated and that during the 1980s and early 1990s the message was clearly one of abstinence, beautifully depicted in the slogan, "Just Say No!" Nearly ten years ago Congress appropriated money for the development of abstinence education programs, and since then abstinence-based programs like *Sex Respect* have been adopted in several states (*Wall Street Journal*, 1992). Many school districts have adopted such programs in the belief that traditional types of programming have not been effective. Students are schooled in the virtues of chastity and are taught that premarital sex can lead to emotional turmoil, disease, pregnancy, and guilt. The *Sex Respect* curriculum includes a chart that marks a prolonged kiss as "the beginning of danger" and the course uses the slogan, "No petting if you want to be free" (*Wall Street Journal*, 1992). Students are encouraged to create bumper stickers that read, "Control Your Urgin'/Be A Virgin," and to consider alternative activities to sex, such as bicycling, dinner parties, and playing Monopoly (*Time*, 1993).

Opponents of abstinence curricula argue that such an approach does little but cause extremely negative ideas about sex. In addition, because such curricula do not include information about preventing pregnancy, HIV infection, and STIs, they may have disastrous effects on sexual behavior. In 1993 Planned Parenthood of Northeast Florida and local citizens in Duval

County, Florida, sued the local school board for rejecting a broad-based sex education curriculum in favor of an abstinence-only program from Teen-Aid of Spokane. Also, in Shreveport, Louisiana, a district judge ruled that the abstinence-only text of *Sex Respect* was biased and inaccurate, ordering its removal from the Caddo Parish junior high schools (*Time*, 1993).

It is ironic that as the new millenium begins, when sexuality education may be playing a part in helping to increase contraceptive usage in general (also, specifically at first intercourse) and decrease the rate of teenage abortions, a major, politically driven economic initiative has developed aimed at ensuring the survival and promotion of abstinence-only sex education. Congress fueled the continuation of this movement with a $50 million yearly allocation in federal funds for abstinence-only-until-marriage programs each year for federal fiscal years 1998 to 2002. State matching funds are expected to increase the amount of funding for abstinence-only sex education to a figure of half a billion dollars over a five-year period. This is a classic example that serves to illustrate for new health educators how many policy decisions are made based on political agendas rather than existing scientific data. While educational curriculum decisions are ordinarily made at the local level, such large federal funds are difficult for states to turn down. A political groundswell occurred based on the unfounded premise that if talking about sex has caused all the previously mentioned teenage sexual pathologies, then talking *only* about abstinence must surely decrease the problems. Debra Haffner, the president of SIECUS, fittingly comments:

> If the Congress and the states are serious about helping young people delay sexual behaviors and grow into healthy, responsible adults, they will support a comprehensive approach to sexuality education that has a proven track record in accomplishing these goals. There are no published studies in the professional literature indicating that abstinence-only-until-marriage programs will result in young people delaying intercourse. (SIECUS, 1998).

In 1998 all but two states accepted the federal funding for abstinence-only education, and five states passed state laws requiring that sexuality education programs teach abstinence-only-until-marriage as the standard for school-age children (SIECUS, 1998). It would seem that just as objective indicators appear to demonstrate a positive shift toward more responsible teenage sexual behavior, a multimillion-dollar federally funded abstinence initiative, based solely on political and religious beliefs, has begun to challenge the more comprehensive, inclusive, and evaluated approaches to sexuality education.

**Europe. . .
a Different
Approach**

European sexuality educators should be forgiven if they look across the Atlantic Ocean and shake their heads in disbelief. Western industrialized nations, having lifestyles not substantially dissimilar to that of the United States, seem to take a very different approach to sexuality, and if objective data such as unintended pregnancy and teenage birth rates are anything to go by, their approaches are much more successful. A U.S. fact-finding

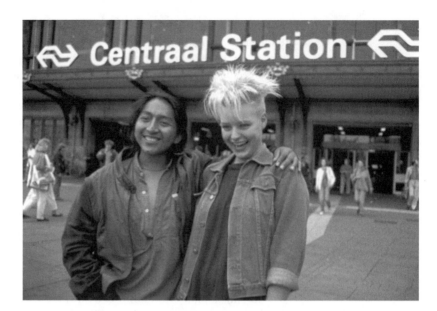

European teen sexuality is characterized by lower rates of pregnancy, births, and abortion.

mission that examined the European approach to teenage sex, characterized by more open attitudes and greater availability of contraception, reported some very interesting findings (Advocates for Youth, 1997). Despite the exposure to more open and often explicit sexual information, European teens tended to *delay* sexual initiation later than their American counterparts. For example, the average age at first intercourse in Holland was 17.0 years, 16.2 in Germany, and 16.8 in France, compared to 15.8 in the United States. In addition, the teen birth rate in the United States of 55 per 1,000 teenage women was found to be much higher than in Germany (13 per 1,000), France (9 per 1,000), or Holland (7 per 1,000) (Advocates for Youth, 1997). Some of the major differences reported between the European countries and the United States with regard to teenage sexuality follow:

- Teen reproductive health is treated as a public health issue, not a political or religious one.
- Research drives public policy to reduce unintended pregnancies, abortion, and STIs.
- Adolescents have convenient, confidential access to contraception and sexual health information and services, which are usually free.
- Teens receive open, honest, consistent messages about sexuality from parents, grandparents, media, schools, and health care providers.
- The governments fund massive, consistent and long-term public education campaigns that utilize television, radio, billboards, discos, pharmacies, and clinics to deliver clear, explicit portrayals of responsible sexual behavior.
- Mass media is a partner, not a problem (Advocates for Youth, 1997).

One of the greatest distinctions that seems to come through when comparing cultures is the *consistency* of messages in European cultures and the *inconsistency* between media messages and political/educational messages in the United States. In referring to the federally funded abstinence-only education, James Wagoner, president of Advocates for Youth, stated, "It is ironic that the United States is the only industrialized nation to have an official government policy of no sex until marriage, yet our teenagers initiate sexual activity at an earlier age than their European counterparts. Instead of encouraging sexual activity, the European openness results in safer and more responsible sexual behavior." (Advocates for Youth, 1997). Clearly, comparing different cultures is a difficult issue, and detractors could suggest that

---

NOTEWORTHY **Why Do Sexuality Education Programs Create Such Controversy?**

Vincent et al. (1999) cite five important factors that seem to add fuel to the fire of sexual controversy:

- *Sexuality education is not a priority in public school education.* This subject is seen as peripheral to the major educational goal of the school, somewhat like art, music, and physical education. In a contemporary atmosphere of time constraints, accountability, and external testing, sexuality education becomes a low priority.
- *Most people have a limited perception about what constitutes sexuality education.* Very few individuals understand the full scope of sexuality education; many fear that their children are being taught *how* to have intercourse.
- *Sexuality education is perceived as direct admonitions by adults.* Adults are often comfortable with the "direct" approach to adolescent/parent interaction ("do as you're told") and expect sexuality education to take the same simplistic and directed approach—an admonition to "just say no." Anything outside this realm is viewed with deep suspicion.
- *Fear of inquiry, objectivity, and development of critical thinking skills.* Teaching students to think critically about sexuality is viewed by many as a sure way to confuse adolescents, undo their values, and usurp parental control. The interesting idea that children "don't need to learn what they shouldn't be doing anyway" falls into this category.
- *Adults have a high degree of discomfort regarding the language of sex, sexual growth and development changes, and their views of appropriate sex role socialization and gender roles.* Most parents have little or no formal training in sexuality and feel distinctly uncomfortable with the whole issue. This discomfort is exacerbated by having to consider their children as sexual beings, making open and honest communication understandably problematic. In addition, much of this informally acquired sexuality education has left some adults with a very negative outlook toward sex in general and a particularly skeptical attitude toward sexuality programming.

European educational approaches would not be equally effective in the United States. Nevertheless, these examples from European countries provide empirical, scientific proof that exposure to openness, access to contraception, and explicit, frank sexuality information do *not* result in greater levels of sexual pathology . . . just the opposite.

Despite any amount of persuasive information that clearly points to the fact that American youth has a problem with both alcohol or other drug abuse, and sexuality issues, the health educator should not be surprised when individuals and groups do not share his or her vision of the situation. Opponents of education on these issues may acknowledge that a national problem exists, but they tend to see the problem in a vacuum—that is, one that does not involve their particular family. To that end, when beginning a program, the cooperation of local experts and respected community leaders who can speak forcefully in favor of programming is absolutely essential. Also, in addition to national statistics, the health educator should make a concerted effort to obtain local data that can be used more effectively to personalize an issue to specific communities.

Developing Goals and Objectives for Sexuality Education

One of the most difficult and sometimes dangerous components of sexuality education is developing meaningful, useful, and attainable objectives. Just what will the program accomplish? What will happen to the students after they experience such a program? Developing unattainable objectives in this area can give the opponents of sexuality programming ammunition with which to challenge the legitimacy of sex education. Reasonable, achievable objectives must be formulated, or the health educator will be literally ensuring failure.

For example, at first glance, the following behavioral objective for a high school sexuality class does not seem unreasonable: *As a result of a recently developed sex education class, there will be fewer pregnancies at All American High School.* In the community setting, developing an objective for HIV education might look like this: *Following a two-hour presentation on "safer sex" the participants will report higher levels of condom usage.* In both cases, the objectives developed are almost certainly doomed to failure.

School   In isolation, very few human sexuality courses have ever been effective enough to significantly reduce rates of unintended pregnancy. So if an objective is written to reduce such rates and no decrease occurs, then the objective has not been reached, and many will judge the class to be a failure. Reducing overall pregnancy rates might be a sound *goal* of any sexuality class, and as such it should be included. Decreased pregnancy rate is not a reasonable, attainable objective under these conditions.

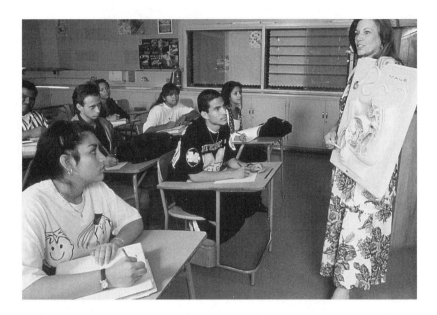

Human sexuality objectives should be both meaningful and attainable.

Community The possibility that condom usage will increase significantly after a two-hour presentation is almost nonexistent! As with most behaviors related to sexuality, condom usage is a complex psychosexual dynamic unlikely to be influenced in such a short period of time. If increased condom usage is written as an objective, then, the likelihood of failure, or not achieving the objective, is almost certain. Again, increased condom usage might be a realistic *goal* to set, but under the present conditions it is a very unrealistic behavioral objective.

So what are some reasonable objectives that can be developed in sexuality education? Some educators have made a definite attempt to avoid the pitfalls just outlined by purposely designing objectives that are *not* easily measurable. For example, Kirby et al. (1979a) suggest the following objectives:

> *To provide accurate information about sexuality.*
> *To facilitate insights into personal sexual behavior.*
> *To reduce fears and anxieties about personal sexual developments and feelings.*
> *To encourage more informed, responsible, and successful decision making.*
> *To encourage students to question, explore, and assess their sexual attitudes.*
> *To develop more tolerant attitudes toward the sexual behavior of others.*
> *To facilitate communication about sexuality with parents and others.*
> *To develop skills for the management of sexual problems.*
> *To facilitate rewarding sexual expression.*
> *To integrate sex into a balanced and purposeful pattern of living.*
> *To create satisfying interpersonal relationships.*
> *To reduce sex-related problems such as venereal disease and unwanted pregnancies.*

The authors of these objectives have cast their net very wide in order to include most of the major facets they consider germane to sexuality education. Under the terminology used in this text these "objectives" would be better characterized as "goals." These goals are obviously a far cry from objectives/goals that might have been generated for the "plumbing" sexuality course. The major advantage to this type of objective/goal is that the educator can promote very generalized aims instead of being restricted to more narrow, specific, and quantifiable projections. This certainly facilitates the avoidance of developing objectives that are unreasonable and likely to remain unattainable. However, this same strength is often viewed by opponents as a definite weakness. If objectives/goals are developed without an eye to some type of evaluation, how is program effectiveness then determined? In times of economic difficulty, particularly in education, accountability has become a crucial factor in funding. As thorough and appropriate as the objectives/goals developed by Kirby et al. might be, most program developers would make an attempt to include objectives that relate to specific sexuality issues and that are quantifiable.

To that end, as in most disciplines, quantifiable behavioral objectives can be confidently written in the cognitive domain. A significant increase in knowledge is often the criteria for evaluating any classroom performance, and human sexuality is no exception.

Examples   1. *The students will be able to list in order of effectiveness four methods of contraception, as described in class.*
   2. *The students will be able to describe three factors that might precipitate date rape, according to the film viewed in class.*

These types of objectives are valid, easily measurable, and attainable. A sound, well-taught class/workshop should be able to achieve objectives like these without much difficulty.

Objectives in the affective domain are more difficult to achieve than their cognitive counterparts. Nevertheless, affective domain objectives should be a reasonable inclusion when planning programs in sexuality. Given that the field of human sexuality has now expanded to be considered more than mere "plumbing," an attempt to consider affective concerns is crucial. One of the simplest ways to evaluate attitudinal changes is by using a pretest/posttest. Give the participants a short questionnaire before the workshop or unit and then have them complete a similar questionnaire at the conclusion of the unit.

Be aware that this procedure raises two important concerns: How valid is the instrument you are using? Won't any changes in attitude that might arise be only short-term in nature? The first concern is of prime importance, but one remedy would be to use an already developed instrument with proven levels of reliability and validity. This is not always possible, but an increasing number of instruments are available as more evaluation is performed in this field (Davis, 1988). In regard to the second concern about short-lived effects on attitude change, it would be unrealistic to assume that as a result of a single unit or workshop any changes would be long-term. Only consistent follow-up programming would be likely to maintain attitude change, and that is not always possible. Health educators have to be prepared to take small gains where they can, and there is nothing wrong with the idea of "planting a seed." Accordingly, writing behavioral objectives that would address only immediate attitude change is not so unreasonable.

Examples
1. As a result of the unit on AIDS, the students will demonstrate higher levels of perceived susceptibility to HIV infection.
2. As a result of the workshop on safer sex, participants will report a higher level of acceptance of using a condom.

Both of these examples reflect affective objectives that are reasonable and attainable. AIDS education should include components intended to personalize the issue to students who fail to see themselves at risk, and one of the most important factors in increasing condom usage is having individuals feel comfortable in accepting condom use. Both these objectives are also measurable, and by using a pretest/posttest questionnaire educators can gain a sense of what might have been accomplished.

As discussed earlier, addressing specific behavioral objectives related to behavior change is a difficult undertaking that might be better written as a less specific program/unit goal. Given the extremely limited time students spend in a sexuality education classroom, or that individuals spend in community workshops, it would not be fair or reasonable to expect changes in sexual behavior such that pregnancy rates or STI rates would dramatically decline. Should a student who has studied French once a week for 50 minutes during one semester be able to pass fluency tests? Suppose the French class was taught by the physical education teacher who had, after all, taken a two-day course in preparation for this teaching assignment! Sexuality educators should try to ensure that their programs are not evaluated by criteria not used to measure other courses. One way to avoid such unfair scrutiny, though, is to avoid writing unreasonable behaviorable objectives that could guarantee failure. One study found that the goals of various school districts were as follows:

- Promoting rational and informed decision making about sexuality—94 percent
- Increasing students' knowledge of reproduction—77 percent
- Reducing the sexual activity of teenagers—25 percent
- Reducing teenage childbearing—21 percent (Hofferth 1981)

It is interesting to note that in this particular study, "plumbing" was superseded by a decision-making focus and much smaller percentages of school districts than before made mention of behavior change, even as goals.

Opposition to Sexuality Education

Even the rivers of igno-
rance contain clever
crocodiles.
—Mohan Singh

Since the inception of widespread sexuality education, opposition groups have attempted to discredit and, in many cases, remove existing programs. A long history of such opposition is beyond the scope of this chapter, but a knowledge of some of the major complaints might prove useful to those planning or maintaining programs. The same principles apply to any area of study.

Majority or Minority?

Many opponents of sexuality education would have us believe that they are in the majority . . . that most Americans oppose sexuality education. Objective barometers of this issue, various national polls, clearly demonstrate that the majority of Americans favor some form of organized sexuality education. One poll carried out in 1986 (Louis Harris & Assoc., 1988) found that 85 percent of U.S. adults favored sexuality instruction in schools, up from 76 percent in 1975 (National Opinion Research Center, 1972–78) and 69 percent in 1965 (Gallup Poll, 1976). Surveys conducted in the 1990s continued to reinforce the large majority of support for comprehensive sexuality education (Gallup Poll, 1991; Clark, Houser, and Powell, 1995). In addition, studies have demonstrated that a large majority of teachers are also in favor of sexuality education in schools (Forrest, 1989). Evidently, opponents of some form of sexuality education have never been in the majority! Unfortunately, as with many other issues, the "squeaky wheel" gathers all the attention, disproportionate to the size of the group. The lesson is clear. Those people in favor of sexuality education should be proactive in order to maintain the gains made over the past 20 years, and should not take for granted what has been achieved.

Common Opposition Arguments

Following is a discussion of some common arguments against sexuality education.

1. *Sex education increases sexual activity.* Perhaps the most common claim made by opponents of sexuality education is that such education will result in and encourage increased sexual behavior. Professional educators, or even those of us with a memory that stretches back to those halcyon days of adolescence, might marvel at the notion that without sex education, teenagers would not think about sex at all! As facile as that idea might seem, many opponents view sex educators as the source of their child's first thought about sex. Opponents view high rates of teen pregnancy, pandemic levels of STIs, and, of course, the AIDS epidemic as clear evidence that sex educators have corrupted today's youth.

Contrary to these subjective and sometimes hysterical beliefs, objective evaluation of sexuality programs does not reveal increased sexual activity. Studies on the effects of sex education demonstrate that it increases knowledge levels of young people, increases the likelihood of contraceptive usage, and in some cases delays the onset of initial sexual intercourse. There is absolutely no empirical evidence that sexuality education encourages young people to initiate or increase sexual activity (Marsiglio, 1986; Dawson, 1986; Zelnik, 1982; Louis Harris & Associates, 1986; Baldo et al., 1993; Sawyer and Gray-Smith, 1996). In addition, how many American teens actually receive regular, consistent dosages of sex education, sufficient to ruin their souls? A large national study performed in the late 1970s placed that figure at no more than 10 percent (Kirby et al., 1979b), and a more recent study showed a modest increase to a maximum of 15 percent (Sonenstein, 1984). Pregnancies and pandemic levels of STIs can hardly be blamed on comprehensive sexuality education when only tiny percentages of American youth are receiving such education!

Figure 10-1 illustrates the many influences related to sexuality experienced by young people today. Note that formalized sex education plays only one small part. Given that all schooling takes up only 8 percent of an individual's life, and that sex education is just a tiny fraction of that amount, the idea that sex education is responsible for a mountain of social ills is not grounded in reality (Finn, 1986).

2. *Sex education doesn't work.* A major criticism leveled at sex education is that it simply doesn't work. Since sex education has become more common in schools in the United States, there has been little reduction in teenage pregnancy and rates of STI transmission. As discussed earlier,

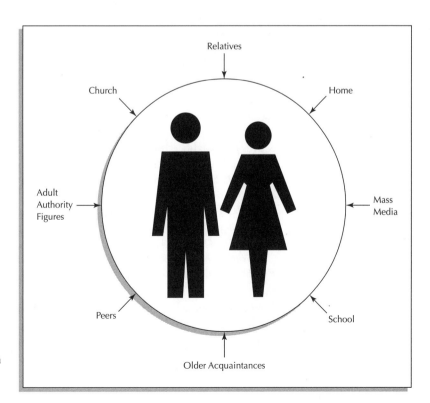

Figure 10-1
Sex education represents only a tiny fraction of all the influences on a teenager's life.

blaming sex education for exacerbating sexual problems is simply not logical when so few children receive any meaningful sex education. However, sex educators need to be able to defend against this type of criticism as programs come under closer scrutiny. Sex educators can help prevent some of this criticism by not promising more than can be realistically delivered. Be extremely cautious about writing behavioral objectives promising to reduce rates of pregnancy and STIs. Sex education on its own will not achieve these objectives.

Individuals who claim that sex education does not work need to be "educated" to the reality that little or no meaningful sex education exists in our schools today, so it is unfair to expect a minimalistic approach to have any meaningful effects. Also, other subjects in school are not held to the same levels of outcome accountability as sex education. Should schools abandon teaching civics because fewer than 50 percent of the population votes in presidential elections and vast numbers of adolescents cannot name the vice-president. One study found that nearly one-half of the nation's 17-year-olds did not know that each state has two senators (National Assessments of Educational Progress, 1976)! Foreign language education provides another fitting example of the double standard to which sexuality education is held. Despite the fact that most students take at least two to three years of a foreign language, usually taught several times a week by a language specialist, how many students can hold a reasonable conversation in that foreign tongue, let alone reach levels of fluency? How, therefore, can we expect sexuality education taught a few times a week for a total of about three weeks (often taught by an unqualified individual) to result in some type of complex behavior change! Obviously, very few people would suggest that American schools discontinue teaching civics or foreign languages because of these dismal findings, but the unfairness and disparity in how programs are evaluated should be noted.

A more tangential but valid response to this criticism would be that objectives of sexuality education are about more than just pregnancy, STI, and AIDS prevention. For example, the Sex Information and Education Council of the U.S. (SIECUS) defines sexuality this way:

> *Human sexuality encompasses the sexual knowledge, beliefs, attitudes, values and behaviors of individuals. It deals with the anatomy, physiology, and biochemistry of the sexual response system; with roles identity and personality; with individual thoughts, feelings, behaviors, and relationships. It addresses ethical, spiritual, and moral concerns, and group and cultural variations.*

Obviously, such a broad definition suggests an educational experience in which sexual health plays only one particular role. Even a cursory glance at the position statement formulated by SIECUS to address sex education (see the box) affords a good example of how education in this area is not concerned with sexual health alone.

NOTEWORTHY   ## SIECUS Position Statement

Sexuality education is a lifelong process that begins at birth. Parents, family, peers, partners, schools, religion, and the media influence the messages people receive about sexuality at all stages of life. These messages can be conflicting, incomplete, and inaccurate.

All people have the right to comprehensive sexuality education that addresses the biological, sociocultural, psychological, and spiritual dimensions of sexuality from the cognitive domain (information), the affective domain (feelings, values, and attitudes), and the behavioral domain (communication and decision-making skills).

Parents are—and ought to be—their children's primary sexuality educators, but they may need help and encouragement to fulfill this important role. Religious leaders, youth and community group leaders, and health and education professionals can complement and augment the sexuality education that takes place at home.

Source: Copyright © Sex Information and Education Council of the U.S., Inc., 130 West 42nd Street, Suite 350, New York, NY 10036. Reprinted by permission.

3. *Abstinence education curricula work.* In 1981 the American Family Life Act was passed, creating Title XX funds that were intended to develop abstinence-based sexuality programs that were expected to result in delaying the onset of sexual activity. Despite rhetoric to the contrary, in five studies of the major abstinence-until-marriage programs (Sex Respect, Success Express, and An Alternative National Curriculum on Responsibility), students who had participated in the programs one to two years earlier showed no significant increases in maintaining abstinence over a control group (Christopher and Roosa, 1990; Weed and Olsen, 1990). A more recent study of the abstinence curricula confirmed earlier findings that such programs have not been found to have consistent or significant effects on the onset of intercourse (Kirby, 1997).

4. *Mixing abstinence education with curricula that includes contraceptive information and skills building ("abstinence plus") gives students a "mixed message" and encourages sexual behavior.* In studies of "abstinence plus" programs (Postponing Sexual Involvement, Reducing the Risk, and Skills for Life), students surveyed one to two years after the programs maintained levels of abstinence longer than students in a control group (Vincent et al., 1987; Howard and McCabe, 1990; Kirby, 1991).

5. *Teaching about contraception encourages students to become sexually active.* There is empirical evidence to suggest that historically many teenagers have sexual intercourse for the first time *before* using contraception and in fact only begin contraceptive use because of a pregnancy or

pregnancy scare. The length of time of unprotected sex before contraceptive use can range from 6 to 18 months (Pollack, 1992). Additionally, no evidence supports the idea that making contraceptives available hastens or increases sexual activity (Kirby, 1997).

6. *Teaching students about contraception increases the likelihood that they will become pregnant.* There is clear evidence to the contrary, particularly in European countries, where educators routinely include contraceptive information in school sexuality programming. U.S. teens initiate sexual activity at earlier ages than their European counterparts and also experience higher rates of pregnancy and births (Guttmacher Institute, 1994; Advocates for Youth, 1997).

7. *Because contraceptives fail so frequently, we should simply teach abstinence.* Although the rate of teenage sexual activity has increased significantly over the past few decades, the rate of pregnancy among 15–19-year-olds has declined by 19 percent, mostly because of more effective use of contraceptives (Guttmacher Institute, 1994).

8. *Condoms have a high failure rate and so are minimally effective.* Most of the failure associated with condoms is related to *user* failure and not any flaw in the condom itself. For example, many individuals reporting condom failure only use them sporadically, only put them on after they have had intercourse but immediately prior to ejaculation, leave no room at the tip to collect semen, or don't hold them during withdrawal. Condom failure rates are likely to hover around the 2 percent mark, with the vast majority of failure owing more to lack of education or motivation than to manufacturing defects (CDC, 1993).

9. *Sex education should be done in the home.* Many opponents of sex education vehemently state that sex is a private matter and children should be educated in the home by the parents. A sex educator would be foolish to deny such a claim, and indeed the statement prepared by SIECUS (see the box) clearly endorses parental responsibility in this area. However, the fact remains that although many parents do a wonderful job of educating their children about sexuality, some parents pass on harmful myths and partial truths, and some parents do nothing. The ideal sex education is one that begins at home and is then augmented by many individuals and agencies, one of which is the school. The reality of the situation is that for some children, the *only* sexuality education they receive is performed by the school (Sawyer and GraySmith, 1996).

10. *People who teach sex education are not qualified.* Unfortunately, this is one area where sexuality education does seem vulnerable to criticism. Although there are numerous well trained, qualified individuals currently teaching human sexuality, there are also too many others who have unwillingly accepted responsibility for this area, lacking both enthusiasm and expertise. There is little or no consistency nationally in the type of preparation individuals receive to teach human sexuality.

One of the few examples of an attempt to standardize sexuality education training is the American Association of Sex Educators, Counselors, and

There is something I don't know that I am supposed to know I don't know what it is I don't know. And yet I am supposed to know. And I feel I look stupid if I seem both not to know it and not know what it is I don't know. Therefore I pretend I know it. This is nerve-racking since I don't know what I must pretend to know. Therefore I pretend to know everything. I feel you know what I am supposed to know but you can't tell me what it is because you don't know that I don't know what it is. You may know what I don't know, but not that I don't know it, and I can't tell you. So you will have to tell me everything.
—R.D. Laing (1972)
(Reprinted by permission)

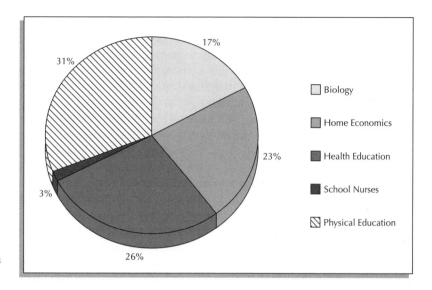

Figure 10-2
Sex Education Teachers
by Specialty.

Therapists (AASECT), which developed standards for granting certification to sex educators. The Guttmacher Institute performed a large survey to identify who is teaching sex education in our schools (Guttmacher Institute, 1989). It is interesting to note that this study identified the greatest proportion of sex education teachers as primarily physical education specialists. Figure 10-2 indicates the breakdown by responsibility area. This study revealed that about 60 percent of sex education teachers are women, half are over 40 years old, and nearly half have been teaching sex education for at least eight years. The majority of these individuals have received some type of preparation to teach sex education, although any type of state or local certification in human sexuality education is rare. Thus, a good proportion of sex education teachers are mature and experienced individuals who have received professional preparation. However, given that there is little quality control in the types of preparation available, school districts and individual schools would be very wise to ensure that any individuals who are asked to teach sex education have adequate training in this field and that they teach within the accepted curricular framework. To do any less than this would make a school and/or school district extremely vulnerable to complaint and criticism, and ultimately jeopardize an entire program.

Obstacles to Teaching Sex Education

Although sexuality education has now existed for quite some time, and despite the fact that the AIDS epidemic has legitimized the need for sex education for at least some people, many obstacles still exist that impede the development and implementation of comprehensive programming. More than one in five sex education teachers report that they face curriculum limitations. A similar proportion report that they experience negative pressure from parents and community groups. One in three feels that their school administration is nervous about negative community reactions, and one in five believes that their school administrators do not support them (Guttmacher Institute, 1989).

On the surface, with more states mandating AIDS education it would seem that sexuality is now an accepted part of educational programming and that obstacles are diminishing. However, the concerns of the teachers just mentioned clearly paint a different picture—a picture of an uneasy and potentially volatile truce between (1) school administrators, who have to do *something* because of the new mandates, and (2) the opponents of sexuality education, who are ever vigilant for mistakes that could provide ammunition for their cause. Often the result of such a situation is that the administrator, in an attempt to avoid offending anyone, restricts and dilutes the sexuality curriculum to the degree that it becomes ineffectual.

Another way to effectively "lose" sex education is to have small segments taught in various classes by regular classroom teachers. This way state requirements are met and yet no one actually realizes that sex education took place . . . and given the level of expertise by many teachers unprepared in this area, sex education did not take place!

Peter Scales identifies five major barriers that sex educators must overcome now or in the future in order to make sexuality education flourish (Scales, 1989).

Barrier 1. Taking a narrow view of sexuality education.
Within this context Scales describes how sex educators must avoid the temptation to "oversell" the impact of sexuality education. As described earlier, sex education in isolation cannot achieve major behavioral changes, and these changes should not be expected.

Sexuality education should not be evaluated solely on the basis of its short-term *measurable* impact. Instead, included in an assessment of the value of sexuality education should be a component of sex education's intrinsic value to the development of the total human being. This would necessitate an acceptance that sex education plays a fundamental role in defining a holistic viewpoint of "being educated."

Instead of a "back to basics" approach, Scales believes educators need to move forward in order to prepare children for a different and complex world. Children will need to develop critical thinking skills to cope with a new and challenging world environment.

Barrier 2. Failure to understand the importance of self efficacy.
Although sex educators have historically held the opinion that self-esteem is pivotal in sexual decision making, Scales argues that perhaps a more relevant component for behavioral change is self-efficacy. However, Scales would argue that neither self-esteem or self-efficacy can really be taught, so educators and policymakers should attempt through social action to create conditions in which self-efficacy can flourish.

Barrier 3. Failure to resolve the role of public schools as "surrogate parents." Schools today are asked to do much more than the "three R's" of education. As we adapt to new demands and pressures, sexuality education must also change to contribute more to students' broader education. Scales describes how sexuality education must go beyond mere pregnancy prevention to tackle issues of sexism, racism, homophobia, and social action.

Barrier 4. AIDS and the decline of pluralism. AIDS prevention of late has included a rather anti-sex message, which Scales argues is causing a decrease in a national acceptance of pluralism and diversity. Acceptance of different ideas and values are seen as a central premise to modern sexuality education, and Scales suggests that all sex educators, whether conservative or liberal, should strive to maintain a flexible and pluralistic approach to the field.

Barrier 5. Inadequate political skills. Although the political savvy of sex educators has improved over the years, Scales sees much room for improvement in the three following areas: translating beliefs into budgets, setting the right agenda, and speaking for ourselves. These areas speak to the importance of realizing that political battles are about resource allocation and that educators must translate ideas and beliefs into funding; that the "right agenda" is much more than just having greater numbers of better trained sex educators; and, finally, that sexuality education advocates must be proactive and not just allow others to say what they think advocates believe.

The observations of Scales are a far cry from the early concerns of sexuality educators and certainly reflect a wider and more visionary perspective of sexuality education. There is no doubt, though, that the politicization of issues like abortion, contraception, AIDS, and sexual orientation will necessitate that teachers of human sexuality be continuously aware that their educational efforts will receive a unique form of public scrutiny. To that end, political awareness should now be considered a prerequisite for teachers involved in sexuality education.

There is no doubt that the implications of making mistakes while implementing a sexuality curriculum can be far more severe than making errors in other subject areas. Even minor examples of poor judgment could compromise an entire program, particularly when administrators might exhibit little or no support for sexuality education.

Avoiding Trouble in Sexuality Education

Sources of problems in implementing sexuality education follow:

1. *Inadequate knowledge and background.* Just as with any subject, an ill-prepared teacher or presenter will inevitably experience great difficulty in providing solid, correct information in a meaningful way. However, the implications of poor preparation in human sexuality are potentially disastrous for the recipients of the program, the teacher/facilitator, and the program

itself. In the school setting, where the participants are often immature and impressionable, incorrect information could lead to disastrous consequences. Then the entire program will very quickly lose credibility, and the next step will be the abandonment of the program.

Ideally, individuals teaching in this area should have the utmost preparation and strive to keep "current" in a field that is always changing. Pragmatically, particularly in the school situation, it is unlikely that this ideal situation will occur. Teachers are often coerced into teaching sex education or have an interest in the area but have very little professional background. If programs are to survive, administrators must ensure that they select individuals who at least have an interest in the subject, and that these individuals receive sufficient training to enable them to be effective. This means they need to be able to attend continuing education workshops and courses that will keep them up to date on new information and teaching methods.

Community health sexuality educators need to be no less qualified and prepared. The organizations they represent, whether they are private or public agencies, will be judged by the response to their presentations, and community groups can be every bit as critical and volatile as parent groups in the school setting. Whenever possible, school and community sex educators should not accept assignments for which they know they are unprepared. The damage could be irreparable.

2. *Unrealistic curriculum goals and objectives.* As mentioned earlier, a major criticism by sex education opponents is that sex education simply does not work. To minimize such attacks, sexuality educators must be very prudent when designing course goals and objectives. Do not write behavioral objectives that are unrealistic. Most sex educators would laugh if a fellow educator wrote as an objective for a 10-week course that their students would discover a cure for AIDS! And yet some of these same sex educators will happily promise to miraculously reduce unintended pregnancy as the result of a once-a-week, for 10 weeks, sex education course. By all means write broad, generalized, **long-range goals** that might include pregnancy reduction or higher rates of condom usage. However, specific behavioral objectives, which must all be *measurable*, should be far more realistic and attainable. Objectives promising knowledge gains, for example, are entirely appropriate. Sexuality educators should not promise what they have no hope of producing.

3. *Not being prepared to defend the program.* Unlike other areas of school curriculum or community health topics, sexuality education is consistently placed under the microscope of scrutiny. Despite the publicity and awareness surrounding the AIDS epidemic, sexuality education remains in many communities a commodity to be either grudgingly tolerated or viewed with intense suspicion. Although studies mentioned earlier in this chapter clearly demonstrate that opponents of sexuality education are in the minority, these groups continue to be a voluble and persistent nuisance. Therefore, both sex educators and administrators of such programs should be prepared to defend programming in the face of intense criticism. Preparation should include a

knowledge of the major opposition arguments (these have not changed greatly over the years), a rebuttal to these arguments, a developed support system within the community to help bolster acceptance of the program, and a major effort to ensure that the sex educators are well trained and teaching within the accepted curriculum guidelines. Of course, not all criticism of programming will be irrational and unreasonable. Administrators should be honest enough to accept valid criticism and be prepared to alter program guidelines in an attempt to improve programming standards and overall quality.

4. *Inappropriate materials or assignments.* More ammunition for opponents of sexuality education and a very quick way to lose program credibility is for the sex educator to use inappropriate materials. The difficulty here is with the definition of "inappropriate." There may be nothing intrinsically wrong with the materials themselves, but it is the setting in which they are to be used that will determine appropriateness. The school setting allows for less discussion than the community environment, as most school districts have fairly strict policies about "sensitive" materials. A committee will preview a film or videotape and determine its acceptibility. Of course, frustration occurs when the teacher feels that the material is acceptable and useful, but the committee in its infinite wisdom thinks otherwise! The teacher has little choice but to accept the committee's decision, other than perhaps approaching the committee members individually to lobby for their support and a possible re-review. Most school districts have a catalogue or list of accepted materials that is well publicized and to which the area teachers must conform.

The community health situation is much less regulated, and if the sex educator is at all uncertain about the acceptability of materials, then people living in or familiar with the targeted community should preview them and provide feedback before any presentations are made. If the community health educator is actually working as a guest speaker in a classroom, it is most important to ensure that materials and content are acceptable in that particular school.

The question of appropriateness is obviously more relevant to school health but could also occur in a community health environment. Asking students to visit a drugstore to purchase condoms is one example of an assignment that would likely cause an uproar with many parents and school administrators. Setting the same assignment for a youth or church group in a community setting would inspire a similar negative reaction. The point is that the assignment itself is perhaps not a bad one, but it is simply inappropriate in many settings. Problems like this can be minimized if the sexuality educator consults administrators or community leaders *before* the damage is done. Also, many of these problems would not arise if all or even most sexuality educators were professionally trained and adequately prepared (see #1).

5. *Using materials without preview.* Using materials without previewing them is never a good idea in school or community health. At least in the school situation, if the educator is using materials from the approved catalogue, the worst that might happen is the students would not understand the

material or, more likely, would become incredibly bored. Of course, using nonapproved sexuality materials in the school with or without preview is grounds for dismissal, so such an action could have severe implications. In the community setting—again, where few regulations exist—the sexuality educator certainly needs to preview the materials to evaluate their appropriateness and usefulness. Beware of using something recommended by a friend or colleague without evaluating it yourself (see Chapter 7). Once the sex educator has previewed the materials, having students or any intended audience also preview the materials can provide useful feedback. Educators can easily fall into the trap of assuming that because they think materials are great, their audiences will feel the same way . . . not always the case!

6. *Inappropriate guest speakers.* Just as certain materials will be deemed by communities and organizations to be "inappropriate," using guest speakers can potentially raise the same concerns. For example, if a school sex educator is fortunate enough to be able to explore sexual orientation as a topic, how will the school and community react if the teacher invites a homosexual or lesbian to speak to the class? How will the community church group react when the sex educator schedules a panel on AIDS that includes a bisexual, a prostitute, and a drug abuser who are all HIV-positive? As valuable and educational as both these examples might be, are they worth potentially placing the programs in jeopardy?

As stated before, experience in this field usually prevents this type of problem from occurring, but there are some simple safeguards the sex educator can take. In the school setting, the teacher can check to see if there is a list of approved guest speakers already in existence. If not, or the desired speaker is not on the list, the teacher should consult a school administrator to seek official approval. In this way, if there is any fallout following the guest speaker's presentation the teacher has protected him/herself and the administrator will handle the conflict. In the community setting there will be few, if any, formal regulations. As with materials discussed above, the community sex educator should consult a few community leaders in an attempt to solicit their opinions regarding the guest speaker. Individuals within the community setting will have a much more accurate reading on how their peers will react to certain types of speakers than will the health educator.

Regardless of the setting, the educator should always discuss with the speaker beforehand just what the speaker is going to present. Similarly to previewing audiovisual materials, ideally the educator should have heard the guest speaker present before an invitation was extended. An important concern should not only be *what* the individual is going to say but *how well* he or she is going to say it! There are many health experts or individuals who have important messages to send who are such poor speakers that the value of their presence is minimized. In the school setting, where attention spans are often very short, a stunningly boring speaker will quickly be "tuned out" regardless of the quality of the information.

7. *Personal bias in teaching.* All teachers and communicators have some types of biases, no matter how subtle. This is a crucial issue for sexuality ed-

ucators to consider, as biases related to so many sensitive issues could potentially cause major problems for the educator and overall program. For example, the sex educator who is "pro-choice" in the volatile abortion issue, and provides a one-sided and very subjective view of the issue, can cause many problems. Obviously, those participants who would describe themselves as "pro-life" will be greatly offended by a pro-choice speaker, as perhaps would those individuals who are undecided. Many school sexuality education programs do not allow any discussion about abortion, but for those that do, if the sex educator merely promotes his or her own subjective views, the school will quickly hear about it! Once again, sexuality educators must take great care not to do anything that might place the entire program at risk. There is nothing wrong with having personal biases, and there are very few human beings who have none. The important point is that the well-prepared sexuality educator should be aware of and sensitive to his or her own biases and ensure that they do not influence how material is presented. The well-prepared and experienced sexuality educator should have achieved this higher level of self-awareness.

8. *Using slang.* For many students and participants, both in the school and community setting, using correct clinical terms to describe reproductive anatomy and sexual behavior will be a new experience. The sexuality educator will play an important role in modeling and normalizing the use of correct terminology, particularly in the school setting. Because there are so many different cultures in the United States, slang terminology will be extremely varied; therefore, if slang is used, communication becomes very complicated. There is nothing wrong with addressing the slang issue early in the class or presentation, where "translations" can be made and the correct terminology established. But for the sake of accuracy and consistency, correct terminology should be used whenever possible. Community health educators, when dealing with specific subcultures, might argue that correct terminology is only an unnecessary diversion, and to some extent that might be true. For example, in regard to a single inner-city, ethnic minority student who is an intravenous drug abuser, to insist that the educator use the correct terminology in attempting to encourage condom usage would seem overzealous, and quite possibly dysfunctional. Community sexuality educators must therefore use their best judgment, using correct terminology whenever possible, but being sensitive to the need for exceptions.

9. *Sharing personal sexual experience.* A more generalized term for this issue might be *self-disclosure.* How much of his or her own experiences does the sexuality educator share? At first glance this would appear to be a simple issue — the sexuality educator should *never* disclose any personal information. But perhaps we are defining *sexual experience* in too narrow a fashion. Look at the following examples, and consider whether or not the disclosures are appropriate:

A female sex educator while teaching about menstruation to a class of sixth grade girls relates how she had felt about her own period beginning.

A male sex educator while discussing relationships in a coed senior high school class describes how he felt when his "first love" ended their relationship in high school.

A female sex educator presenting a workshop for community youth on becoming sexually active describes her own fears of having sex for the first time when she was a teenager.

A female sex educator describes her own experience with inorgasmia *(inability to orgasm) to an adult community group interested in sexual dysfunction.*

A male peer sexuality educator during a workshop on date rape explains how he had previously had sex with a women after she had said "No."

Clearly, the gratuitous use of graphic depictions of personal sexual experiences have no place in sexuality education. However, as you consider the preceding examples, you might gain a sense that not all personal revelation in the area of sexuality needs to be viewed as negative and forbidden. There is no doubt that in many instances, self-revelation by the educator places the participants at greater ease, thus encouraging more meaningful contributions. Self-disclosure allows the participants to perceive the "expert" or educator as not being so different from them, and the environment for participant disclosure as being safe.

Again, experience and training will help the educator avoid trouble, and a good rule of thumb, particularly in the school setting, is that if there is any doubt as to the appropriateness of the disclosure, decide against it. Do not feel duty bound to answer every question that you are asked.

For example, suppose that while discussing decision-making skills related to becoming sexually active, a student asks, "How old were you when you had sex for the first time?" How should you respond? This is probably not an appropriate question, nor an appropriate issue about which to self-disclose. A possible reply might be, "That is a personal issue which I would prefer to remain private. I will respect your privacy about such issues and I won't ask you personal questions, and I'd be grateful if you would respect me in the same way." In the school setting students will always ask inappropriate questions . . . that's their job! The sexuality educator, therefore, must always be alert to possible problems that might arise from impulsive self-disclosure, and be prepared to politely but firmly decline to answer certain questions.

10. *Behind closed doors.* All individuals who work with youth are placed in a position of trust—a trust that they will not abuse by using their positions of power to take advantage, in any way, of young persons placed in their care. To many individuals, sexuality educators are a little "suspect" anyway, as a result of the sensitive nature of the material that they teach. Ironically, students often view the sexuality educator as a warm, caring individual and one of few adult figures with whom they can discuss personal concerns and problems. There is no question that in the school setting, good, effective sexuality educators will frequently be consulted by students on many diverse

issues. Some of the issues may be simple clarification of fact; others may range from disclosure of the students about unintended pregnancy, STIs, and even sexual abuse. There is no simple formula or recipe for dealing with these issues, but the sexuality educator must balance genuine concern for the student with an awareness of the dangers that advising students on personal matters may pose to the educator's professional reputation and the integrity of the entire program.

To minimize the potential for problems, do not meet students in "private places" outside class. There is nothing wrong with having a private conversation, but have it in an office or classroom, where the wrong assumptions are less likely to be made. If a student wants to relate something in confidence, explain that there are certain issues that the law requires an educator to report, child sexual abuse, for example. Many sexuality educators, because of the types of individuals they are, can provide an incredibly important outlet for student concerns, and this invaluable service should not be compromised. However, the educator needs to be aware of potential misinterpretations and take preventive measures against them.

Assumptions to Avoid

Mary Krueger (1993) provides an interesting and thought-provoking list of *assumptions to avoid* when discussing sex education, particularly in the classroom. Some of the following ideas may seem obvious, but they are definitely worthy of our attention:

1. *All students come from traditional families.* With divorce rates of over 50 percent, the "traditional" family is no longer the norm. Make no assumptions about home situations.

2. *All students are heterosexual.* Whatever the rate of homosexuality/bisexuality in our society, alternate sexual orientations certainly exist. Include all segments of society in the educative process.

3. *All students are sexually involved.* Not all young people are sexually active, so do not present information as if being a virgin is somehow abnormal and undesirable.

4. *No students are sexually involved.* Alternatively, avoid the assumption that *no one* is sexually active, which often leads to an emphasis on abstinence, a concept to which some sexually active individuals might have difficulty relating.

5. *All students' sexual involvements are consensual.* Given the prevalence of sex abuse in our society, particularly with school-aged individuals, an educator should assume that some students/participants are experiencing or have experienced sexual exploitation. Sexuality educators can expect to be approached about this type of issue and should be prepared to give aid and advice.

6. *Students who are "sexually active" are having intercourse.* There are many different forms of sexual behaviors that do not include penis/vagina intercourse. Therefore, discussion should not be confined to preventing pregnancy and STD/HIV transmission but should incorporate other behaviors

such as masturbation, mutual masturbation, oral sex, petting, and kissing and hugging.

Establishing Curriculum or Program in Controversial Area

Whether you are establishing a potentially controversial program in sexuality, drug education, nutrition, or any other subject matter, it is important to follow procedures that will minimize complaints and address the standards of the environment you are working. Following the procedures previously discussed in conducting a needs assessment will be very important. Establishing a process to ensure that representatives of the community are involved and that community standards are represented is vital to the success of any program. A common method that has proved successful for developing a curriculum or program involves the establishment of two committees. In this **two-committee system,** one committee is made up of professionals who are charged with writing the curriculum, and the other is advisory in nature to give some guidance and reaction to the first committee's work before it is presented to a school board or community agency.

Writing Committee   The *writing committee* should be composed of professionals in the area of study. If this is a school curriculum, this committee should be made up of employees of the school district only. The size is very important, since the charge of the committee is to write or adapt materials for use. Therefore, it is recommended that the committee never exceed eight members, with the optimal size being six members. The writing committee has final say on what is submitted to the supervising board for approval. School districts generally have a school board, and health agencies have some type of board of directors.

Advisory Committee   The *advisory committee* is to be composed of citizens from the community who have an interest in the subject matter to be addressed. The charge is to react to materials developed by the writing committee and to make suggestions. This can be a large committee, since it is advisory in nature and reacts to the work of the professional committee. Care should be taken in membership to ensure proportionate representation of the community. It is generally a good idea to place a representative of the opposition on the committee. This will demonstrate there is nothing secret and there is a willingness to listen to all sides. However, it is important not to let this person or group dominate the discussions; the selection of a strong chair can help with this issue. This is a lay advisory group but might include ministers or other religious leaders, physicians, and other appropriate members of the medical community, parents, community leaders, police, and community organization leaders.

Political Correctness and the Health Educator

Political correctness (PC) . . . myth or reality, fact or fiction? Does any such phenomenon exist, or is PC just an epithet used to describe an imaginary influence? The term PC certainly seems to have become part of everyday life, and those two letters can be frequently heard, particularly in the enclaves of education. But what does PC mean? Is it good or bad? Should we embrace the positive, worthwhile tenets of the PC movement (if, of course, it exists), or should we struggle to free ourselves from the ties of such a stifling, censorial monster? A chapter on controversial topics would not be complete without a mention of this phenomenon, which has actually become a controversial topic in its own right.

A 1991 study by the American Council on Education surveyed university administrators on campus trends and suggested that "reports of widespread efforts to impose politically correct thinking on college students and faculty appear to be overblown" (Dodge, 1991). Reinforcing these data is the sentiment of UCLA professor Alexander Astin that "the PC thing is a kind of Christmas tree the Right has chosen to hang on all the things it doesn't like about higher education today . . . there's no thought control occurring" (Daniels, 1991). An opposite position was taken by Yale president Benno Schmidt, who stated when discussing the effects of PC, "The most serious problems of freedom of expression in our society exist on our campuses" (Cheney,1992). Even presidents have voiced an opinion related to this issue. When ex-president Bush addressed the graduates of Michigan University in 1991, he warned that "the notion of political correctness replaces old prejudices with new ones. It declares certain topics off-limits, certain expressions off-limits, even certain gestures off-limits. What began as a crusade for civility has soured into a cause of conflict and even censorship" (Daniels, 1991).

Unlike education in general, very little attention has been paid to PC in the field of health education, which, given the sensitivity of many health-related topics, is somewhat surprising. One area of PC that is particularly relevant to health education is the use of language. Zola (1993) reflected on the power and importance of language in an article that discussed the linguistics of disability. Zola compares the linguistic terms used in regard to the disability issue and describes the negative connotations and inferences that some of the terms carry. Zola also decries the overt criticism suffered by individuals who use the "wrong" or un-PC terminology, and suggests that such reactions are unproductive (Zola, 1993). In addition to disability, use of appropriate language is often scrutinized in the areas of ethnicity, gender, and sexual orientation.

Undergraduate students, for example, often full of youthful zeal and desperate for others to embrace their cause, often seem oblivious to the fact that their ideas, values, concepts, and approach will not be uniformly accepted. When the nonacceptance accelerates to a personal challenge against the type of health education message or the messenger's style of delivery, the neophyte health educator risks intimidation and bewilderment. Conceding that most of us have found that experience (albeit painful) is the best teacher, protecting students from unnecessary criticism and harm through professional preparation would seem the ethical thing to do. After polling both graduate and undergraduate health education majors, it became clear to this author (RGS) that there was absolutely no consensus as to the definition of PC or whether or not the whole concept of PC was positive or negative. Perhaps arriving at an agreed-upon definition, or even establishing whether or not such a phenomenon exists, is less important than ensuring that students at least consider the possible implications that PC might hold in the practice of health education.

For example, as someone who has taught human sexuality for a number of years, this author has observed a definite decline in willingness to share ideas and attitudes that do not conform to what has been recognized as the PC position. Specifically, very few males in sexuality and communication presentations are willing to publicly voice any sentiments that might be labeled "traditionally male." Some of the men sheepishly shuffle up to the teacher after the presentation to say that they would have liked to have contributed during the discussion, but they were tired of being ridiculed and berated for their opinions. When program participants all adhere to the "party line" and keep their real opinions to themselves, we achieve nothing save a sanitized and hollow version of what could have been a meaningful, honest, and open discussion. However, one could argue against that position by stating that maybe men's attitudes have really changed. Another argument might be that men are not feeling comfortable enough to deliver what could be construed as sexist, misogynistic comments is actually a positive thing because their silence demonstrates society's successful lack of tolerance for "antisocial" speech. The important point here is not who is right or wrong, PC or un-PC, but rather that the health educator be aware of the potential presence of "outside influences" when planning and conducting programs.

Case Study Exercise: Paul

Paul, a newly qualified health educator, has been tasked with designing a date rape workshop for college students. Being fresh out of college, Paul remembers his "methods" course and vaguely recalls that such a topic might include some sensitive issues that he should consider. Before sitting down to write objectives and consider appropriate strategies, Paul decides to develop a list of any potential PC issues that might be relevant to this particular situation.

Before seeing what Paul came up with, why don't you jot down some issues that you consider might have some relevance here, then compare your list with Paul's thoughts. When you are ready, see Case Studies Revisited page 320.

For more information and tools related to this chapter visit www.jbpub.com/healtheducation.

EXERCISES

1. You have been asked by your rather reluctant high school principal to design a one-semester human sexuality course that may become mandatory for all 10th-grade students. Consider what you think is feasible, then construct relevant goals and objectives that you will present to the principal.

2. You have been given the onerous task of speaking for the development of a human sexuality program in the local school system. The public evening meeting is expected to be volatile and opposition to the proposed program very vocal. Describe the steps you will take in preparing your presentation and on which points you will focus your discussion.

3. Anystate University, where you are employed as a health educator, has an obvious alcohol problem. You have been asked by your supervisor to design a workshop for incoming freshmen about alcohol use and abuse. Consider your own philosophy, likely university administration philosophy, and the current political climate before briefly describing your approach to such a workshop. Which goals and objectives would you choose? What types of strategies/methods would you utilize?

4. You are a community health educator responsible for designing and implementing a sexuality program for a local youth group (aged 14–16 years). While you are describing the program to the parents of the prospective participants, one parent becomes extremely antagonistic and demands to know why "responsible sex" is even mentioned, as abstinence is the only message that should be given. Briefly describe how you would respond to such an attack, and justify your reasoning.

5. You are a community health educator working in an inner city clinic that deals mostly with unintended pregnancy, STD, treatment and HIV testing. A 13-year-old girl tells you that she has been having sexual intercourse regularly during her period and cannot understand why she has not become pregnant. She explains that she "needs" to get pregnant in order to keep her boyfriend, who has threatened to leave her unless she has his baby. You try the predictable counseling route of the difficulties of a 13-year-old raising a baby, not finishing school, the boyfriend leaving anyway . . . all the rational reasons why she should not get pregnant. None of these arguments makes a difference, and the girl demands to know what she is doing wrong. How will you respond? Will you help her to become pregnant, or is it ethically all right to suggest that she keep having sex during her period? Does the end truly justify the means? Respond briefly to this situation, and justify your answers.

6. One of your 10th-grade students comes to you after class, visibly upset. She confides in you that she is pregnant and needs information about having an abortion but is uncertain where to go for help. Despite your encouragement to discuss this with her parents, the girl is adamant that she cannot involve them. You are the only person she felt comfortable enough to approach, and she needs your help. What are you going to do? Carefully think through the issue, and then briefly describe and justify your actions.

Responding to these last two exercise questions will not be easy. Health education students must realize that because they deal with sensitive issues, they will invariably become involved in real-life, personal problems, not just the abstract design of objectives or workshop protocols. Thinking through your own ideas and listening to the philosophies of others will prepare you, at least in some small way, to handle extremely difficult situations.

CASE STUDIES REVISITED

Case Study Revisited: Todd

Todd had allowed his own belief and enthusiasm in sex education to blind him to the realization that many individuals are extremely opposed to the inclusion of sex education in the school curriculum. Setting up new programs is one of the most difficult facets of sex education, and health educators who are involved in any controversial programming should be as prepared as possible to defend against a sometimes vociferous opposition. As health educators we sometimes forget that although responses to health concerns appear obvious to us, many individuals will greet our propositions with great skepticism. To that end, an ever increasing role played by the health educator is that of politician, who must carefully prepare the ground for innovative ideas that might be met by strong public opposition. Support for programming must be carefully but consistently developed with influential community individuals, and opposition arguments must be anticipated and appropriate responses prepared. (See page 287.)

Case Study Revisited: Paul

- Use of language — "women" rather than "girls."
- Inclusion — if designing scenarios of sexual situations, include a same-gender situation.
- Stereotypes — consider including scenarios that are not so stereotypical, such as a woman pressuring a man to have sex.
- Gender — does the gender of the presenter(s) influence the presentation, and if so, how? Is there a preferred format with regard to gender?
- Many men tend not to actively participate in such discussions for fear of criticism. What can you do to draw them out?
- This topic might stimulate some students to be very "political" in their interaction. How would you handle that?

This list is by no means exhaustive, but generating the list might be useful in helping health educators realize that even the most straightforward assignments can be fraught with potential problems. Once the potential difficulties have been established, possible responses or solutions can be developed. (See page 318.)

SUMMARY

1. There are many controversial issues within the discipline of health education.

2. Sexuality education and drug education have traced parallel paths with regard to the evolution of teaching strategies.

3. An ever increasing number of "canned," or commercially prepared, programs are being utilized in both the drug and sexuality areas.

4. Health educators must be prepared to defend the existence of programming in controversial areas.

5. The accurate development of feasible, attainable objectives is of crucial importance when developing programs in controversial areas.

6. Health educators must be knowledgeable about the existence and tactics of opposition groups.

7. Health educators must be aware of the major obstacles to developing a sexuality education program.

8. Health educators must be aware of and avoid some of the more common pitfalls in teaching/presenting sex education.

9. The current struggle in sex education, particularly in the schools, is the adoption of abstinence-versus-responsibility curricula.

10. Developers of potentially controversial programs should consider the two-committee strategy of development.

11. Political correctness is an issue that health educators should consider, regardless of individual definitions or even disagreements over actual existence.

REFERENCES

Advocates for Youth (1997). Differing European/US approaches to teen sex show surprising results. Press release. Retrieved April 16, 1999 from the World Wide Web: http://www.advocatesforyouth.org/estretur.htm

Anderson, P. (1973). The Pot Lobby. *New York Times Magazine*, January 21, 8–9.

Baldo, M., Aggleton, P., & Slutin, G. (1993). *Does Sex Education Lead to Earlier or Increased Sexual Activity in Youth?* Geneva: World Health Organization Global Programme on AIDS.

Battjes, R.J. (1985). Prevention of Adolescent Drug Abuse. *International Journal of Addiction, 20,* 1113–1134.

Botvin, G.J. (1983). Prevention of adolescent substance abuse through the development of personal and social competence. In Glynn, T. Leukefeld, C., & Ludford, J.P. (Eds.), *Preventing Adolescent Drug Abuse: Intervention Strategies.* Rockville, MD: NIDA.

Centers for Disease Control and Prevention (1992). *HIV/AIDS Prevention Newsletter, 3* (1), 4 (Atlanta, GA).

Centers for Disease Control and Prevention (1993). Update: Barrier protection against HIV infection and other sexually transmitted diseases: Editorial note. *Morbidity and Mortality Weekly Report, 42,* 590.

Centers for Disease Control and Prevention (1995). National College Health Risk Behavior Survey. Retrieved April 27, 1999 from the World Wide Web: http://www.cdc.gov.

Centers for Disease Control and Prevention (1997). Youth Risk Behavior Surveillance. Retrieved April 27, 1999 from the World Wide Web: http://www.cdc.gov.

Centers for Disease Control and Prevention (1998). Trends of sexual risk taking among high school students. *Morbidity and Mortality Weekly Report,* September 18.

Cheney, L.V. (1992). Beware the PC police. *Executive Educator, 14,* 31–34.

Christopher, F.S., & Roosa, M.W. (1990). An evaluation of an adolescent pregnancy prevention program: Is 'just say no' enough? *Family Relations, 39,* 68–72.

Clark, J.E., Houser, C.M., Powell, K.D. (1995). *We the people* Charlotte, N.C.: Pregnancy Prevention Coalition of North Carolina, p. 5.

Daniels, L.A. (1991). Diversity, correctness, and campus life. *Change,* September/October, 16–20.

Davis, C.M., Davis, S.L., & Yarber, W.L. (Eds.) (1988). *Sexuality Related Measures: A Compendium.* Lake Mills, IA: Graphic Publications Co.

Dawson, D.A. (1986). The effects of sex education on adolescent behavior, *Family Planning Perspectives 18,* July/August.

Dodge, S. (1991). Few colleges have had "Political correctness" controversies, study finds. *Chronicle of Higher Education 37(47),* A23–A24.

Finn, C. (1986). Educational excellence: Eight elements. *Foundations News, 27(2),* 40–45.

Forrest, J.D., & Silverman, J. (1989). What public school teachers teach about pregnancy prevention and AIDS," *Family Planning Perspectives 21,* March/April.

Gallup Poll (1976). *Growing Number of Americans Favor Discussion of Sex in the Classroom.* News release, Princeton, NJ, January 23.

Gallup Poll Monthly (1991). Sex in America, 56:1–9, 71.

Gilbert, G.G. (1979). Easy ways of getting into trouble when teaching sex education. *Health Education,* September/October.

Greenberg, J.S., & Bruess, C.E. (1981). *Sex Education; Theory & Practice,* Wadsworth Publishing Co., Belmont, CA.

Guttmacher Institute (1989). *Risk and Responsibility* (p. 7). New York: Alan Guttmacher Institute.

Guttmacher Institute (1994). *Sex and America's Teenagers* (p. 76). New York: Alan Guttmacher Institute.

Guttmacher Institute (1998). *Teen sex and pregnancy.* From "Facts in Brief." Retrieved February 16, 1999 from the World Wide Web: http://www.agi-usa.org/pubs/fb_teen_sex.

Hofferth, S.L. (1981). Effects of number and timing of births on family well-being over the life cycle. Final report to National Institute of Child Health and Human Development (Contract # 1-HD-82850).

Holmes, S.A. (1996). Public cost of teenage pregnancy is put at $7 billion this year. *New York Times.* July 13, 1996, A19.

Howard, M., & McCabe, B. (1990). Helping teens postpone sexual involvement. *Family Planning Perspectives, 22,* 21–26.

Jones, E.F., et al. (1986). *Teenage pregnancy in industrialized countries,* Yale University Press, New Haven.

Kirby, D., Alter, J., & Scales, P. (1979a). An analysis of U.S. sex education programs and evaluation methods. Springfield, VA. National Technical Information Service.

Kirby, D., Alter, J., & Scales, P. (1979b). "Executive Summary" in An Analysis of U.S. Education Programs and Evaluation Methods. Atlanta, GA.: U.S. Department of Health, Education and Welfare.

Kirby, D., et al. (1991). "Reducing the Risk: Impact of a new curriculum on sexual risk taking." *Planning Perspectives, 23,* 253–262.

Kirby, D. (1997). No easy answers: Research findings on programs to reduce teen pregnancy. Washington DC: National Campaign to Prevent Teen Pregnancy.

Laing, R.D. (1972). *Knots* (p. 56). New York: Random House.

Louis Harris & Associates (1986). American teens speak: Sex, myth, T.V. and birth control, New York.

Louis Harris & Associates (1988). Public attitudes toward teenage pregnancy, sex education & birth control (p. 24). H. Quinley of Yankelovich Clancy Shulman, memorandum to all data users regarding Time/Yankelovich Clancy Shulman Poll Findings on Sex Education, November 17, 1986.

Marsiglio, W., & Mott, F.L. (1986). The impact of sex education on sexual activity, contraceptive use and premarital pregnancy among American teenagers, *Family Planning Perspectives, 18,* July/August.

Means, R.K. (1962). A *History of Health Education in the U.S.* Lea & Febiger, Philadelphia.

NARAL (1998). *A State by State Review of Abortion and Reproductive Rights.* Washington, DC: NARAL Foundation.

National Assessment of Educational Progress (1976). *Bicentennial Citizenship Survey.* Denver.

National Institute of Drug Abuse (1986). *National Survey on Drug Abuse.* DHHS Pub. No. (ADM) 84-1356. Washington, DC.

National Institute of Drug Abuse (1991). *High School Senior Survey.* Washington, DC.

National Opinion Research Center (1982). *General Social Surveys, 1972–1978: Cumulative Code Book,* Chicago.

Pollack, A.E. (1992). Teen contraception in the 90s. *Journal of School Health, 62,* 288–293.

Popham, W.J. (1993). Wanted: AIDS Education that Works. *Phi Delta Kappan,* March, 559–562.

Ringwalt, C., Ennett, S.T., & Holt, K.D. (1991). An Outcome Evaluation of Project DARE. *Health Education Research,* 6(3), 327–337.

For a more complete discussion of political correctness see Sawyer and Anastasi's (1988) article on the subject. Sawyer, R.G., & Anastasi, M.C. (1998). Political correctness and the professional preparation of health educators. *Journal of Health Education* 29(4), 240–243.

Sawyer, R.G., & Gray-Smith (1996). A survey of situational factors at first intercourse among college students. *American Journal of Health Behavior, 20(4),* 208–217.

Scales, P. (1989). Overcoming future barriers to sexuality education, Theory into practice, *Health Education, 28(3),* 172–176.

SIECUS (1999). Position statement on human sexuality. Retrieved May 5, 1999 from the World Wide Web: http://www.siecus.org.

SIECUS (1998). *Between the Lines: States' Implementation of the Federal Government's Section 510(b) Abstinence Education Program in Fiscal Year 1998.* SIECUS, New York.

Sonenstein, F.L., & Pittman, K.J. (1984). The availability of sex education in large school districts. *Family Planning Perspectives 16,* 19–25.

Taqi, S. (1972). The Drug Cinema. *Bulletin on Narcotics, 24,* 19–24.

Time (1993). How should we teach our children about sex? May, 60–66.

U.S. Department of Health & Human Services (1984). *Highlights from the National Survey on Drug Abuse.* DHHS Pub. No. (ADM) 83-1277. Washington, DC.

Vincent, M.L., Clearie, A.F., & Schlucter, M.D. (1987). Reducing adolescent pregnancy through school and community-based education. *Journal of the American Medical Association, 257,* 3382–3386.

Vincent, M.L., Berne, L.A., Lammers, J.W., & Strack, R. (1999) Pregnancy prevention, sexuality education, and coping with opposing views. *Journal of Health Education* 30(3), 142–149.

Wall Street Journal (1992). Schools teach the virtues of virginity, February 20, B1.

Weed, S.E., & Olsen, J.A. (1990). Evaluation report of the Sex Respect program: Results for the 1989–1990 School Year. Salt Lake City: Institute for Research and Evaluation, 19–25.

Zelnik, M., & Kim, Y.J. (1982). Sex education and its association with teenage sexual activity, pregnancy and contraceptive use, *Family Planning Perspectives, 14,* May/June.

Zola, I.K. (1993). Self, identity and the naming question: Reflections on the language of disability. *Social Science and Medicine,* 36(2), 167–173.

Resources

Entry-Level and Graduate-Level Health Educator Competencies Addressed in This Appendix

Responsibility VI: Acting as a Resource Person in Health Education

Competency A: Utilize computerized health information retrieval systems effectively.

Competency B: Establish effective consultative relationships with those requesting assistance in solving health-related problems.

Competency C: Interpret and respond to requests for health information.

Competency D: Select effective resource materials for dissemination.

Responsibility VII: Communicating Health and Health Education Needs, Concerns, and Resources

Competency C: Select a variety of communication methods and techniques in providing health information.

Note: The competencies listed here are both entry-level and graduate-level competencies by the National Commission for Health Education Credentialing, Inc. They are taken from *A Framework for the Development of Competency-Based Curricula for Entry Level Health Educators* by the National Task Force on the Preparation and Practice of Health Educators, Inc., 1985.

KEY ISSUES

Entry-level health educator competencies

Graduate-level health educator competencies

Code of ethics for the health profession

Professional organizations

Additional readings

Method Selection in Health Education

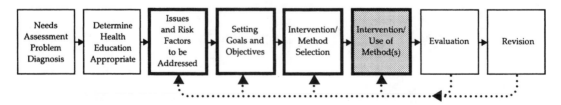

Heavy-bordered boxes indicate subjects addressed in this text; shaded boxes indicate subject(s) of current chapter.

Entry-Level Health Educator Competencies

Responsibility I: **Assessing Individual and Community Needs for Health Education**
Competency A: Obtain health-related data about social and cultural environments, growth and development factors, needs, and interests.
Competency B: Distinguish between behaviors that foster and those that hinder well-being.
Competency C: Infer needs for health education on the basis of obtained data.

Responsibility II: **Planning Effective Health Education Programs**
Competency A: Recruit community organizations, resource people, and potential participants for support and assistance in program planning.
Competency B: Develop a logical scope and sequence plan for a health education program.
Competency C: Formulate appropriate and measurable program objectives.

Responsibility III: **Implementing Health Education Programs**
Competency A: Exhibit competence in carrying out planned educational programs.
Competency B: Infer enabling objectives as needed to implement instructional program in specified settings.
Competency C: Select methods and media best suited to implement program plans for specific learners.
Competency D: Monitor educational programs, adjusting objectives and activities as necessary.

Responsibility IV: **Evaluating Effectiveness of Health Education Programs**
Competency A: Develop plans to assess achievement of program objectives.
Competency B: Carry out evaluation plans.
Competency C: Interpret results of program evaluation.
Competency D: Infer implications from findings for future program planning.

Responsibility V: **Coordinating Provision of Health Education Services**   Administer
Competency A: Develop a plan for coordinating health education services.
Competency B: Facilitate cooperation between and among levels of program personnel.
Competency C: Formulate practical modes of collaboration among health agencies and organizations.
Competency D: Organize in-service training programs for teachers, volunteers, and other interested personnel.

Responsibility VI: **Acting as a Resource Person in Health Education**
Competency A: Utilize computerized health information retrieval systems effectively.
Competency B: Establish effective consultative relationships with those requesting assistance in solving health-related problems.
Competency C: Interpret and respond to requests for health information.
Competency D: Select effective resource materials for dissemination.

Responsibility VII: **Communicating Health and Health Education Needs, Concerns, and Resources**
Competency A: Interpret concepts, purposes, and theories of health education.
Competency B: Predict the impact of societal value systems on health education programs.
Competency C: Select a variety of communication methods and techniques in providing health information.

Graduate-Level Health Educator Competencies

The following is taken from A *Competency-Based Framework for Graduate Level Health Educators* AAHE/NCHEC/SOPHE, 1999.

Responsibility I: **Assessing Individual and Community Needs for Health Education**

Competency A: Obtain health related data about social and cultural environments, growth and development factors, needs, and interests.

Competency B: Distinguish between behaviors that foster and those that hinder well-being.

Competency C: Infer needs for health education on the basis of obtained data.

Competency D: Determine factors that influence learning and development.

Responsibility II: **Planning Effective Health Education Programs**

Competency A: Recruit community organizations, resource people, and potential participants for support and assistance in program planning.

Competency B: Develop a logical scope and sequence plan for a health education program.

Competency C: Formulate appropriate and measurable program objectives.

Competency D: Design education programs consistent with specified program objectives.

Competency E: Develop health education programs using social marketing principles.

Responsibility III: **Implementing Health Education Programs**

Competency A: Exhibit competency in carrying out planned programs.

Competency B: Infer enabling objectives as needed to implement instructional program in specified settings.

Competency C: Select media and methods best suited to implement program plans for specific learners.

Competency D: Monitor educational programs and adjust objectives and activities as necessary.

Responsibility IV: **Evaluating Effectiveness of Health Education Programs**

Competency A: Develop plans to assess achievement of program objectives.

Competency B: Carry out evaluation plans.

Competency C: Interpret results of program evaluation.

Competency D: Infer implications from findings for future program planning.

Responsibility V: **Coordinating Provision of Health Education Services**

Competency A: Develop a plan for coordinating health education services.

Competency B: Facilitate cooperation between and among levels of program personnel.

Competency C: Formulate practical modes of collaboration among health agencies and organizations.

Competency D: Organize in-service training for teachers, volunteers, and other interested personnel.

Responsibility VI: **Acting as a Resource Person in Health Education**

Competency A: Utilize computerized health information retrieval system effectively.

Competency B: Establish effective consultive relationships with those requesting assistance in solving health-related problems.

Competency C:	Interpret and respond to requests for health information.
Competency D:	Select effective educational resource materials for dissemination.
ResponsibilityVII:	**Communicating Health and Health Education Needs, Concerns, and Resources**
Competency A:	Interpret concepts, purposes, and theories of health education.
Competency B:	Predict the impact of societal value systems on health education programs.
Competency C:	Select a variety of communication methods and techniques in providing health information.
Competency D:	Foster communication between health care providers and consumers.
Responsibility	**VIII: Apply Appropriate Research Principles and Methods in Health Education**
Competency A:	Conduct thorough reviews of literature.
Competency B:	Use appropriate qualitative and quantitative research methods.
Competency C:	Apply research to health education practice.
Responsibility IX:	**Administering Health Education Programs**
Competency A:	Develop and manage fiscal resources.
Competency B:	Develop and manage human resources.
Competency C:	Exercise organizational leadership.
Competency D:	Obtain acceptance and support for programs.
Responsibility X:	**Advancing the Profession of Health Education**
Competency A:	Provide a critical analysis of current and future needs in health education.
Competency B:	Assume responsibility for advancing the profession.
Competency C:	Apply ethical principles as they relate to the practice of health education.

For a complete set of graduate level competencies, including subcompetencies, contact NCHEC, 944 Marcon Blvd., Suite 310, Allentown, PA 18103. (Ph. 1-888-624-3248).

Code of Ethics for the Health Education Profession

PREAMBLE

The Health Education profession is dedicated to excellence in the practice of promoting individual, family, organizational, and community health. Guided by common ideals, Health Educators are responsible for upholding the integrity and ethics of the profession as they face the daily challenges of making decisions. By acknowledging the value of diversity in society and embracing a cross-cultural approach, Health Educators support the worth, dignity, potential, and uniqueness of all people.

The Code of Ethics provides a framework of shared values within which Health Education is practice. The Code of Ethics is grounded in fundamental ethical principles that underlie all health care services: respect for autonomy, promotion of social justice, active promotion of good, and avoidance of harm. The responsibility of each health educator is to aspire to the highest possible standards of conduct and to encourage the ethical behavior of all those with whom they work.

Regardless of job title, professional affiliation, work setting, or population served, Health Educators abide by these guidelines when making professional decisions.

Article I: Responsibility to the Public

A Health Educator's ultimate responsibility is to educate people for the purpose of promoting, maintaining, and improving individual, family, and community health. When a conflict of issues arises among individuals, groups, organizations, agencies, or institutions, health educators must consider all issues and give priority to those that promote wellness and quality of living through principles of self-determination and freedom of choice for the individual.

Section 1: Health Educators support the right of individuals to make informed decisions regarding health, as long as such decisions pose no threat to the health of others.

Section 2: Health Educators encourage actions and social policies that support and facilitate the best balance of benefits over harm for all affected parties.

Section 3: Health Educators accurately communicate the potential benefits and consequences of the services and programs with which they are associated.

Section 4: Health Educators accept the responsibility to act on issues that can adversely affect the health of individuals, families, and communities.

Section 5: Health Educators are truthful about their qualifications and the limitations of their expertise and provide services consistent with their competencies.

Section 6: Health Educators protect the privacy and dignity of individuals.

Section 7: Health Educators actively involve individuals, groups, and communities in the entire educational process so that all aspects of the process are clearly understood by those who may be affected.

Section 8: Health Educators respect and acknowledge the rights of others to hold diverse values, attitudes, and opinions.

Section 9: Health Educators provide services equitably to all people.

Article II: Responsibility to the Profession

Health Educators are responsible for their professional behavior, for the reputation of their profession, and for promoting ethical conduct among their colleagues.

Section 1: Health Educators maintain, improve, and expand their professional competence through continued study and education; membership, participation, and leadership in professional organizations; and involvement in issues related to the health of the public.

Section 2: Health Educators model and encourage nondiscriminatory standards of behavior in their interactions with others.

Section 3: Health Educators encourage and accept responsible critical discourse to protect and enhance the profession.

Section 4: Health Educators contribute to the development of the profession by sharing the processes and outcomes of their work.

Section 5: Health Educators are aware of possible professional conflicts of interest, exercise integrity in conflict situations, and do not manipulate or violate the rights of others.

Section 6: Health Educators give appropriate recognition to others for their professional contributions and achievements

Article III: Responsibility to Employers

Health Educators recognize the boundaries of their professional competence and are accountable for their professional activities and actions.

Section 1: Health Educators accurately represent their qualifications and the qualifications of others whom they recommend.

Section 2: Health Educators use appropriate standards, theories, and guidelines as criteria when carrying out their professional responsibilities.

Section 3: Health Educators accurately represent potential service and program outcomes to employers.

Section 4: Health Educators anticipate and disclose competing commitments, conflicts of interest, and endorsement of products.

Section 5: Health Educators openly communicate to employers, expectations of job-related assignments that conflict with their professional ethics.

Section 6: Health Educators maintain competence in their areas of professional practice.

Article IV: Responsibility in the Delivery of Health Education

Health Educators promote integrity in the delivery of health education. They respect the rights, dignity, confidentiality, and worth of all people by adapting strategies and methods to the needs of diverse populations and communities.

Section 1: Health Educators are sensitive to social and cultural diversity and are in accord with the law, when planning and implementing programs.

Section 2: Health Educators are informed of the latest advances in theory, research, and practice, and use strategies and methods that are grounded in and contribute to development of professional standards, theories, guidelines, statistics, and experience.

Section 3: Health Educators are committed to rigorous evaluation of both program effectiveness and the methods used to achieve results.

Section 4: Health Educators empower individuals to adopt healthy lifestyles through informed choice rather than by coercion or intimidation.

Section 5: Health Educators communicate the potential outcomes of proposed services, strategies, and pending decisions to all individuals who will be affected.

Article V: Responsibility in Research and Evaluation

Health Educators contribute to the health of the population and to the profession through research and evaluation activities. When planning and conducting research or evaluation, health educators do so in accordance with federal and state laws and regulations, organizational and institutional policies, and professional standards.

Section 1: Health Educators support principles and practices of research and evaluation that do no harm to individuals, groups, society, or the environment.

Section 2: Health Educators ensure that participation in research is voluntary and is based upon the informed consent of the participants.

Section 3: Health Educators respect the privacy, rights, and dignity of research participants, and honor commitments made to those participants.

Section 4: Health Educators treat all information obtained from participants as confidential unless otherwise required by law.

Section 5: Health Educators take credit, including authorship, only for work they have actually performed and give credit to the contributions of others.

Section 6: Health Educators who serve as research or evaluation consultants discuss their results only with those to whom they are providing service, unless maintaining such confidentiality would jeopardize the health or safety of others.

Section 7: Health Educators report the results of their research and evaluation objectively, accurately, and in a timely fashion.

Article VI: Responsibility in Professional Preparation

Those involved in the preparation and training of Health Educators have an obligation to accord learners the same respect and treatment given other groups by providing quality education that benefits the profession and the public.

Section 1: Health Educators select students for professional preparation programs based upon equal opportunity for all, and the individual's academic performance, abilities, and potential contribution to the profession and the public's health.

Section 2: Health Educators strive to make the educational environment and culture conducive to the health of all involved, and free from sexual harassment and all forms of discrimination.

Section 3: Health Educators involved in professional preparation and professional development engage in careful preparation; present material that is accurate, up-to-date, and timely; provide reasonable and timely feedback; state clear and reasonable expectations; and conduct fair assessments and evaluations of learners.

Section 4: Health Educators provide objective and accurate counseling to learners about career opportunities, development, and advancement, and assist learners secure professional employment.

Section 5: Health Educators provide adequate supervision and meaningful opportunities for the professional development of learners.

(Adopted by the Coalition of National Health Education Organizations, November 1999.)

Professional Organizations

Organization	Publication	Address	Abbreviation	Approximate Membership
American School Health Association	*Journal of School Health*	7263 Route 43 P.O. Box 708 Kent, OH 44240 (330) 678-1601 asha@ashaweb.org http://www.asha.web.org	ASHA	4,500
American Public Health Association	*American Journal of Public Health* Umbrella organizations include PHES and SHES	800 I St. NW Washington, DC 20005 (202) 777-2742 comments@msmail.apha.org http://www.apha.org	APHA	50,000
APHA–Public Health Education Section	Newsletter	800 I St. NW Washington, DC 20005 202-777-2742	PHES	
APHA–School Health Education and Services Section	Newsletter	800 I St. NW Washington, DC 20005	SHES	

Organization	Publication	Address	Abbreviation	Approximate Membership
American College Health Association	*Journal of American College Health*	P.O. Box 28937 Baltimore, MD 21240 (410) 859-1500 acha@access.digex.net http://www.acha.org	ACHA	2,500
American Alliance for Health, Physical Education, Recreation, and Dance	Umbrella organization includes AAHE	1900 Association Dr. Reston, VA 22091 703-476-3404 membshp@aahperd.org http://www.aahperd.org	AAHPERD	30,000
American Association for Health Education	*Journal of Health Education*	1900 Association Dr. Reston, VA 22091 703-476-3437 aahe@aahperd.org http://www.aahperd.org	AAHE	10,000
Eta Sigma Gamma	*The Gamman*	2000 University Ave. Ball State University Muncie, IN 47306 (800) 715-2559# etasigmagam@bsu.edu http://www.cast.ilstu.edu/ temple/esg.htm		3,000
National Commission for Health Education Credentialing, Inc.	Newsletter	944 Marcon Blvd Suite 310 Allentown, PA 18103 1-888 624-3248 www.nchec.org	The Commission	Membership through examination
Society for Public Health Education	*Health Education Quarterly*	1015 15th St. NW Suite 410 Washington D.C. 20005 (202) 408-9804 sopheauld@aol.com www.sophe.org	SOPHE	4,000

Glossary

Entry-Level Health and Graduate-Level Educator Competencies Addressed in This Chapter

Responsibility VI: Acting as a Resource Person in Health Education
  Competency A: Utilize computerized health information retrieval systems effectively.
  Competency B: Establish effective consultative relationships with those requesting assistance in solving health-related problems.
  Competency C: Interpret and respond to requests for health information.
  Competency D: Select effective resource materials for dissemination.

> Note: The competencies listed above are both entry-level and graduate-level competencies by the National Commission for Health Education Credentialing, Inc. They are taken from *A Framework for the Development of Competency-Based Curricula for Entry Level Health Educators* by the National Task Force on the Preparation and Practice of Health Educators, Inc., 1985.

Method Selection in Health Education

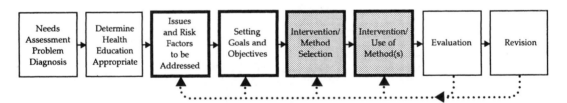

Heavy-bordered boxes indicate subjects addressed in this text; shaded boxes indicate subject(s) of current chapter.

American sign language The native language of most culturally deaf Americans, this is a visually based language that bears little relationship to English, particularly in grammar and syntax.

Behavioral capability Individual possesses the knowledge and skill to perform a behavior.

Blindisms Movements, often of the head and upper body of a blind individual, thought to result from a deprivation of visual stimulation.

Block plan This is a term used by educators regarding the organizing of educational activities into "blocks" of time. They are presented as sequential "blocks" with only minimal discription. The details are found in the methods section of a unit plan.

CD-ROM Compact disk read-only memory.

Certified Health Education Specialist (CHES) An individual who is credentialed as a result of demonstrating competency based on criteria established by the National Commission for Health Education Credentialing, Inc. (NCHEC). (1990 Joint Committee on Health Education Terminology)

Community health education The application of a variety of methods that result in the education and mobilization of community members in actions for resolving health issues and problems that affect the community. These methods include, but are not limited to: group process, mass media, communication, community organization, organization development, strategic planning, skills training, legislation, policy making, and advocacy. (1990 Joint Committee on Health Education Terminology)

Community health educator A practitioner professionally prepared in the field of community/ public health education who demonstrates competence in the planning, implementation, and evaluation of a broad range of health-promoting or health enhancing programs for

community groups. (1990 Joint Committee on Health Education Terminology)

Comprehensive school health program The development, delivery, and evaluation of a planned curriculum, preschool through 12, with goals, objectives, content sequence, and specific classroom lessons. It includes, but is not limited to, the following major content areas:

> Community health
> Consumer health
> Environmental health
> Family life
> Mental and emotional health
> Injury prevention and safety
> Nutrition
> Personal health
> Prevention and control of disease
> Substance use and abuse

(1990 Joint Committee on Health Education Terminology)

Contact time The time spent with a target group as part of a health education intervention.

Cooperative learning Broad category of learning experiences that center on learning from fellow participants.

Cultural competency An attempt to optimize the likelihood that individuals from all cultures, ethnicities, and races will receive appropriate and sensitive health care.

Curriculum A planned set of lessons or courses designed to lead to competence in an area of study.

Deaf A hearing impairment so severe that an individual is impaired in processing linguistic information through hearing. (Federal Register, 1977)

Demographics Information such as ages, ethnicity, gender, and other characteristics that describe a population and may impact objectives and method selection.

Diffusion The process of making innovations/ methods available and understandable to practicing health educators.

Disability A total or partial behavioral, mental, physical, or sensorial loss of functioning. (Mandell & Fiscus, 1981)

DVD Digitized video disc.

Exceptional A label usually associated with an individual whose performance is atypical and often deviates from what is expected. The performance could be superior or inferior to what is expected. (Mandell & Fiscus, 1981)

Expectancy As applied to social learning theory. Is the value an individual places on a particular outcome.

Facilitator The leader or teacher of a method or strategy.

Failure cycle Common among children with learning disabilities. A child fails to master a skill and consequently avoids the activity, guaranteeing that he or she will never achieve competency.

Family life Also known as family living, human sexuality, sex education. Scope and depth of information can vary in the extreme, according to the specific situation.

Fidelity The degree to which a lesson, program or curriculum is implemented according to the original intention of the developers.

Gatekeepers Used to describe the key leaders in a community that either get things done, allow things to get done or prevent action.

Goal A broad statement of direction used to present the overall intent of a program or course. Unlike an objective, it does not need to be stated in measurable terms.

Guided imagery A mental journey led by a guide or leader in person or on tape. Often used in stress management and in seeking behavior change

Handicap Environmental restrictions placed on a person's life as a result of a disability or exceptionality. (Mandell & Fiscus, 1981)

Hard of hearing A hearing impairment, either permanent or fluctuating, which adversely affects an individual's educational performance. (Federal Register, 1977)

Health advising A process of informing and assisting individuals or groups in making decisions and solving problems related to health. (1990 Joint Committee on Health Education Terminology)

Health education (1) A discipline dedicated to the improvement of the health status of individuals and the community. (2) The process of favorably and voluntarily influencing the health behavior of others.

Health education administrator A professional health educator who has the authority and responsibility for the management and coordination of all health education policies, activities, and resources within a particular setting or circumstance. (1990 Joint Committee on Health Education Terminology)

Health education coordinator A professional health educator who is responsible for the management and coordination of all health education policies, activities, and resources within a particular setting or circumstance. (1990 Joint Committee on Health Education Terminology)

Health education field The multi-disciplinary practice concerned with designing, implementing, and evaluating educational programs that enable individuals, families, groups, organizations, and communities to play active roles in achieving, protecting, and sustaining health. (1990 Joint Committee on Health Education Terminology)

Health education process The continuum of learning that enables people, as individuals and as members of social structures, to voluntarily make decisions, modify behaviors, and change social conditions in ways that are health enhancing.

Health education program A planned combination of activities developed with the involvement of specific populations and based on a needs assessment, sound principles of education, and periodic evaluation using a clear set of goals and objectives. (1990 Joint Committee on Health Education Terminology)

Health educator A practitioner professionally prepared in the field of health education who demonstrates competence in both theory and practice, and who accepts responsibility to advance the aims of the health education profession. (1990 Joint Committee on Health Education Terminology)

Health information The content of communications based on data derived from systematic and scientific methods as they relate to health issues, policies, programs, services, and other aspects of individual and public health, which can be used for informing various populations and for planning health education activities. (1990 Joint Committee on Health Education Terminology)

Health literacy The capacity of an individual to obtain, interpret, and understand basic health information and services and the competence to use such information and services in ways that are health enhancing. (1990 Joint Committee on Health Education Terminology)

Health promotion and disease prevention The aggregate of all purposeful activities designed to improve personal and public health through a combination of strategies, including the competent implementation of behavioral change strategies, health education, health protection measures, risk factor detection, health enhancement and health maintenance. (1990 Joint Committee on Health Education Terminology)

Healthy lifestyle A set of health-enhancing behaviors shaped by internally consistent values, attitudes, beliefs and external social and cultural forces. (1990 Joint Committee on Health Education Terminology)

Hispanic A classification of national background. A Hispanic person may be from any ethnic group.

Implementation The carrying out of or operationalizing of a plan of action.

Innovation An educational tool or method perceived as being new to potential users.

Intervention The total overall strategy to achieve our objectives.

Lesson/presentation plan The organized plan for a presentation.

Locus of control Expectations of reinforcement. The sense of whether or not a person feels in control of their life. Often characterized as external—under the control of outside forces—or internal—under the individual's personal control.

Long-range goals The very broad outcome intentions for the unit. These are optimal behaviors the educator hopes to achieve; they need not be easily measurable.

Mass media Refers to media capable of reaching large audiences. Television and national magazines are examples.

Method One component of the intervention such as an educational game or a health fair. We use the term interchangeably with strategy.

Normative belief Subjective norm—see definition.

Objective A precise statement of intended outcome; it must be stated in measurable terms.

Official health agency A publicly supported government organization mandated by public law and/or regulation for the protection and improvement of the health of the public.

Panel Several people who are invited to speak together on a topic. They may be selected due to expertise, political reasons or as representatives.

Pedagogy The art and science of teaching.

Post-secondary health education program A planned set of health education policies, procedures, activities, and services that are directed to students, faculty and/or staff of colleges, universities, and other higher education institutions. This includes, but is not limited to:

general health courses for students
employee and student health promotion activities
health services
professional preparation of health educators and other professionals
self-help groups
student life

(1990 Joint Committee on Health Education Terminology)

Postlingual deafness Deafness that occurs after spoken language has been developed.

Prelingual deafness Deafness that occurs before spoken language skills have been developed.

Private health agency A profit or nonprofit organization devoted to providing primary, secondary, and/or tertiary health services which may include health education. (1990 Joint Committee on Health Education Terminology)

Problem solution technique A discussion technique where a scenario is provided with discussion items of possible contributing factors. It is deliberately set up to cause disagreement and related discussion.

School health education One component of the comprehensive school health program which includes the development, delivery, and evaluation of a planned instructional program and other activities for students preschool through grade 12, for parents and for school staff. It is designed to influence positively the health knowledge, attitudes, and skills of individuals. (1990 Joint Committee on Health Education Terminology)

School health educator A practitioner who is professionally prepared in the field of school health education; meets state teaching requirements; and has demonstrated competence in the development, delivery, and evaluation of curricula for students and adults in the school setting that enhance health knowledge, attitudes, and problem-solving skills. (1990 Joint Committee on Health Education Terminology)

School health services That part of the school health program provided by physicians, nurses, dentists, health educators, other allied health personnel, social workers, teachers and others to appraise, protect and promote the health of students and school personnel. These services are designed to ensure access to and appropriate use of primary health care services, prevent and control communicable disease, provide emergency care for injury or sudden illness, promote and provide optimum sanitary conditions in a safe school facility and environment, and provide concurrent learning opportunities which are conducive to the maintenance and promotion of individual and community health. (1990 Joint Committee on Health Education Terminology)

Self-efficacy Belief or expectation by an individual that he or she can carry out the desired behavior.

Service learning Is offering or requiring hours of service for students either for academic credit or as part of some other requirement such as a general graduation requirement.

Sex educator An individual who teaches about human sexuality. Although professional certification can be obtained through AASECT (American Association of Sex Educators, Counselors & Therapists), many individuals may have little or no training.

Simulation The simulation is contrived experience used to expose someone to a certain prescribed set of circumstances based on a model. It has the appearance of some real-life phenomenon.

Social cognitive theory Social learning theory

Strategy One component of the intervention such as an educational game or a health fair. We use the term interchangeably with method.

Subjective norm The norm or social standard set by the common practice of a group. Example bell bottom pants become the most common pants in school due to the establishment of a subjective norm. Sometimes referred to as normative belief.

Target population The population for whom we are targeting our health education intervention.

Theory (heath) The presentation of a system to explain and predict health behaviors given identified variables.

Two-committee system A system designed to minimize complaint and maximize community involvement when developing materials and programs that might be viewed as controversial.

Unit plan An orderly self-contained collection of activities designed to meet a set of given objectives.

URL Uniform resource locators, an Internet site address.

Value clarification As the name implies is a method designed to help people clarify how they feel about issues and how they reach decisions.

Visually impaired Individuals who have defective or impaired vision. Definitions of impairment or blindness can be either legally or educationally based. (Meyen 1978)

Voluntary health organization A nonprofit association supported by contributions dedicated to conducting research and providing education and/or services related to particular health problems or concerns. (1990 Joint Committee on Health Education Terminology)

REFERENCES

Federal Register (Part IV). (1977). Washington DC: Department of Health, Education, and Welfare, 42 (163).

Mandell, C.J., & Fiscus, E. (1981). *Understanding Exceptional People.* St. Paul, MN: West Publishing Co.

Meyen, E.L. (1978). *Exceptional Children and Youth.* Denver: Love Publishing Co.

Report of the 1990 Joint Committee on Health Education Terminology (1991). *Journal of Health Education,* 22(2).

Photo Credits

Index